"Understanding the biological underpinnings of human mental functioning as seen through the lens of psychoanalytic observations was, of course, an initial goal of Sigmund Freud. This challenging, but intriguing task has been the focus of neuropsychoanlaysis. This updated edited text by Salas, Turnbull and Solms summarizes in a very interesting manner the evolution of this field of study over the last twenty years. In addition, it provides several useful clinical examples of how psychological work with brain dysfunctional individuals have utilized psychodynamic insights. It is a book that both informs and inspires and is especially helpful in understanding the subjective experiences of some brain dysfunctional individuals."

— **George P. Prigatano**, *Ph.D., Barrow Neurological Institute*

"This book is a must-read for anyone interested in, or working with, the mysteries of human minds. You will find new hypotheses, discussions, suggestions and examples of clinical cases from the interdisciplinary work of neuropsychoanalysis. This is a young but very important and innovative field proposing a new vision for studying and clinically approaching mental functions. A pleasure to read, it poses engaging, exciting and innovative questions."

— **Cristina M. Alberini**, *Professor of Neuroscience, New York University*

W0113606

Clinical Studies in Neuropsychoanalysis Revisited

In the past few decades, we have accumulated an impressive amount of knowledge regarding the neural basis of the mind. One of the most important sources of this knowledge has been the in-depth study of individuals with focal brain damage and other neurological disorders. This book offers a unique perspective, in that it uses a combination of neuropsychology and psychoanalytic knowledge from diverse schools (Freudian, Kleinian, Lacanian, Relational, etc.), to explore how damage to specific areas of the brain can change the mind.

Twenty years after the publication of *Clinical Studies in Neuro-Psychoanalysis*, this book continues the pioneering work of Mark Solms and Karen Kaplan-Solms, bringing together clinicians and researchers from all over the world to report key developments in the field. They present a rich set of new case studies, from a diverse range of brain injuries, neuropsychological impairments and even degenerative and paediatric pathologies.

This volume will be of immense value to those working with neurological populations that want to incorporate psychoanalytic ideas in case formulations, as well as for those who want to introduce themselves in the neurological basis of psychoanalytic models of the mind and the broader psychoanalytic community.

Christian Salas is a clinical neuropsychologist and psychoanalytic psychotherapist from Santiago, Chile. He is Assistant Professor at the Centre for Human Neuroscience and Neuropsychology and Director of the Clinical Neuropsychology Unit in Diego Portales University. He is also a staff member at the Dynamic Psychotherapy Unit, J. Horwtiz Barak Psychiatric Institute. He is co-author of *Addressing Brain Injury in Under-Resourced Settings*.

Oliver Turnbull is a neuropsychologist and clinical psychologist with an interest in emotion and its many consequences for mental life, as well as a Professor of Neuropsychology at Bangor University, where he is Deputy Vice Chancellor. He is the author of many scientific articles and co-author of *The Brain and the Inner World*.

Mark Solms is Co-Chair of the International Neuropsychoanalysis Society, Research Chair of the International Psychoanalytical Association and Science Director of the American Psychoanalytic Association. He is Director of Neuropsychology at the Neuroscience Institute of the University of Cape Town.

The Brain Injuries Series
Dr Giles N. Yeates and Dr Fergus Gracey (Series Editors)

This series is dedicated to psychological therapies, social interventions and psychosocial issues following acquired brain injury, emphasising both theoretical exploration and the 'how-to' of therapeutic work. These titles stand in contrast with previous clinical titles in the brain injury literature that have been assessment-focused and offered little in the way of intervention. Every jobbing clinician and therapist working with survivors of brain injury and their significant others should have this series on their shelves.

Previous titles in the series:

Practical Neuropsychological Rehabilitation in Acquired Brain Injury
A Guide for Working Clinicians
Edited by Gavin Newby, Rudi Coetzer, Audrey Daisley and Stephen Weatherhead

Narrative Approaches to Brain Injury
Edited by Stephen Weatherhead and David Todd

Psychological Therapy for Paediatric Acquired Brain Injury
Innovations for Children, Young People and Families
Edited by Jenny Jim and Esther Cole

Headaches and Mild Brain Trauma
A Practical Therapy Guide
Birgit Gurr

Clinical Studies in Neuropsychoanalysis Revisited
Edited By Christian Salas, Oliver Turnbull and Mark Solms

For further information about this series please visit: www.routledge.com/The-Brain-Injuries-Series/book-series/KARNACBI

Clinical Studies in Neuropsychoanalysis Revisited

Edited by Christian Salas,
Oliver Turnbull and Mark Solms

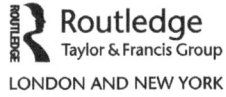
Routledge
Taylor & Francis Group

LONDON AND NEW YORK

First published 2022
by Routledge
2 Park Square, Milton Park, Abingdon, Oxon OX14 4RN

and by Routledge
605 Third Avenue, New York, NY 10158

Routledge is an imprint of the Taylor & Francis Group, an informa business

British Library Cataloguing-in-Publication Data
A catalogue record for this book is available from the British Library

Library of Congress Cataloging-in-Publication Data
Names: Salas, Christian (Clinical neuropsychologist), editor. | Turnbull, Oliver, 1964– editor. | Solms, Mark, editor.
Title: Clinical studies in neuropsychoanalysis revisited / edited by Christian Salas, Oliver Turnbull & Mark Solms.
Description: Milton Park, Abingdon, Oxon;
New York, NY: Routledge, 2021. |
Series: The brain injuries series | Includes bibliographical references and index.
Identifiers: LCCN 2021002587 (print) | LCCN 2021002588 (ebook) | ISBN 9781032036939 (hardback) | ISBN 9781032036878 (paperback) | ISBN 9781003188551 (ebook)
Subjects: LCSH: Psychoanalysis—Case studies. | Neurosciences—Case studies. | Nervous system—Diseases—Case studies.
Classification: LCC RC506 .C55 2021 (print) | LCC RC506 (ebook) | DDC 616.89/17—dc23
LC record available at https://lccn.loc.gov/2021002587
LC ebook record available at https://lccn.loc.gov/2021002588

ISBN: 978-1-032-03693-9 (hbk)
ISBN: 978-1-032-03687-8 (pbk)
ISBN: 978-1-003-18855-1 (ebk)

Typeset in Times New Roman
by codeMantra

"The aims of this book are modest but far reaching"

Kaplan-Solms & Solms, 2000

Contents

Contributors

Ariane Bazan, Ph.D., is Professor of Clinical Psychology and Psychopathology at the Université libre de Bruxelles (Belgium) and at the Université de Lorraine (France). She is author of *Des fantômes dans la voix: une hypothèse neuropsychanalytique sur la structure de l'inconscient* (Liber, 2007). She is affiliated with the Interpsy laboratory at the Université de Lorraine and has a private psychoanalytic practice.

Sahba Besharati, Ph.D., is a neuropsychologist and Senior Lecturer in Cognitive Neuroscience at the Department of Psychology at the University of the Witwatersrand (Wits, South Africa). She is the co-founder and joint leader of Wits NeuRL, a cross-disciplinary research laboratory that aims to advance the practice and research of social-affective-cognitive neuroscience in the Southern African context.

Diana Caine is a psychoanalyst and consultant clinical neuropsychologist at the National Hospital for Neurology and Neurosurgery (London, UK). Her published research has focused on the neuropsychology of dementia, disorders of autobiographical and semantic memory and delusions of misidentification. More recently, she has drawn on psychoanalytic theory to re-think the implications of neurological damage for subjectivity.

Richard Cheston, Ph.D., is a Professor of Dementia Research at the University of the West of England (UK). He is a clinical psychologist and psychotherapist, and provides a weekly clinic for people living with dementia and their carers. His research interests focus on how people respond to the existential threats to their identity that dementia creates.

Francisco Cruz-Quintana, Ph.D., is a psychoanalyst and Full Professor of Psychology at the University of Granada (Spain). He is the Director of the End of life and Bereavement Lab in the Mind, Brain and Behavior Research Centre.

Amy Duncan, Ph.D., is a neuropsychologist from Cape Town, South Africa. She is currently applying these skills from a learning experience design perspective for Sea Monster Entertainment, South Africa's leading company in animation and serious games for social impact. Her research interest focuses on euphoria and multiple sclerosis.

Manuel Fernández-Alcántara, Ph.D., is an Associate Lecturer at the Department of Health Psychology at the University of Alicante (Spain); expert in Applied Psychoanalysis by the University of Granada; coordinator of the Master of Active and Healthy Ageing at the University of Alicante; Associate Editor in *Death Studies and Plos One.*

Aikaterini Fotopoulou, Ph.D., is a Professor in Psychodynamic Neuroscience at University College London, a psychotherapist and chartered psychologist in private practice. Her research focuses on the mental-physical health interface. She is the co-founder of the *International Association for the Study of Affective Touch* (IASAT) and editor of the book *From the Couch to the Lab: Trends in Psychodynamic Neuroscience.*

Pamela Klonoff, PhD., is a board-certified clinical neuropsychologist specializing in neurorehabilitation. She is the Clinical Director of the Center for Transitional Neuro-Rehabilitation at Barrow Neurological Institute, St Joseph's Hospital and Medical Center, in Phoenix, Arizona. She is the author of *Psychotherapy after Brain Injury: Principles and Techniques* and *Psychotherapy for Families after Brian Injury.*

Carolina Laynez-Rubio, Ph.D., is a psychoanalyst and clinical psychologist specialized in neuropsychology. She works at the Neuropsychology Unit in the San Cecilio Hospital, Granada, Spain.

Paul Moore is a psychoanalytic psychotherapist from Carlow (Ireland). He is an Assistant Professor and Director of the Psychoanalytic Psychotherapy Training Programme at the Department of Psychiatry at the School of Medicine at Trinity College Dublin.

Juan Francisco Navas, Ph.D., is an Assistant Professor of the Department of Clinical Psychology at the Complutense University of Madrid. His research focuses on the study of the behavioral and neural correlates of emotional processing dysfunction in people with addictive behaviors.

Aonghus Ryan is a clinical neuropsychologist who has specialised in Intensive Short-Term Dynamic Psychotherapy (ISTDP). He works in neurological rehabilitation at the Oxford Centre for Enablement, UK. His research focuses on applying affective neuroscience concepts in understanding apathy after brain injury.

Kobi Tiberg is a rehabilitation psychologist and a neuropsychologist, working in private practice in Tel-Aviv, Israel. He has written and lectured widely in the field of neuropsychoanalysis. Currently, he is writing a PhD thesis at Tel-Aviv University on complex trauma from a neuropsychoanalytic perspective.

Gertrudis Van de Vijver is Professor of Philosophy at Ghent University where she works on issues in the history of philosophy, epistemology and philosophy of science. She is affiliated to the Centre for the History of Philosophy and Continental Philosophy (HICO). She has a private psychoanalytical practice in Ghent.

Dr Giles Yeates is a consultant clinical neuropsychologist, and Series Editor of the *Brain Injuries* and *Neuro-Disability & Psychotherapy* series (Routledge). He holds an academic position at the Centre for Movement, Occupational and Rehabilitation Sciences (MOReS) at Oxford Brookes University (UK). Dr Yeates is the Chair of the Thames Valley Brain Injury Forum. He is the co-author of *A Relational Approach to Rehabilitation: Thinking about Relationships after Brain Injury.*

Maggie Zellner is the Executive Director of the Neuropsychoanalysis Foundation in New York City. She is a psychoanalytic psychotherapist in private practice, and is the Managing Editor of *Neuropsychoanalysis*, an interdisciplinary journal for psychoanalysis and the neurosciences.

Series editors' foreword

This is a timely and significant addition to Routledge's Brain Injuries Series, one that we are very honoured to host. We know this will make serious waves within the neuropsychoanalytical world, that's a given, and justly-deserved, given the quality, range and intellectual vibrancy of the chapters. In an echo of the concluding chapter by Christian Salas, Oliver Turnbull and Mark Solms, we wanted here to situate the unique ideas from these neuropsychoanalytical writers within a broader neuropsychological rehabilitation setting. This will not be via a literature review, but a reflection of a personal story and a formative time between the two of us series editors.

It is 2000–2003. Giles Yeates is a trainee clinical psychologist thrilled to be undertaking a specialist placement in holistic neuropsychological rehabilitation at the Oliver Zangwill Centre in Ely, UK. Fergus Gracey is a recently-qualified clinical psychologist at the centre, who has agreed to supervise Giles' placement, along with Jonathan Evans (now a Professor of Clinical Neuropsychology at the University of Glasgow). Giles had been inspired by Oliver Sacks' famous works and was committed to work as a clinical neuropsychologist with the subjectivity of survivors as centre-stage. He was as inspired by relational, family systems ideas as Prigatano's (1999) vision of a phenomenological-focused rehabilitation remit. Fergus was developing his core ideas on identity work with survivors of brain injury and supporting adjustment through the interdisciplinary, holistic, intensive neuropsychological rehabilitation process (the Y-Shaped Model, Gracey et al., 2009).

Giles' curiosity was peaked by a Karnac Books flyer in Kaplan-Solms and Solms (2000) now seminal *Clinical Studies in Neuro-psychoanalysis: Introduction to a Depth Neuropsychology*. In this mysterious text, formulation of the impact of different neuro-anatomical lesions was constructed through neuro-imaging, psychometric testing *and* counter-transference reflections – what it *feels* like to work with patients with different lesion types. This blew Giles' mind, yet was so obvious and in resonance with his early clinical experiences. The chapter on perisylvian lesions that presented a post-Freudian and Kleinian conceptualisation of simultaneous cognitive, emotional and relational phenomena that were all different aspects of the same neuropsychological mechanism (a narcissistic collapse of neuropsychologically-constructed allocentric space) was the icing and the cherry on the NPSA-cake. Giles couldn't experience this clinical world and work the same way ever again.

Adding Freud and Klein to the existing supervision discussion with Fergus did not phase him one bit, and he and Jonathan Evans took these ideas in their stride (perhaps with a degree of amused curiosity), typical of their pioneering and flexible approach to clinical work. Jung had already been introduced by Prigatano (1999) into neuropsychological rehabilitation's frame of reference. In the final year of clinical training and the first year postqualification, Giles deepened his interest in Klein and Bion during a week of group analysis at the Tavistock Clinic in London, and started to find a way into Lacanian psychoanalysis, via helpful introductory lectures by Darian Leeder, and the psychosocial work of Wendy Hollway and Stephen Frosch. Giles also attended a local psychoanalytical group in Norwich that met in a park hall to watch a video series on NPSA by Mark Solms. Giles' first attendance at a neuropsychoanalysis congress was in Rome in 2004, where the centrality of these dual-aspect monist ideas and identification with the NPSA community as a whole was cemented forever in his practice.

At the congress, Giles presented work from his thesis on awareness of difficulties following brain injury, again supervised by Fergus and Jonathan Evans. Giles was supported by the Oliver Zangwill Centre to go to Rome, to contribute and find a place in the NPSA community. Social constructionism and neuropsychological models were hastily supplemented by Klein and Lacan in the 11th hour prior to submission for training in 2003, and these new ideas, with NPSA being a linking nodal point for all traditions, had been digested and developed in a year of post-qualification clinical practice, with Fergus' thoughtful mentorship and containment.

Fergus' main clinical psychotherapeutic orientation is cognitivebehavioural (Gracey et al., 2016), but was drawing beyond CBT to find adequate schemes to conceptualise cognitive-emotion interactions and meet brain injury survivors where they needed to be met in the therapy room: to explore and assist at the level of identity and personal meaning.

We were using different ideas, but were approaching the same phenomena. We both equally dismayed at the typical trends of the day in clinical neuropsychology handbooks – dry tomes filled with chapters on testing, some on cognitive rehabilitation and barely a dreg of a chapter towards the end, as if an afterthought, on emotion. Books and chapters by Ben-Yishay, Prigatano and Ylvisaker were rare exceptions, and our clinical neuropsychology professional development events in the UK were similarly bereft of training events on working with emotion, identity and relationships following neuro-disability in a psychotherapeutic manner. So in London in 2005,

we both co-hosted a one day conference on psychological therapies following brain injury. The same case was formulated in different ways using different orientations. This event, novel for the UK, hosted presentations from
clinical neuropsychologists working from Gestalt, cognitive-behavioural,
systemic orientations, including Mark Solms presenting a neuropsychoanalytical formulation for the first time to the UK's clinical neuropsychology
community (we remember it came straight after a preceding talk on neu-
ro-behavioural approaches!). It was warmly accepted by many.

For those not working within a psychodynamic orientation within neurorehabilitation, NPSA ideas still make an important epistemological contribution – they act as a thought-experiment that shows that a strikingly-different
array of metaphors and assumptions can be usefully brought to bear on the
phenomenology of experience and need in those with neurological conditions.
This difference forces clinicians to question lazy, boxes and arrow models as
sufficient for intellectual and applied progress in our fields.

In the last 15 years, in many countries psychotherapy of all kinds has
become a more central element of the clinical neuropsychologist's core competencies if they are working in neuro-rehabilitation and community services. There are still parts of the world where separate training routes for
clinical psychology, psychotherapy and clinical neuropsychology result in
a lack of dialogue and compartmentalised practices, but these are reassur-
ingly becoming the exceptions. Where there is dialogue, a new wider field of
neuropsychotherapy is born, and as noted in the last chapter of this book,
this convergence will in-turn stimulate future innovations in psychoanalytical practice in the face of neurological difficulties and differences. More
professional events, chapters, books, journals such as *Neuro-Disability &*
Psychotherapy and *Neuropsychoanalysis*, plus book series such as this one,
signify a growing and burgeoning field, with NPSA playing an important
role alongside other psychotherapies and meta-psychologies. The diversity
of need and experience in neuro-disability populations means that no one
therapy approach or model of clinical phenomena will be optimal for all
service users, so the pluralism in the neuropsychotherapy field is warmly
welcome. In this same vein, the pluralism of this book, a successor from
the original Kaplan-Solms work that is a 3D development of the pioneering
beginning, serves to make NPSA a vital element of wider clinical neurorehabilitation and care, in particular as it evolves to offer support commen-
surate with the complex emotional, relational and psychosocial needs of
survivors in the long-term.

We hope the reader will forgive this very long and indulgent personal introduction by both of us. If we take our story up until the present in 2020,
and the two decades that this account now spans, we have both worked
apart in different parts of the country, in different sectors, different service
models and on different writing projects. We have both enjoyed working

closely in writing and dissemination with all three editors of this book, and are inspired by the developing scope of their work. Set-up by Ceri Bowen in 2009, Giles developed this very book series to be the antithesis of those dry academic clinical neuropsychology tomes that were affect-phobic, and through poetic circularity, Fergus recently partnered as series co-editor in 2018.

The reason for this lengthy disclosure is to provide a context for how honoured we are to include *Clinical Studies in Neuropsychoanalysis Revisited* as the latest edition of the series, of how the traditions and scope in the following pages have played an important role in our working relationship as series editors over the last two decades. Regardless of your theoretical orientation and biases, enjoy the pages ahead, be inspired, change your perspective.

Giles Yeates (Series Editor) and Fergus Gracey
(Series Co-Editor), February 2020

Introduction

Chapter 1

Great expectations

Oliver Turnbull, Christian Salas and Mark Solms

Any field which has modest beginnings will inevitably dream of what it might become. Viewed with hindsight, what would success look like? If we may use a metaphor from ecology, the field would begin with a few small plants in one corner of a landscape. Successful evolution would involve, firstly, plants spreading across *more* of the landscape; secondly, plants evolving into different *species* that are better able to promote diversity; and finally, plants setting down *deeper roots* in an enriched soil to consolidate permanence. With this metaphor in mind, we ponder whether neuropsychoanalysis has developed these properties of health across the past two decades, as showcased in this book. We will consider four themes as reflecting the growth of neuropsychoanalysis: the people involved in the process, the methods used by the field, the theoretical underpinnings and the objects of study. In each case, we lay out the trajectory of growth, from the *Clinical Studies* book (Kaplan-Solms & Solms, 2000), and contrast this with the situation two decades later in the present volume.

1 People

The original *Clinical Studies* volume was the work of two individuals working in relative social and geographical isolation: Karen Kaplan-Solms and Mark Solms. The foundational clinical work was carried out in the 1980s and 1990s, before the setting up of the International Neuropsychoanalysis Society (2000), the foundation of the journal *Neuropsychoanalysis* (1999), the First International Congress of the Society (2000) and the publication of the popular introductory work *The Brain and the Inner World* (Solms & Turnbull, 2002). Over the past two decades, the Society has grown to a membership of many hundreds, together with the formation of some 40 regional groups, across all five continents. The Society, and other sources, has also contributed towards many funded research grants for early career scientists. The Congress has continued to be an annual gathering of this community, now in its 20th year, hosting several hundred regular and local attendees per year. It has also spread from a small group of invited speakers to an event which hosts multiple parallel research sessions and poster presentations, typically by early career clinicians (psychiatrists, neurologists, psychologists, neuropsychologists) and scientists (Salas & Palmer-Cancel, 2019). The *Clinical Studies* and *The Brain and the Inner World* books have each been translated into more than a dozen languages. Finally, the journal has continued a regular publication schedule, across a series of editors (from Mark Solms and Edward Nersessian, through Oliver Turnbull, Yoram Yovell, Maggie Zellner and Richard Kessler, to Iftah Biran), and is now indexed in the peer-reviewed citation database Scopus. This book is then, in one respect, a reflection of the maturity of the field and the diversity and scale of this growth. We have chapters written by psychologists, neuropsychologists and psychoanalysts, and from North and South America, Europe and Africa. In sum, neuropsychoanalysis is growing.

2 Methods

The original *Clinical Studies* volume was based on a small number of patients with focal brain lesions, who were investigated in a setting of psychoanalytic psychotherapy for a limited number of sessions (sometimes fewer than ten). The rationale of the methodology employed by Kaplan-Solms and Solms was a blend of the syndrome approach at the heart of dynamic neuropsychology (Luria, 1966) and the free-association technique developed by Freud. Kaplan-Solms and Solms were explicit that this combined technique was the optimal one for bridging the third-person perspective (the brain) and the first-person perspective (subjective experience) (Turnbull & Solms, 2004). The *Clinical Studies* book then outlined a series of formulations about the possible neural architecture of the psychodynamic "mental apparatus". However, it was always clear that the testing of these ideas would require not only a larger sample of patients but also the use of more conventional methods in experimental psychology, neuropsychology and neuroscience (Solms & Turnbull, 2002).

How has the field responded to these challenges? There has been a wide range of empirical research which has built upon these foundational ideas (see Fotopoulou, Pfaff & Conway, 2012). Further studies of patients with brain lesions have been carried out, using more conventional experimental methods (e.g. Fotopoulou et al., 2011; Turnbull, Fotopoulou & Solms, 2014, for reviews see Turnbull, Lovett, Chaldecott & Lucas, 2014; Turnbull & Salas, 2017), including investigations of brain-injured patients in the context of long-term psychotherapy (Moore, Salas, Dockree & Turnbull, 2017; Salas & Yuen, 2016). We might also have hoped that there would be growth in the use of modern neuroscience technology (e.g. neuroimaging and event-related potentials [ERP]), and this area has also been productive (Anderson et al., 2004; Besharati et al., 2014; Kim, Fonagy, Allen & Strathearn, 2014; Nolte et al., 2013; Schmeing et al., 2013; Shevrin et al., 2013). Interestingly, a direction of travel which was *not* anticipated in the *Clinical Studies* book was the link with animal work and affective neuroscience. This relationship, mediated primarily by the remarkable Jaak Panksepp, also proved fruitful, generating many interesting proposals, and even pharmacological intervention studies (Zellner et al., 2011, Yovell et al., 2016), and dramatically changing the theoretical landscape of neuropsychoanalysis (Panksepp & Solms, 2012; Solms & Panksepp, 2012). The present volume reflects many of these trends, but has intentionally sought to focus on clinical case studies, the better to observe continuities with the original *Clinical Studies* book. Novel developments in this volume include reports of much longer term psychotherapies (Chapter 9 by Moore) and work with new populations such as dementia and developmental disorders (Chapter 10 by Cheston and Chapter 11 by Fernández-Alcántara and colleagues). We are also pleased to report that the methodological rigour of case studies is demonstrated in the convergence and "dense description" of clinical history and neuropsychological assessment (Chapter 8 by Ryan and Yeates), following case-study guidelines suggested by authors in the field (Salas, Casassus & Turnbull, 2016). In sum, neuropsychoanalysis is diversifying.

3 Theory

The original *Clinical Studies* was heavily influenced by Freudian and Kleinian ideas, particularly related to metapsychological concepts linked to three brain regions: (1) the left perisylvian cortex and its role in word versus thing presentation; (2) the right perisylvian cortex and its relationship with mourning and object/self-representation; and (3) the medial frontal lobe and its relevance to sustaining a balance between the pleasure and reality principles. Across the past two decades, the range of theoretical influences has greatly expanded, often reflecting the conceptual background of a diverse community of scientists and clinicians. This includes understanding the brain/mind in the light of post-Freudian psychoanalytic schools, such as Jung (George Prigatano), Kohut (Pamela Klonoff), Lacan (Arianne Bazan) and relational psychoanalysis (Giles Yeates). Another important theoretical development of the field has been the influence of animal work, and its associated ethological perspective, through the lens of affective neuroscience (Jaak Panksepp). This interface has been especially relevant in reconceptualizing drive and motivation, as well as understanding the relationship between emotional systems, psychiatric disorders and their associated pharmacological treatment (Panksepp 2015, 2016; Panksepp & Yovell, 2014; Wright & Panksepp, 2011; Zellner, Watt, Solms, & Panksepp, 2011). A major new development in more recent years has been the increasing influence of predictive coding and the free energy principle of Karl Friston (Solms, 2018, 2019; Solms & Friston, 2018). The present volume especially reflects this diversity of tongues, with chapters from Freudian (Zellner), relational (Yeats and Salas), Lacanian (Bazan, Van de Vijver and Caine) and Kohutian (Klonoff) perspectives. Here, again, neuropsychoanalysis is diversifying.

4 Objects of study

The original *Clinical Studies* volume was focused on three classes of disorders: denial of deficit (anosognosia), various forms of language impairment (fluent and nonfluent aphasias) and confabulation and delusional beliefs. These were presented as "proofs of concept" that the neuropsychoanalytic method could be successful, but, of course, it did not exclude the idea of other neuropsychological disorders yielding further knowledge on the neural basis of complex mental processes. A number of papers have been written in relation to these *initial* disorders, consolidating and refining these findings (for review see Salas & Yuen, 2016; Turnbull, Fotopoulou & Solms, 2014; Turnbull and Salas, 2017).

However, there have also been a number of *new* developments, based on neuropsychological disorders that did not appear in the original volume, contributing to the understanding of other mental processes. These include dysexecutive impairment (Yeates et al., 2008), amnesia (Moore, Salas, Dockree & Turnbull, 2017; Turnbull, Zois, Kaplan-Solms & Solms, 2006), confabulation (Tiberg, 2014; Turnbull, Jenkins & Rowley, 2004), emotion dysregulation (Salas et al., 2014), interoception (Fotopoulou & Tsakiris, 2017) and sexuality (Turnbull et al, 2014). The present volume reflects advances in several of these strands, such as confabulation (Tiberg), memory (Moore), language (Bazan, Van de Vijver and Caine) and interoception and touch (Besharati and Fotopoulou), and new themes such as an investigation of locked-in syndrome (Duncan) and post-stroke adynamia (Ryan and Yeates). This forms a final strand of evidence that neuropsychoanalysis is diversifying and consolidating.

In short, the present volume reflects an impressive and substantial range of developments in the recent history of neuropsychoanalysis. Existing concepts, such as the interpretation of confabulation and anosognosia, have been strengthened by two decades of experimental research, with greater scientific rigour and novel experimental methods. New topics, reflecting new aspects of the mind and uninvestigated clinical disorders and subjects, have allowed an expansion of the field beyond the focus of the original book. This has been achieved by a larger group of clinician/scientists, spread across the world. In several senses, then, the hopes and ambitions of the original text have been achieved. However, we have no doubt that all of those involved are aware that this is merely the beginning of an ambitious endeavour: to link together two large disciplines and better understand the nature of woefully under-investigated aspects of the mind and its feelings. We hope that this book represents a helpful milestone in that journey.

March, 2019
Vicuña, Chile / Cape Town, South Africa

References

Anderson, M. C., Ochsner, K. N., Kuhl, B., Cooper, J., Robertson, E., Gabrieli, S. W., Glover, G. H., & Gabrieli, J. D. (2004). Neural systems underlying the suppression of unwanted memories. *Science, 303*(5655), 232–235.

Besharati, S., Forkel, S. J., Kopelman, M., Solms, M., Jenkinson, P. M., & Fotopoulou, A. (2014). The affective modulation of motor awareness in anosognosia for hemiplegia: Behavioural and lesion evidence. *Cortex, 61*, 127–140.

Fotopoulou, A., Jenkinson, P. M., Tsakiris, M., Haggard, P., Rudd, A., & Kopelman M. (2011). Mirror-view reverses somatoparaphrenia: Dissociation between first- and third-person perspectives on body ownership. *Neuropsychologia, 49*, 3946–3955.

Fotopoulou, A., Pfaff, D., & Conway, M. A. (Eds.). (2012). *From the couch to the lab: Trends in psychodynamic neuroscience.* Oxford: Oxford University Press.

Fotopoulou, A., & Tsakiris, M. (2017). Mentalizing homeostasis: The social origins of interoceptive inference. *Neuropsychoanalysis, 19*(1), 3–28.

Kaplan-Solms, K., & Solms, M. (2000). *Clinical studies in neuro-psychoanalysis: Introduction to a depth neuropsychology.* Karnac Books: London.

Kim, S., Fonagy, P., Allen, J., & Strathearn, L. (2014). Mothers' unresolved trauma blunts amygdala response to infant distress. *Social Neuroscience, 9*, 352–363.

Luria, A. (1966). *Higher cortical functions in man.* Tavistock Publications Limited: London.

Moore, P. A., Salas, C. E., Dockree, S., & Turnbull, O. H. (2017). Observations on working psychoanalytically with a profoundly amnesic patient. *Frontiers in Psychology, 8*, 1418.

Nolte, T., Bolling, D. Z., Hudac, C. M., Fonagy, P., Mayes, L., & Pelphrey, K. A. (2013). Brain mechanisms underlying the impact of attachment-related stress on social cognition. *Frontiers in Human Neuroscience, 7*, 816.

Panksepp, J. (2015). Affective preclinical modeling of psychiatric disorders: taking imbalanced primal emotional feelings of animals seriously in our search for novel antidepressants. *Dialogues in Clinical Neuroscience, 17*(4), 363.

Panksepp, J. (2016). The psycho-neurology of cross-species affective/social neuroscience: Understanding animal affective states as a guide to development of novel psychiatric treatments. In M. Wöhr & S. Krach (Eds.) *Social behavior from rodents to humans* (pp. 109–125). Springer: Cham.

Panksepp, J., & Solms, M. (2012). What is neuropsychoanalysis? Clinically relevant studies of the minded brain. *Trends in Cognitive Sciences, 16*(1), 6–8.

Panksepp, J., & Yovell, Y. (2014). Preclinical modeling of primal emotional affects (SEEKING, PANIC and PLAY): Gateways to the development of new treatments for depression. *Psychopathology, 47*(6), 383–393.

Salas, C. E., Casassus, M., & Turnbull, O. H. (2016). A neuropsychoanalytic approach to case studies. *Clinical Social Work Journal, 45*(3), 201–214.

Salas, C. E., & Palmer-Cancel, S. J. (2019) Neuropsychoanalysis 20 years later: an interview with Oliver Turnbull. *Neuropsychoanalysis,* doi:10.1080/15294145.2019.1631039.

Salas, C. E., Radovic, D., Yuen, K. S., Yeates, G. N., Castro, O., & Turnbull, O. H. (2014). "Opening an emotional dimension in me": Changes in emotional reactivity and emotion regulation in a case of executive impairment after left fronto-parietal damage. *Bulletin of the Menninger Clinic, 78*(4), 301–334.

Salas, C. E., & Yuen, K. S. (2016). Revisiting the left convexity hypothesis: Changes in the mental apparatus after left dorso-medial prefrontal damage. *Neuropsychoanalysis, 18*(2), 85–100.

Schmeing, J. B., Kehyayan, A., Kessler, H., Do Lam, A. T., Fell, J., Schmidt, A. C., & Axmacher, N. (2013). Can the neural basis of repression be studied in the MRI scanner? New insights from two free association paradigms. *PLoS One, 8*(4), e62358.

Shevrin, H., Snodgrass, M., Brakel, L. A., Kushwaha, R., Kalaida, N. L., & Bazan, A. (2013). Subliminal unconscious conflict alpha power inhibits supraliminal conscious symptom experience. *Frontiers in Human Neuroscience, 7*, 544.

Solms, M. (2018). The neurobiological underpinnings of psychoanalytic theory and therapy. *Frontiers in Behavioral Neuroscience, 12*, 294. doi:10.3389/fnbeh.2018.00294

Solms M. (2019). The hard problem of consciousness and the free energy principle. *Frontiers in Psychology, 10*: 2714. doi:10.3389/fpsyg.2018.02714

Solms, M., & Friston, K. (2018). How and why consciousness arises: Some considerations from physics and physiology. *Journal of Consciousness Studies, 25*: 202–238.

Solms, M., & Panksepp, J. (2012). The "Id" knows more than the "Ego" admits: Neuropsychoanalytic and primal consciousness perspectives on the interface between affective and cognitive neuroscience. *Brain Sciences, 2*(2), 147–175.

Solms, M., & Turnbull, O. (2002). *The brain and the inner world: An introduction to the neuroscience of subjective experience.* Karnac Books: London.

Tiberg, K. (2014). Confabulating in the transference. *Neuropsychoanalysis, 16*(1), 57–67.

Turnbull, O. H., Fotopoulou, A., & Solms, M. (2014). Anosognosia as motivated unawareness: The 'defence' hypothesis revisited. *Cortex, 61*, 18–29.

Turnbull, O. H., Jenkins, S., & Rowley, M. L. (2004). The pleasantness of false beliefs: An emotion-based account of confabulation. *Neuropsychoanalysis, 6*(1), 5–16.

Turnbull, O. H., Lovett, V. E., Chaldecott, J., & Lucas, M. (2014). Reports of intimate touch: Erogenous zones and somatosensory cortical organization. *Cortex, 53*, 146–154.

Turnbull, O. H., & Salas, C. E. (2017). Confabulation: Developing the 'emotion dysregulation' hypothesis. *Cortex, 87*, 52–61.

Turnbull, O. H., & Solms, M. (2004) Depth psychological consequences of brain damage. In J. Panksepp (Ed.) *Textbook of biological psychiatry* (pp. 571–595). Wiley-Liss: New Jersey.

Turnbull, O. H., Zois, E., Kaplan-Solms, K., & Solms, M. (2006). The developing transference in amnesia: Changes in interpersonal relationship, despite profound episodic-memory loss. *Neuropsychoanalysis, 8*(2), 199–204.

Wright, J. S., & Panksepp, J. (2011). Toward affective circuit-based preclinical models of depression: sensitizing dorsal PAG arousal leads to sustained suppression of positive affect in rats. *Neuroscience & Biobehavioral Reviews, 35*(9), 1902–1915.

Yeates, G., Hamill, M., Sutton, L., Psaila, K., Gracey, F., Mohamed, S., & O'Dell, J. (2008). Dysexecutive problems and interpersonal relating following frontal brain injury: Reformulation and compensation in cognitive analytic therapy (CAT). *Neuropsychoanalysis*, *10*(1), 43–58.

Yovell, Y., Bar, G., Mashiah, M., Baruch, Y., Briskman, I., Asherov, J., Lotan, A., Rigbi, A., & Panksepp, J. (2016, May 1). Ultra-low-dose buprenorphine as a time-limited treatment for severe suicidal ideation: A randomized controlled trial. *American Journal of Psychiatry 173*(5), 491–498.

Zellner, M. R., Watt, D. F., Solms, M., & Panksepp, J. (2011). Affective neuroscientific and neuropsychoanalytic approaches to two intractable psychiatric problems: why depression feels so bad and what addicts really want. *Neuroscience & Biobehavioral Reviews*, *35*(9), 2000–2008.

Chapter 2

From depth neuropsychology to neuropsychoanalysis

A historical comment 20 years later

Mark Solms

Clinical Studies in Neuro-Psychoanalysis was the second of three foundational texts in the nascent field of neuropsychoanalysis. The first was *The Neuropsychology of Dreams* (Solms, 1997a) and the third was *The Brain and the Inner World* (Solms and Turnbull, 2002). What separates the second and third of these texts is that the *Clinical Studies* gave no hint of the huge influence that Jaak Panksepp was going to have on the field. His influence became apparent only gradually in my own publications, culminating in 'The Conscious Id' (Solms, 2013) which, in turn, led to a series of publications on the implications of neuropsychoanalysis for the ordinary practice of psychotherapy, with patients in whom there is no question of neurological disease (e.g., Solms, 2017, 2018a, 2018b; Smith and Solms, 2018).

A further major development – one which has taken place since *The Brain and the Inner World* – is the growing influence of the 'predictive coding' framework and 'free energy principle' of Karl Friston (see Solms and Friston, 2018; Solms, 2019). This development, combined with a recognition of the importance of 'reconsolidation' (Solms, 2015), contributed to some re-thinking of the mode of action of psychoanalytic therapy (mainly through the realization that repressed 'wishes' are prematurely automatized *predictions*). However, as far as I am concerned, the most important implication of the free energy principle concerns our understanding of *consciousness itself*. On this basis, I have recently launched an approach to the 'hard problem' that will culminate in a book which has just appeared (Solms, 2021). This development is the culmination of my life's work and, dare I say it, a personal attempt to complete Freud's *Project for a Scientific Psychology* (see also Solms, 2020).

In this chapter, I would like to say something about both of these developments. But first, let me say something about the origins of the field as a whole. Although the *Clinical Studies* was published in 2000, in the same year that our Society was formed and a year after the word 'neuropsychoanalysis' first appeared in print, the work leading up to them began long before the turn of the century.

1 Neuropsychoanalysis: then and now

It was in 1985 that I wrote my first 'neuropsychoanalytic' article (Solms and Saling, 1986), started my dream research, and began the work with Karen Kaplan-Solms that became the *Clinical Studies*. The most important thing that has happened to the field since then is the very fact that neuropsychoanalysis is a 'thing'. It has an established presence in both psychoanalysis and the neurosciences. I do not mean to imply that neuropsychoanalysis now represents the *mainstream* of these fields; but it is definitely part and parcel of them, and even of biological psychiatry (see for example Turnbull and Solms, 2007; Zellner, Watt, Solms and Panksepp, 2011; Panksepp and Solms, 2012). I was very surprised by the hostility with which *psychoanalysts* initially received our efforts – see for example the infamous article by Blass and Carmeli (2007). Their resistance was far greater than what I experienced at the hands of neuroscientists. The small group of analysts who received me warmly in New York (led by Arnold Pfeffer) was very much the exception. But all that has changed now. Today, neuropsychoanalysis has a respectable place in almost every major psychoanalytic centre, with the possible exception of Paris.

I am not sure how many people realise how *odd* it was to envisage such a thing in the 1980s. It was in a sense fortunate that we began in such a remote and isolated place, because it is highly doubtful that the consultant neurologists and neurosurgeons and professors of neuropsychology in the hospitals and universities of more developed countries would have tolerated it. The same applies to institutional psychoanalysis, of course, but it didn't exist in South Africa in the 1980s. In short, nobody told Karen and me that the sort of thing we were doing was not what one is supposed to do, because they didn't know it wasn't. Our medical colleagues simply assumed that neuropsychologists do things like that. They didn't know, to paraphrase Oliver Sacks (1984), that 'official' neuropsychology excluded the psyche. To me, what Karen and I did was the obvious thing for neuropsychologists to do, so we did it. Now, happily, it is the obvious thing for hundreds of colleagues too.

I am not going to say much here about the many reasons that happened. The most clear and demonstrable reasons were, above all, the way in which our *Clinical Studies* led to far more systematic research into the psychodynamic components of 'neurocognitive' disorders. The research of Oliver Turnbull and Katerina Fotopoulou (on confabulation and anosognosia) was pivotal in this regard. Something similar can be said for the way in which my dream research was followed up by others, by experimentalists like Perrine Ruby and Sophie Schwartz. My co-editors have already covered these topics in their introductory chapter. So, if you will indulge me, I would prefer to say something here (extracted from Solms, 2021) about the *very* early years of neuropsychoanalysis.

In fact, the true origins of it were even more obscure than most people know. I was born on the Skeleton Coast of the former German colony of Namibia, where my father administered a diamond mine. The holding company, De Beers, had created a virtual country within a country, known as the *Sperrgebiet* ('prohibited area'). Its sprawling alluvial mines extended from the sand dunes of the Namib Desert down to the Atlantic Ocean floor, several kilometres out to sea. As small children, my older brother Lee and I used to play at diamond mining, using toy earth-moving machines, recreating in our garden the impressive engineering feats we witnessed at our father's side when he took us to see the open-cast mines in the desert. (We were, of course, too young to know about the less impressive aspects of his industry.)

One day, in 1965, when I was five years old, my parents were yachting at the Cormorant Yacht Club, as they often did, and I was left playing in the clubhouse with Lee. I wandered from the cool interior of the three-storey building down to the water's edge. What I remember next is three snapshots. Firstly, the sound of something like a watermelon cracking open. Next, the image of Lee lying on the ground whimpering about a sore leg. Lastly, my aunt and uncle telling me that they would be looking after my sister and me while our parents travelled to the hospital with Lee. The bit about a sore leg must be a confabulation: the medical records state that my brother lost consciousness upon impact with the concrete paving.

Lee needed specialist care of a kind that our local hospital could not provide. He was flown by helicopter to Groote Schuur Hospital in Cape Town, 800 km away. The Neurosurgery Department was then housed in an impressive block built in the Cape Dutch style, the very building that today houses the Neuroscience Institute in which I work. Lee's skull had fractured and he suffered an intracranial haemorrhage. Fortunately, the haematoma resolved itself and he returned home after a few weeks.

Apart from the fact that he had to wear a helmet after the accident to protect his fractured skull, Lee looked no different. As a person, however, he was profoundly altered. The most obvious way in which he was changed was that he lost his developmental milestones, such as reliable bowel control. What I found more disturbing was the fact that he seemed to *think* differently from before. It felt as if Lee was there but not there at the same time. He also seemed to have forgotten many of the games we played. Now our diamond mining game became simply digging holes. Its imaginative and symbolic aspects no longer spoke to him. He was no longer Lee.

He failed that year at school – his first year. The thing I remember most from those early days after the accident was trying to reconcile the fact that my returned brother looked the same with the fact that he was not the same. I wondered where the earlier version of him had gone to.

Over the years following his accident, I fell into a depression. I remember not being able to muster the energy to put on my shoes in the morning, to go to school. I couldn't find the energy because I couldn't see the point of it. If our very being depended upon the functioning of our brains, then what would become of me when *my* brain died, with the rest of my body? If Lee's mind and personality were somehow reducible to a bodily organ, then, surely, mine were too. This meant that I – my sentient being – would exist only for a relatively short period of time. Then I would disappear.

That is how it all began. I wanted to understand what happened to my brother and what would in time happen to me, and to all of us. I wanted to understand what our biological existence as *experiencing beings* amounted to. In short, I wanted to understand the relationship between the brain and subjectivity. That is why I eventually became a neuropsychologist; I thought *that* was what 'neuropsychology' was about!

The state of neuropsychology in the 1980s (when I entered the field) explains why behaviourists made such a seamless transition from learning theory to cognitive neuroscience. The neuropsychology of that time might as well have been called 'neurobehaviourism'. The more I was taught about functions like perception, memory and language, the more I realised that the field was about something other than what I had signed up for. It was about the functional tools *used* by the mind, rather than the mind itself. I was dismayed.

That was when I read Oliver Sacks's book *A Leg to Stand On* (1984), in which he wrote:

> Neuropsychology, like classical neurology, aims to be entirely objective, and its great power, its advances, come from just this. But a living creature, and especially a human being, is first and last active – a subject, not an object. It is precisely the subject, the living 'I', which is being excluded. Neuropsychology is admirable, but it excludes the psyche – it excludes the experiencing, active, living 'I'.

That last line captured my disappointment perfectly. Upon reading it, I entered into a correspondence with Oliver Sacks, which continued until his death in 2015. What drew me to him was the fact that he took so seriously the subjective experience of his patients. *A Leg to Stand On* described his own experience of a nervous system injury. Shortly thereafter, he published *The Man Who Mistook His Wife for a Hat* (1985), which brought him lasting fame.

These books were quite unlike my neuropsychological textbooks, which dissected brain functions as we would the functions of any other bodily organ. Was the brain really no different from the stomach and lungs? The obvious thing that set it apart was the fact that there is *something it is like* to be a brain. This does not apply to any other part of the body. Surely this highly distinctive property of brain tissue – the capacity to sense, feel and think things – exists for a reason. This property appears to *do* something. And if it does, then we will be led badly astray if we omit it from our scientific accounts. Yet that is precisely what was happening in the 1980s. At no point did my lecturers say anything about *what it is like* to comprehend speech or retrieve a memory, let alone *why* it feels like anything at all.

Those who did take the subjective perspective into account were not taken seriously by proper neuroscientists. I am not sure how many people know that Sacks's publications were widely derided by his colleagues at the time. One commentator went so far as to describe him as 'The man who mistook his patients for a literary career'. This caused him a good deal of distress. How can you describe the inner life of human beings without telling their personal *stories*? As Freud had lamented a century before in relation to his own clinical reports:

> It still strikes me as strange that the case histories I write should read like short stories and that, as one might say, they lack the serious stamp of science. I must console myself with the reflection that the nature of the subject is evidently responsible for this, rather than any preference of my own.
>
> (Freud and Breuer, 1895, p. 160)

Sacks was delighted when I sent him this quotation.[1] For my own part, when I first read his work, I realised that I was not alone in having entered neuropsychology with the hope that it would enable me to learn how the brain generates subjectivity. One is quickly disabused of this notion. You are warned not to pursue such intractable questions – they are 'bad for your career'. And so, most students of neuropsychology gradually forget why they entered the field and come to identify with the dogmas of behaviourism or cognitivism.

The one aspect of consciousness that *was* a respectable scientific topic in the 1980s was the brain mechanism of wakefulness versus sleep. In other words, the quantitative 'level' of consciousness was a respectable topic but not its phenomenal 'contents'. So, I decided to focus my doctoral research on an aspect of sleep. But I chose to focus upon the subjective aspect of sleep, namely the brain mechanisms of dreaming. Dreaming, after all, is nothing but a paradoxical intrusion of 'wakefulness' into sleep. Amazingly, there was a huge gap in the literature on this topic: nobody had systematically described how damage to different parts of the brain affected dreaming. So this is what I set out to do.

The Department of Neurosurgery at the University of the Witwatersrand, Johannesburg, had wards in two teaching hospitals: Baragwanath Hospital and Johannesburg General Hospital. Baragwanath was a sprawling ex-military hospital, set in the 'non-European' township of Soweto. Bearing in mind that this was during the height of Apartheid, it was a sea of human misery. The Johannesburg General Hospital, by contrast, was reserved for 'Europeans'; it was a state-of-the-art academic hospital; a monument to racial inequality. The Neurosurgery Department also had beds in the Brain and Spine Rehabilitation Unit at Edenvale General Hospital, which was in an old colonial building set in the middle of Johannesburg's suburbia. Starting in 1985, I worked across all three sites, examining hundreds of patients per year. I included 361 of them in my dream research, which extended over the next five years.

I simply asked neurological and neurosurgical patients at the bedside about changes in their dreams, and then followed them up over days, weeks and months. This is how I proceeded to investigate whether the experience of dreams was systematically affected by localised damage to different parts of the brain. Despite the dubious reputation of dream reports, I assumed that if patients with damage to the same brain area claimed the same change, there was every reason to believe them. This method is, of course, good old 'clinico-anatomical correlation': the standard method of neuropsychology in those days, which had been systematically applied decades before to all the major cognitive functions, such as perception, memory and language. But it had not yet been applied to dreams.

At first, I was a little uneasy about talking to such seriously ill people about their dreams. Many of them were facing, or had just undergone, life-threatening brain surgery, and in the circumstances I feared they might consider my questions frivolous. But, as I am sure many of my colleagues have observed, serious illness can bring out the best in people. The patients were extremely willing to describe the changes in their dreams that their brain diseases had brought about, especially if this meant they might be contributing something to science.

When I first reported that dreaming was obliterated by damage in different parts of the brain from the part that generates rapid eye movement (REM) sleep, I took pains to stress that the critical areas were *not in the brainstem* (see Solms, 1995). This was because I wanted to emphasise the *mental* nature of dreaming, which was being disputed by Allan Hobson (see Hobson, 1988). We all 'knew' that mental life resided in the cortex: the organ of the mind. My error was politely pointed out to me by Allen Braun, who had just done the first major positron emission tomography (PET) study of the dreaming brain (Braun et al., 1997). In the context of my scientific disagreement with Allan Hobson, Braun wrote:

> The curious thing is that, after making a case that forebrain structures must play a critical role in the dream system, Solms ends up by suggesting that it is the dopaminergic afferents to these regions that [generate dreams] – *thereby placing the dream instigator back in the brainstem.*
> (Braun, 1999, p. 196)

Braun concluded: "It sounds to me like these gentlemen are approaching common ground." In the 1990s, in common with the rest of neuropsychology,

I assumed that the cortex was the organ of the mind, so I focused on the fact that the white matter tracts that interested me were located in the frontal lobes, which is where the damage in the most scientifically interesting of my non-dreaming cases was located. But, of course, all the core nuclei of the brainstem send long axons upwards into the forebrain. This underpins the main *arousal* function of the reticular activating system. It was these (mesocortical–mesolimbic dopamine) activating pathways that were damaged in my patients, and in the hundreds of documented non-dreaming leucotomy patients that preceded them.

From 1999 onwards, partly inspired by Braun's comments about the implications of my discovery, I directed my attention to the other arousal systems of the brainstem. The most interesting work in this area was being done by Jaak Panksepp, whose encyclopaedic book *Affective Neuroscience* (1998) laid out in exquisite detail a vast array of evidence for his view that these supposedly mindless systems, responsible for regulating only the 'level' of consciousness, generated a 'content' of their own. This would turn out to be highly significant, as it laid the groundwork for the seminal role that he would play from then onwards, not only in my own scientific life but in the whole development of neuropsychoanalysis.

2 The influence of Jaak Panksepp

The most important thing to remember about the work of Jaak Panksepp is that he was *not a psychoanalyst*. He was not a psychotherapist of any kind. We therefore had to *apply* his ideas to our field, rather than incorporating them into it. Unlike Antonio Damasio, who is at least a clinician – a behavioural neurologist – Panksepp knew next to nothing about the distinctive features of the human mind in health and disease. That is not to say that he knew nothing about people – Jaak was a true Mensch, and he had a lovely way with people – but he had no clinical expertise.

I recall, on one of the occasions that he visited me in Cape Town, taking him into the wards of the famous Groote Schuur Hospital and demonstrating various neuropsychological symptoms and signs to him – while examining some of the patients I thought he might find interesting. I was amazed by how little he understood of what he saw. For example, after demonstrating a textbook instance of denial of illness in a case of dense left hemiplegia following a massive infarction of the right hemisphere (i.e., anosognosia), I asked Jaak if he would like to discuss anything with the patient. "Yes", he replied, and then, turning to her, he kindly asked: "How do you *feel?*". To this she replied, as any good anosognosic would, "I feel fine, thank you". Jaak seemed totally stumped by this response, and he could think of nothing further to say. So we moved on to the next bed. He seemed genuinely to have expected that, although this patient was denying her illness *in words*, the truth would shine through in her feelings!

Jaak's one and only interest in the universe (scientifically speaking) was feelings. He wanted to carve affect at its natural joints. To do this, he used a variety of methods, but mostly he used deep brain stimulation, followed by localized pharmacological probes and lesion studies. For obvious ethical reasons, you cannot do this sort of research on human beings. Jaak's model species, therefore, were (mainly) rodents. He also studied dogs and birds in his early years, but the vast bulk of his research was conducted on laboratory rats.

On this basis, his great contribution to science – for which he will be long remembered – was the anatomical and chemical mapping of seven 'basic emotion' command systems in the rodent brain, which generate seven distinctive sets of instinctual behaviours: LUST, SEEKING, RAGE, FEAR, PANIC/GRIEF, CARE and PLAY. (The capitalization of the terms refers to the fact that they denote whole functional systems, not merely the feelings or behaviours which they give rise to; see Panksepp, 1998.) Extending outwards from there, Jaak was able to show that the very same seven systems could be found in every mammalian species. The same cell groups, located in the same places, connected in the same ways, using the same neurotransmitters and modulators, did roughly the same things in all mammals. This means that the seven basic emotional drives of human beings are at least 200 million years old, since that is how long ago we mammals shared a common ancestor. (I say 'at least' because many of these systems are found in birds too, and some are found in all vertebrates.)

This is news. Really important news. When I first came across Jaak's work (Panksepp, 1985), belatedly, I realized immediately that it had enormous implications for psychoanalysis. Freudian 'instinct' theory had always been the foundation of our metapsychology (since instinctual life clearly represents the bedrock of intentionality), but it was also the most dubious part of it, as Freud himself freely admitted. The reason for this doubt was plain for all to see; how on earth can you expect to identify the basic biological forces driving the human brain just by listening to people saying whatever comes into their heads? Those days, Freud had no choice; neurobiology had not yet developed better methods to answer these questions. Hence, Freud's famous words, when he published his final stab at an instinct theory (I do not say *human* instinct theory, because Freud knew as well as any scientist does that instincts are deeply conserved things, and therefore very ancient)[2]:

> Biology is truly a land of unlimited possibilities. We may expect it to give us the most surprising information, and we cannot guess what answers it will return in a few dozen years. […] They may be of a kind which will blow away the whole of the artificial structure of our hypotheses.
>
> (Freud, 1920, p. 60)

When I read Jaak's (1985) paper, shortly before I read his (1998) magnum opus, I realized that the "few dozen years" that Freud referred to had now passed, of course, and that we finally were in a position to "blow away the whole of the artificial structure" of his hypotheses. From 1999 onwards, therefore, with the aim of developing a new drive theory for psychoanalysis, Jaak became my closest scientific collaborator. He wrote the inaugural paper for our new journal, *Neuropsychoanalysis* (Panksepp, 1999); he also (together with Damasio and Oliver Sacks) delivered one of the keynote addresses at our first annual neuropsychoanalytic congress in 2000 – and he never missed a single one of them after that – and he was elected co-chair (with me) of the International Neuropsychoanalysis Society – a position that he retained until his death in 2017.

Why was Jaak so keen on neuropsychoanalysis? The simple answer is: human beings can 'declare' their subjective mental states. Jaak was traumatized from the very beginning of his scientific career by the injunction that one should not 'anthropomorphise' animal behaviour and, more specifically, that one should not attribute subjective mental states to non-speaking animals – since they are in no position to confirm or deny one's attributions. What Jaak saw in neuropsychoanalysis, therefore, was the opportunity to confirm that the systems he had identified in other mammals led not only to roughly the same behaviours in all of them but also to the specific feelings that he had inferred from the behaviours.

To this end, to mention just one example, after we developed an integrated neuropsychoanalytic view of *depression*, which combined his animal findings with our psychoanalytic ones (Solms and Panksepp, 2010), he participated in studies in which the SEEKING system was activated through deep brain stimulation in humans with depression (Coenen et al., 2019) and in which their PANIC/GRIEF systems were de-activated through novel pharmacological interventions (Yovell et al., 2016). The findings were extremely promising, and they provided proof of concept: the 'despair' phenotype in other mammals is indeed the equivalent of 'depression' in human beings.

These findings were very important for psychoanalysis, too, for the reasons I have just mentioned. We were sorely in need of a new drive theory. That is why, in the wake of the above-mentioned studies (not only on depression but on a host of other psychopathologies, too, and on normal human mental functioning), I set about elaborating a new theory (e.g., Solms and Zellner 2012a, 2012b, Solms and Panksepp, 2012, Solms 2013, Solms, 2018a). These efforts have now culminated in Solms (in press).

However, since this involves an *application* of neuroscientific knowledge to the psychoanalytic situation, the new drive theory could not be elaborated on the basis of an armchair synthesis. It required actual research which (among other things) explicitly involved the psychoanalytic method itself, which necessarily meant clinical research. One of the ways I set about doing this was a double-blind study in which I pharmacologically manipulated various neuromodulators implicated in Jaak's drive theory (Pantelis, unpublished). The results of this study have not yet been published, so I will say nothing more about it here. Another was to establish a study group in Cape Town, in which we considered ordinary psychoanalytical clinical material through two lenses. First we considered the cases through the lens of Freudian instinct theory (in its most developed form, as elaborated by Melanie Klein), and then we re-considered the same material through the lens of Panksepp's instinct theory. Our questions were: (1) does Panksepp's classification of the instincts enable us to see new things that we did not see before? (2) does it prevent us from seeing things we could see before? (3) does this new understanding lead us to a different formulation of the psychopathology? (4) does this different formulation suggest new interventions? (5) does this different understanding and the interventions it leads to yield better outcomes? This group has been meeting monthly for eight years now, and I have since established similar groups in other cities (e.g., in Lima, Tel Aviv, Chicago, Vienna, Buenos Aires, Leeds and Cambridge); and over the past four years I have also held weekend workshops in about 20 cities around the world in which we have used this same method (with two cases being presented by local colleagues in each workshop).

What have our findings been? In short, the consistent answer to four of the above five questions was 'yes' – the exception being question (2). But that is by no means all that we found using this simple method. The other thing we learnt (which was obvious, in retrospect) is that you cannot understand psychopathology – or the psychoanalytic treatment process – using instinct theory alone! To put it as bluntly as I can (again): Jaak Panksepp – God bless him – had no conception of things like RAGE and PANIC/GRIEF coming into *conflict* with one another in depression. He therefore had no conception of the role in depression of the incredibly common (albeit 'secondary') emotion called *guilt*. Moreover, he had no conception of what human beings do when they find themselves in the grip of such insoluble conflicts; that is, he had no conception of the 'solutions' that we in psychoanalysis call *defences*. How can you understand psychopathology without recourse to the concept of defence? And the same applies to a whole host of other highly relevant processes which are absolutely essential to understanding human mental life and psychopathology, such as symbolization, to mention just the most obvious example.

This is no doubt why our psychoanalytic colleague Lucy Biven was driven to distraction when she tried to co-author a book with Jaak on the implications of his work for psychotherapists (Panksepp and Biven, 2012), so much so that they eventually parted ways, and Jaak concluded their book with some infamous 'recommendations' for psychotherapists that no self-respecting psychoanalyst would want to touch with a bargepole. I am not being indiscrete; I said these things to Jaak himself, repeatedly, and in public too. I said:

> Jaak, we love you, and we have an enormous amount to learn from you, but when it comes to psychotherapy, you don't know what you are talking about. So, please stop making all those recommendations; they are

embarrassing! Your giving advice to psychoanalysts about how to do their work is as silly as them giving you advice about how to design your rat experiments. Let each side stick to what it knows, then we can both learn from each other.

Jaak took it all on the chin. But it didn't stop him from making more of his wild recommendations; I think it was all just too much fun for him.

Anyway, the point is that the process of applying Panksepp's findings to psychoanalysis will be a slow and complicated one, if it is going to be done properly. (The same applies to Damasio's findings, of course.)[3] But it deserves every effort. The rewards to psychoanalysis are enormous, as we slowly renew our evidence base, re-establish our empirical credentials and rejoin the family of mental sciences (see Solms, 2018b).

The greatest contribution that Panksepp made to science (and the greatest service he performed for psychoanalysis) perhaps boils down to just this: he demonstrated, using the most rigorous of scientific methods, that feelings *mean* something.

To understand where my own thinking has gone since the *Clinical Studies*, the publications cited above are the most important. But this is in the direction of psychopathology (i.e., 'non-neurological' disorders). The other major direction has been to use what we have learnt from neurological and psychological disorders, both, as well as from the experimental research that we mention above in the introduction, to deepen our understanding of *normal* brain functioning. That takes us even further afield.

3 The influence of Karl Friston

You will recall that what interested me in the first place was the question: where does subjective experience come from? Jaak Panksepp's work had pointed me to the brainstem. He (and later, Antonio Damasio) had made it apparent that subjective feelings were somehow a product of *homeostasis*. This eventually led me to the realization that Freud's (1915) definition of 'drive' as "a measure of the demand made upon the mind for work in consequence of its connection with the body" was nothing other than a definition of what we would now call homeostatic 'error' signals. This took me back to the foundational insights of Freud's 'Project', namely that bodily needs are the driving force of mental life – what he there called "the mainspring of the psychical mechanism" – and that the forebrain is merely a "sympathetic ganglion" monitoring and regulating drive needs. Homeostatic settling points are, of course, a living organism's *expected* states. This meant that feelings were, at bottom, *prediction error* signals.

I only realized this after Katerina Fotopoulou first brought Karl Friston's work to my attention in 2010. This was just after the publication of a remarkable article in the neurological journal *Brain*: Carhart-Harris and

Friston (2010). I knew Robin Carhart-Harris because he had attended several neuropsychoanalytic meetings in London, but, believe it or not, I had barely heard of Karl Friston before. He is (objectively) the most influential neuroscientist in the world today (Friston's h-index is 243). His original claim to fame was 'statistical parametric mapping' which enabled the analysis of functional neuroimaging, but his work on predictive coding and the free energy principle has brought him much more fame.

His paper with Carhart-Harris argued that Freud's conception of drive energy (i.e., 'psychical energy') is consistent with the free energy principle. Freud had readily admitted that he was "totally unable to form a conception" of how bodily needs could become a mental energy. He also wrote that psychical energy is capable of increase, diminution, displacement and discharge, and therefore possesses all the characteristics of a quantity, "though we have no means of measuring it" (Freud, 1894). Considering that Freud's original (abandoned) intention had been to "represent psychical processes as *quantitatively determinate* states", Carhart-Harris and Friston's paper was big news.

I therefore immersed myself in Friston's earlier publications and sought him out. We met several times over the subsequent years, in London and Frankfurt. The main topic of our conversations was the role of affect in mental life, because Friston's work at that time was, like most everyone's, still heavily cortico-centric. The predictive mechanisms he outlined in his publications concerned *cognition* almost exclusively. That is why, for example, his celebrated paper showing how predictive coding explains the way in which neurons communicate with each other was entitled 'A Theory of *Cortical* Responses' (Friston, 2005). The same applied even to his article with Carhart-Harris, which begins like this:

> Freud's descriptions of the primary and secondary processes are consistent with self-organized activity in hierarchical *cortical* systems and [...] his descriptions of the ego are consistent with the functions of the default-mode and its reciprocal exchanges with subordinate brain systems. This neurobiological account rests on a view of the brain as a hierarchical inference or Helmholtz machine. In this view, large-scale intrinsic networks occupy supraordinate levels of hierarchical brain systems that try to optimize their representation of the sensorium. This optimization has been formulated as minimizing a free-energy; a process that is formally similar to the treatment of energy in Freudian formulations.
> (Friston and Carhart-Harris, p. 1265, emphasis added)

I must confess: I never fully understood Friston's more technical publications. This is because the equations in them made me dizzy. In 2017, though, he was invited to be the keynote speaker at our annual Neuropsychoanalysis Congress (which was held in London that year). If I was going to make my usual 'closing remarks' without embarrassing myself, I *had to* master the physics. Among many of Friston's other publications, therefore, I carefully re-read a highly technical article of his in one of the journals of the Royal Society. It was entitled 'Life As We Know It' (Friston, 2013). With great effort, I properly understood it for the first time. This article aimed at nothing less than reducing to mathematical equations the basic laws that distinguish living from non-living things. What are those laws? Well, they are the laws governing *homeostasis* of course. The tendency of living things to resist entropy through homeostasis is the very basis of how we stay alive. The implications were electrifying. I suddenly realised that Friston's equations might provide the breakthrough Freud was looking for in 1895.

Immediately after our scientific exchanges at the congress, therefore, I sent him the following email:

Dear Karl,

I am writing to you in the wake of the London NPSA congress. As you will have noticed – and as was the case at our Frankfurt meeting – I am trying to combine my own thoughts about the nature of consciousness with your fundamental insights into the physical-mathematical laws governing self-organizing dynamical systems. I am increasingly convinced that this combination of ideas yields a solution to Chalmers's 'hard problem' [...] I am busy drafting a book-length explication of my proposed solution, under the title *Consciousness Itself,* but I feel uncomfortable about piggy-backing half of my argument on your work without involving you. I therefore want to suggest that we start by writing something together – a brief article along the lines of 'Why and How Consciousness Arises'. [I then outlined the ideas that eventually became our joint paper, and the book, incidentally, ended up being titled *The Hidden Spring*.] The question is: should we write a joint paper along these lines?

With all good wishes, and enormous respect,

Mark

Friston replied by return:

Dear Mark,

I would be honoured to write a joint paper with you. If it helps, Graham Horswell (the editor in chief of the *Journal of Consciousness Studies*) has requested an inaugural paper after I joined the editorial board earlier this year. If you thought this was a useful forum, I am sure that he would be delighted to receive a paper from us.

With very best wishes – Karl

The *Journal of Consciousness Studies* was where David Chalmers (1995) first articulated the 'hard problem', the Holy Grail of modern neuroscience. The rest, as they, is history.

It turns out that the fundamental driving force of all life forms is that they are obliged to minimise their free energy. This principle governs everything they do. It is a homeostatic principle, but it also goes deeper than that: it explains 'self organisation' (Ashby, 1962), which is the mechanism whereby homeostasis arose from the primal soup in the first place. Not to put too fine a point on it, self-organisation is also how 'selfhood' comes about (through the formation of something called a 'Markov blanket'). Now Friston had reduced self-organisation to a simple law. I call it Friston's law (see below). Armed with this law, everything that we call mental life becomes mathematically tractable, and reducible to physics: to the laws of thermodynamics (and behind that, statistical mechanics) to be exact. I was beside myself with excitement. I recalled Freud's famous words to Wilhelm Fliess:

> In the course of a busy night [...] the barriers were suddenly raised, the veils fell away, and it was possible to see through from the details of the neuroses to the determinants of consciousness. Everything seemed to fit together, the gears were in mesh, the thing gave one the impression that it was really a machine and would soon run of itself. The three systems of neurons [φ, ψ and ω], the free and bound conditions of quantity [Q], the primary and secondary processes, the main trend and the compromise trend of the nervous system, the two biological rules of attention and defence, the indications of quality, reality and thought, the state of the psychosexual groups, the sexual determination of repression, and, finally, the determinants of consciousness as a perceptual function – all this fitted together and still fits together! Of course, I cannot contain myself with delight.

Soon after, however, Freud realised that the gears were not in mesh after all, the thing had not completely fitted together. He then abandoned the project. When Carhart-Harris and Friston's article – and all that it led to – resurrected it, I remembered Freud's poignant remark: "the thing gave one the impression that it was really a machine and would soon run of itself".

I will close these historical musings with a brief synopsis of the argument contained in the book that I announced to Friston, in the letter quoted above. This argument represents the culmination of my life's work and therefore of my part in what has come to be known as neuropsychoanalysis:

1 The great 19th-century physiologist Johannes Müller believed that animate organisms "contain some non-physical element or are governed by different principles than are inanimate things". His students (Helmholtz, Brücke, Du Bois-Reymond, Ludwig and others) disagreed; they were certain that "no other forces than the common physical and chemical ones are active within the organism". Brücke's pupil, Sigmund Freud, tried to establish a natural science of the mind on this basis, in

which mental life could be reduced to "quantitatively determinate states of specifiable material particles". He failed in his project, lacking the methods, and abandoned it in 1896.

2   A century later, the pioneering biologist Francis Crick (1994) declared that "you, your joys and your sorrows, your memories and your ambitions, your sense of personal identity and free will, are in fact no more than the behaviour of a vast assembly of nerve cells and their associated molecules". He exhorted us to try again to discover the neural correlates of consciousness, and he attempted to do so himself. Unfortunately, however, he used *visual* consciousness as his model example.

3   In response, the philosopher David Chalmers (1995) argued that Crick's search for the neural correlates of consciousness was an 'easy' problem – a correlational rather than a causal task – the solution of which could explain *where* but not how and why consciousness arises. For Chalmers, the 'hard' problem of consciousness was: "How and why do neurophysiological activities produce the experience of consciousness?". For him (and his philosophical predecessor Thomas Nagel, 1974) the problem revolved around the something-it-is-likeness of experience: "An organism has conscious mental states if and only if there is something that it is like to *be* that organism – something it is like *for* the organism". The hard problem, therefore, is this: how and why does the subjective quality of experience arise from objective neurophysiological events?

4   To ask how objective things *produce* subjective things is to speak loosely; it risks making the hard problem harder than it needs to be. Objectivity and subjectivity are observational perspectives, not causes and effects. Neurophysiological events can no more produce psychological events than lightning can produce thunder. They are parallel manifestations of a *single underlying process*. The underlying cause of lightning and thunder (both) is electricity, the lawful mechanisms of which explain them both. Physiological and psychological phenomena can likewise be reduced to unitary causes, but not to each other.

5   We normally describe the underlying causes of biological phenomena in 'functional' terms, which can in turn be reduced to physical laws. For example: what is the functional mechanism of vision? However, Chalmers correctly points out that the functional mechanism of vision does not explain *what it is like* to see. This is because vision is not an intrinsically conscious function. The performance of visual functions (even specifically human ones, like reading) need not feel like anything. Perception readily occurs without awareness of what is perceived, and learning without awareness of what is learned. Therefore, Chalmers reasonably asked: "Why is the performance of these functions accompanied by experience? Why doesn't all this information-processing go on 'in the dark', free of any inner feel?". Science's failure to answer this question suggests that consciousness does not form part of the ordinary causal nexus of the universe.

6 Chalmers's question may reasonably be asked of all cognitive functions, not only visual ones, but the same does not apply to affective functions. How can you have a feeling without feeling it? How can we explain the functional mechanism of affect without explaining why it causes us to experience something? Even Freud agreed on this score:

> It is surely of the essence of an emotion that we should be aware of it, i.e., that it should become known to consciousness. Thus, the possibility of the attribute of unconsciousness would be completely excluded as far as emotions, feelings, and affects are concerned.

7 Against this background, it is of the utmost interest to observe that cortical functions are accompanied by consciousness only if it is 'enabled' by the reticular activating system of the upper brainstem. Damage to 2 mm^3 of this region obliterates all consciousness. Many people believe that this is because the brainstem modulates the quantitative level of consciousness or 'wakefulness', but that view is unsustainable. The consciousness generated by the reticular activating system has qualitative content of its own. This is affect. Since cortical consciousness is contingent upon brainstem consciousness, affect is revealed to be the foundational form of consciousness. *The sentient subject is literally constituted by affect.*

8 The qualitative content of affect hedonically valences biological needs, so that increasing and decreasing deviations from homeostatic settling points (increasing and decreasing prediction errors) are felt as unpleasure and pleasure, respectively. Each category of need – of which there is a great variety – has an affective quality of its own (hunger vs. fear vs. disgust, etc.), and each triggers action programmes which are predicted to return the organism to its viable bounds. These active states – i.e., *intentional* responses to the sensory (affective) states – take the form of innate instincts and reflexes, which are gradually elaborated and conditioned by learning from experience in accordance with the law of affect.[4] Feeling by an organism of fluctuations in its own needs enables *choice* and thereby supports its survival in unpredicted contexts. This is the biological function of experience.

9 Needs cannot all be felt at once. They are prioritised by a midbrain decision triangle, where current needs (residual prediction errors, quantified as free energy) converging on the periaqueductal grey are ranked in relation to current opportunities (displayed in the form of a two-dimensional 'saliency map' in the superior colliculi). This triggers conditioned action programmes, which unfold in expected contexts over a deep hierarchy of predictions (the generative model of the expanded forebrain). The actions that are generated by prioritised affects are *voluntary*, which means they are subject to here-and-now choices rather than pre-established algorithms. Such choices are felt as exteroceptive consciousness, which contextualises affect. The choices are made on

the basis of fluctuating precision weighting (aka modulation, arousal and post-synaptic gain) of the incoming error signals that are rendered salient by prioritised needs, with the aim of minimizing uncertainty (maximising confidence) in a current prediction as to how the needs can be met. This is 'reconsolidation'. As Freud (1920) said: "consciousness arises instead of a memory-trace".

10   Reliably successful choices result in long-term adjustments of sensory-motor predictions. This is learning from experience. Thus, exteroceptive consciousness is predictive work in progress, the aim of which is to establish ever deeper (more certain, less conscious) predictions as to how needs may be resolved. This long-term consolidation – and the transition from 'declarative' to 'nondeclarative' memory systems – requires minimization of complexity in the predictive model, to facilitate generalisability. We aspire to automaticity, but we can never achieve it completely. To the extent that we fail, we suffer feelings. Since we never achieve errorless prediction, the default drive (when all goes well) is what Jaak Panksepp calls SEEKING – positive engagement with uncertainty, with the aim of resolving it in advance. When this affect is prioritised, it is felt as curiosity and interest in the world.

11   These are the causal mechanisms of consciousness – in both its manifestations, physiological and psychological – what it looks like and what it feels like. The underlying abstractions can be reduced to natural laws, such as Friston's law.[5] These laws underwrite self-organisation. They are no less capable of explaining how and why proactively resisting oblivion feels like something to an organism, for an organism, than other scientific laws are capable of explaining other natural things. Consciousness is part of nature and it is mathematically tractable.

This is an apt note on which to end these musings.

I cannot find words to express what a pleasure it has been to read the chapters that make up this volume. Studying the inner world of neurological patients is where neuropsychoanalysis began. It is 'home ground', not only for the field but also for me, personally, as a neuropsychologist. It reminds me of my first encounter with the effects of a traumatic brain injury, when I was just five years old, and it reminds me of the scientific debt I owe to every patient I have encountered since. To see how far this new approach to neuropsychological disorders has been developed, by colleagues all over the world, in just 20 years, is cause for deep satisfaction.

Notes

1   "I *love* the passage from Freud – I am very happy you tracked it down. As you say, generously, something analogous might be said of my own case-histories, and of neurological (at least neuropsychological) case-histories in general. I

have quoted it (tho' I don't know whether it will survive – my manuscript has become far too long and footnotey) in a just-completed, rather general piece ('Scotoma') about forgetting and neglect in science." (Letter from Sacks dated January 2, 1995).

2 Thus Freud developed his (1920) theory starting from observations upon unicellular organisms.

3 See, for example, my criticisms of his conception of anosognosia (Solms, 1997b) which revolved around essentially the same points as I make above about Panksepp, namely his failure to take account of the role of *defence* in symptom formation (see also Turnbull, Fotopoulou and Solms 2014).

4 The law of affect: "If a behaviour is consistently accompanied by pleasure it will increase, and if it is consistently accompanied by unpleasure it will decrease".

5 Friston's law: All the quantities that can change, that is, that are part of the system, will change to minimise free energy.

References

Ashby, W. (1962) Principles of the self-organizing system. In H. von Foerster and G. Zopf (eds.). *Principles of Self-Organization: Transactions of the University of Illinois Symposium*. London: Pergamon Press, pp. 255–278.

Blass, R., and Carmeli, Z. (2007) The case against neuropsychoanalysis. On fallacies underlying psychoanalysis' latest scientific trend and its negative impact on psychoanalytic discourse. *International Journal of Psychoanalysis*, 88: 19–40.

Braun, A. (1999) The new neuropsychology of sleep. *Neuropsychoanalysis*, 1: 196–201.

Braun, A., Balkin, T., Wesenten, N., et al. (1997) Regional cerebral blood flow throughout the sleep-wake cycle. An H2(15)O PET study. *Brain*, 120: 1173–1197.

Carhart-Harris, R., and Friston, K. (2010) The default-mode, ego-functions and free-energy: A neurobiological account of Freudian ideas. *Brain*, 133: 1265–1283.

Chalmers, D. (1995) Facing up to the problem of consciousness. *Journal of Consciousness Studies*, 2: 200–219.

Coenen, V., Bewernick, B., Kayser, S., et al. (2019) Superolateral medial forebrain bundle deep brain stimulation in major depression: a gateway trial. *Neuropsychopharmacology*, 44: 1224–1232.

Crick, F. (1994) *The Astonishing Hypothesis: The Scientific Search for the Soul*. New York, NY: Scribner.

Friston, K. (2005) A theory of cortical responses. *Philosophical Transactions of the Royal Society B*, 360: 815–836.

Friston, K. (2013) Life as we know it. *Journal of the Royal Society Interface*, 10: dx. doi.org/10.1098/rsif.2013.0475

Freud, S. (1894) The neuro-psychoses of defence. *Standard Edition*, 3. London: Hogarth Press.

Freud, S. (1915) Instincts and their vicissitudes. *Standard Edition*, 14. London: Hogarth Press.

Freud, S. (1920) Beyond the pleasure principle. *Standard Edition*, 19. London: Hogarth Press.

Freud, S., and Breuer, J. (1895) Studies on hysteria. *Standard Edition*, 2. London: Hogarth Press.

Hobson, J.A. (1988) *The Dreaming Brain*. New York, NY: Basic Books.

Nagel, T. (1974) What is it like to be a bat? What is it like to be a bat? *The Philosophical Review*, 83: 435–450.

Panksepp J. (1985). Mood changes. In P. Vinken, G. Bruyn, and H. Klawans (eds.), *Handbook of Clinical Neurology*. Amsterdam: Elsevier, pp. 271–285.

Panksepp, J. (1998) *Affective Neuroscience*. New York, NY: Oxford University Press.

Panksepp, J. (1999). Emotions as viewed by psychoanalysis and neuroscience: An exercise in consilience. *Neuropsychoanalysis*, 1: 15–38.

Panksepp, J., and Biven, L. (2012) *Archaeology of Mind*. New York, NY: Norton.

Panksepp, J., and Solms, M. (2012) What is neuropsychoanalysis? Clinically relevant studies of the minded brain. *Trends in Cognitive Science*, 16: 6–8.

Sacks, O. (1984). *A Leg to Stand On*. New York, NY: Simon & Schuster.

Sacks, O. (1985) *The Man Who Mistook His Wife for a Hat*. New York, NY: Simon & Schuster.

Smith, R., and Solms, M. (2018) Examination of the hypothesis that *repression is premature automatization*: A psychoanalytic case report and discussion. *Neuropsychoanalysis*, 19: doi.org/10.1080/15294145.2018.1473045

Solms, M. (1995) New findings on the neurological organization of dreaming: Implications for psychoanalysis. *Psychoanalytic Quartely*, 64: 43–67.

Solms, M. (1997a) *The Neuropsychology of Dreams*. Mahwah, NJ: Lawrence Erlbaum Associates.

Solms, M. (1997b) Review of A. Damasio, 'Descartes' error: Emotion, reason, and the human brain. *Journal of the American Psychoanalytic Association*, 45: 959–964.

Solms, M. (2013) The conscious id. *Neuropsychoanalysis*, 15: 5–85.

Solms, M. (2015) Reconsolidation: Turning consciousness into memory. *Behavioral & Brain Sciences*, 38, 40–41.

Solms, M. (2017) What is "the unconscious," and where is it located in the brain? A neuropsychoanalytic perspective. *Annals of the New York Academy of Sciences*, 1406: 90–97.

Solms, M. (2018a) The neurobiological underpinnings of psychoanalytic theory and therapy. *Frontiers in Behavioral Neuroscience*, 12, 294. doi: 10.3389/fnbeh.2018.00294

Solms, M. (2018b) The scientific standing of psychoanalysis. *British Journal of Psychiatry International*, 15: 5–8.

Solms M. (2019) The hard problem of consciousness and the free energy principle. *Frontiers in Psychology*, 10: 2714. doi.org/10.3389/fpsyg.2018.02714

Solms, M. (2020) New Project for a Scientific Psychology: General Scheme. *Neuropsychoanalysis*, 22: 1-31.

Solms, M. (2021) *The Hidden Spring: A Journey to the Source of Consciousness Itself*. London: Profile Books, New York: WW Norton.

Solms, M. (in press) Revision of drive theory. *Journal of the American Psychoanalytic Association*.

Solms, M., and Friston, K. (2018) How and why consciousness arises: Some considerations from physics and physiology. *Journal of Consciousness Studies*, 25: 202–238.

Solms, M., and Panksepp, J. (2010) Why depression feels bad. In E. Perry, D. Collerton, F. LeBeau and H. Ashton (eds.). *New Horizons in the Neuroscience of Consciousness*. New York, NY: John Benjamins, pp. 169–179.

Solms, M., and Panksepp, J. (2012) The 'Id' knows more than the 'Ego' admits: Neuropsychoanalytic and primal consciousness perspectives on the interface between affective and cognitive neuroscience. *Brain Sciences*, 2: 147–175.

Solms, M., and Saling, M. (1986) On psychoanalysis and neuroscience: Freud's attitude to the localizationist tradition'. *International Journal of Psycho-Analysis*, 67: 397–416.

Solms, M., and Turnbull, O. (2002) *The Brain and the Inner World*. London: Karnac.

Solms, M., and Zellner, M. (2012a) Freudian drive theory today. In A. Fotopoulou, D. Pfaff and M. Conway (eds.). *From the Couch to the Lab: Trends in Psychodynamic Neuroscience*. New York: Oxford University Press, pp. 49–63.

Solms, M., and Zellner, M. (2012b) Freudian affect theory today. In A. Fotopoulou, D. Pfaff and M. Conway (eds.). *From the Couch to the Lab: Trends in Psychodynamic Neuroscience*. New York: Oxford University Press, pp. 133–144.

Turnbull, O., Fotopoulou, A., and Solms, M. (2014) Anosognosia as motivated unawareness: The 'defence' hypothesis revisited. *Cortex*, 61: 18–29.

Turnbull, O., and Solms, M. (2007) Awareness, desire, and false beliefs. *Cortex*, 43: 1083–1090.

Yovell, Y., Bar, G., Mashiah, M., et al. (2016) Ultra-low-dose buprenorphine as a time-limited treatment for severe suicidal ideation: A randomized controlled trial. *American Journal of Psychiatry*, 173: 491–498.

Zellner, M., Watt, D., Solms, M., and Panksepp, J. (2011) Affective neuroscientific and neuropsychoanalytic approaches to two intractable psychiatric problems: Why depression feels so bad and what addicts really want. *Neuroscience & Biobehavioral Reviews*, 35, 2000–2008.

Neuropsychoanalyses

Chapter 3

Freud in the light of neuroscience

The brain in the light of psychoanalysis

Maggie Zellner

I Introduction

Since you are reading this book, you are interested in the mind's relationship to the brain – how the brain mediates what we think, feel, and do. You're also interested in a particular question about the mind–brain relationship: how the mind is affected by brain injury or disease. In that case, you need to learn about the brain and the mind from both directions at once. For clinicians working with neurological patients, knowing some organizing principles about the brain helps us make sense of the complicated mental, emotional, or behavioral changes that can happen after brain injury. Conversely, observing how a person's mind changes after a brain injury helps us learn what the brain does under normal conditions.

Clinical Studies in Neuro-psychoanalysis (Kaplan-Solms & Solms, 2000) was a groundbreaking book on both accounts. First, it was the first major work to lay out a comprehensive correlation between brain function and psychoanalytic concepts. It thereby was an excellent primer for psychoanalytic clinicians who were just learning about the brain. In addition, Solms and Kaplan-Solms made extensive psychodynamic observations about the depth psychological consequences of injury in various regions of the brain. This shed important, and often novel, light on the underlying functions of those brain regions. This current book builds on that foundation, exploring new realms of insight at the intersection between neurology, neuropsychology, and psychoanalysis. Clinicians and researchers bring new insights and elaborate older models, through reflecting on the clinical and metapsychological consequences of brain injury or disease. This chapter is designed to provide a foundation for the dialogue that will follow in the next chapters.

Since you are reading a book about *neuropsychoanalysis*, I also guess that you are interested in subjectivity, and you are curious about the inner world. What makes neuropsychoanalysis different from other areas of neuropsychology is our appreciation of that realm, which includes the subjective experience and the dynamic unconscious. In addition to cognition and behavior, we are interested in the things like identification, projection, repression and defense, memory, dreams, and drives. These processes often operate at a deeper level than has typically been taken seriously in main-stream neuropsychology and cognitive science.

This book provides observations from the "front lines" in clinical neuropsychoanalysis – a perspective based on the assumption that, because the brain is the organ of the mind, anything that affects *brain* function is likely to have both conscious and unconscious effects on *mental* processes. These processes include the subjective sense of self, or one's ability to regulate one's thoughts, feelings, and behavior – not to mention the painful emotions that arise from the experience of being impaired in some irreparable way.

In this vein, my final guess is that you are concerned about what makes people suffer and how to help them. You may be interested in the brain mechanisms of effective psychodynamic therapy – how we help "neurotypical" people resolve the conflicts that cause suffering, so that they can lead more engaged lives. You may provide treatment to survivors of brain injury and want to help them navigate their new circumstances. Or both! Although this book focuses on clinical neuropsychoanalysis – observations and techniques related to survivors of brain injury or disease – there is much that will also enrich everyday psychotherapy practice, as well as our daily exploration of our own mental lives and the mysteries of being human. I hope this chapter helps to light your way.

2 Towards a basic model of the brain and mind

To provide a foundation for exploring the chapters to come in this volume, here I sketch out a big-picture view of the organization of the mind and brain, which is largely informed by the model laid out by Solms, particularly in *Clinical Studies* and his paper "The Conscious Id" (Solms, 2013). I focus on several organizing principles described by Sigmund Freud in his model of the mind, primarily informed by his discussion of the mind in *The Ego and the Id* (1923) and Lecture XXIII of the *New Introductory Lectures* (1933). In a very broad-brushstroke fashion, I connect those organizing principles with a relatively simple overview of the brain, designed for newcomers, to prepare for the nuanced, rich, and more scholarly chapters to follow. In addition to *Clinical Studies*, connections between brain functions and psychoanalytic models have been explored in many recent books and book chapters (see, e.g., Boag, 2014; Carhart-Harris et al., 2008; Carhart-Harris & Friston, 2010; Northoff et al., 2007, 2013; Pally, 2007, 2010; Rizzolatti et al., 2013; Roffman & Gerber, 2009; Solms & Zellner, 2012a, 2012b, 2012c; Watt, 1990; Watt & Panksepp, 2009).

As a broader context for the specific correlations I will be sketching in this chapter, I want to note that quite a number of impressive bodies of evidence have emerged from neuroscience since the 1990s that resonate with long-standing psychodynamic claims. These include the following:

*   Most brain activity is *endogenous* (Raichle et al., 2001) (e.g., self-generated, not responding to external stimuli).
*   Most mental processes are *unconscious* (Bargh, 2006).

- *Affect* plays a central role in mental life (Panksepp, 1998).
- Our central motivations are *libidinal* and/or *aggressive*: survival of the individual and propagation of the species (Panksepp, 1998; Swanson, 2000).
- *Early experience* has long-lasting effects (Meaney, 2001; Suomi, 2011).
- Brain activity is guided by *predictions*, derived from experience, at almost every level (Friston, 2010).
- *Fantasy* (including daydreaming and autobiographical memory) constitutes a large portion of conscious mental activity in adult humans (Andrews-Hanna, Reidler, Huang & Buckner, 2010), and activates sensory circuits (Ishai, 2010; Kosslyn et al., 2001) similar to actual perception.
- Delusions and confabulations are often motivated, indicating the *influence of emotion on perception and cognition* (Turnbull & Solms, 2007).

Each of these claims could be a subject of an entire chapter, if not a whole book. Indeed, there are a number of such books by Solms and Turnbull (2002), Panksepp and Biven (2012), Damasio (2010), Mesulam (2000), Hassin, Uleman and Bargh (2006), Dehaene (2014), and Cozolino (2010). Much of this chapter is informed by these works.

One note about the focus on Freud's model. Among the many streams of contemporary psychoanalysis, some have either implicitly abandoned his models or explicitly rejected it (for an overview, see Eagle, 2011). From those perspectives, any attempt to link Freud's concepts to the brain is an irrelevant exercise. At the extreme end of this spectrum, some have even suggested that the entire neuropsychoanalytic project is dangerous (Blass & Carmeli, 2007). But even among those who accept Freud's basic propositions, neuropsychoanalysis has often been criticized for being too Freud-centric, which I often hear from participants at neuropsychoanalytic meetings. Neuropsychoanalysis is often seen, perhaps rightly so, as too "one person"– not taking object relations, relational psychoanalysis, or other developments into account, for example. Mark Solms has expressed, in relation to those concerns, that drawing correlations with some of the basic principles of Freud's models is a necessary starting point, since Freud's ideas are the foundation of psychoanalytic theory. Since Freud's models were largely a one-person model (although always embedded in an object world), this neuropsychoanalytic exploration thus lays the foundation for further exploration of the complexities of the social relational world. Moreover, exploring the inner workings of one brain or mind is already a complex undertaking; dyadic or social interactions are even more so. In parallel with this, although social neuroscience has recently expanded into dyadic interactions, its paradigms and models are still largely unipersonal because of the theoretical and empirical constraints in research (Hasson et al., 2012).

I hope this chapter addresses readers in both camps. If you think most of Freud's core ideas have been surpassed or disproven, I hope you will see the central essence of his model in the brain's organization – which suggests that

Freud's model is still valid. If you think neuropsychoanalysis is "too Freudian", I hope this overview will show you that a neuropsychoanalytic perspective on the brain can accommodate many post-Freudian contemporary psychoanalytic developments – including object relations theory, self-psychology, attachment theory, and interpersonal, relational, and Lacanian perspectives. Of course, some would argue that Freud's thought planted the seeds for, or is consistent with, all of these later trends, even if they were not fully elaborated in his thinking (Makari, 2008; Pine, 1990). Many chapters in this book are examples of how neuropsychoanalysis has begun to engage with psychoanalytic ideas beyond Freud's metapsychology. I trust you will find many examples of how neuropsychoanalytic exploration creates points of contact between streams of psychoanalytic thought. In short, while it is true that, to date, neuropsychoanalysis has been dominated by Freud, the floor is open for your contributions!

3 The big picture

Here is the essential starting point: both the brain and the mind can be divided into *two major sections*. First, there is an *affective/instinctual core*. Second, this core is regulated by an *inhibitory/cognitive/symbolic overlay*. Importantly, the cognitive overlay is significantly influenced by, and indeed is fundamentally in the service of, the affective instinctual core. This basic division emerges from the proposals of Damasio (2010), Mesulam (2000), Panksepp (1998), and Solms (2013). In this section, I will synthesize some of the main ideas these authors have proposed about this structural and functional division.

In the affective/instinctual core are the circuits which mediate the drives, instincts, and primary emotions that we share with all mammals. Our desires press us to get our needs met. Our basic emotions are evolutionarily "designed" to cope with events that help with our survival. We do not need to learn how to do these things. When activated, they are largely *involuntary* and *deeply embodied*. In contrast, our regulatory functions give us the capacity to inhibit our impulses and reactions, creating the space to plan our behavior. We can learn about new things that are associated with rewards and punishments. Finally, we can think and imagine, so we can consider alternatives, and therefore we can create things that didn't exist before. These regulatory capacities are often more *voluntary*, more *abstract*, and *less embodied*. Moreover, regulation is interwoven with the abstract system that is language, which is involved with self-reflection and consideration.

The affective/instinctual core is mediated subcortically: in the brainstem, hypothalamus, and basal ganglia (although certain ancient areas of cortex are also interwoven in these processes). In contrast, the capacities to inhibit, regulate, think, and imagine are primarily mediated in the cortex. The cerebellum is integrated with virtually every level of the brain, so it plays an important role in both divisions.

In an intact adult human brain, these capacities – involuntary and voluntary, emotional and cognitive, perception and imagination, and so on –
are integrated in complex ways, and at such a fast timescale (on the order
of milliseconds) that it is hard to dissociate them in our lived awareness.
However, it does still seem fair to say that in the broadest terms, the inhibitory and regulatory capacities of the cortex are fundamentally in the service
of managing the sub-cortically mediated emotions and instinctual needs
(Solms, 2013). This integration develops over time, in a profound interaction
between nature and nurture that begins *in utero* (see, e.g., Champagne, 2008;
Uhlhaas & Singer, 2011). Thus, we have a "blueprint" for the nervous system
which, while genetically determined, is intensely influenced by experience
(Krubitzer & Kahn, 2003). This influence is strongest in the first years of life,
when our neural circuits are the most "plastic" (Fox, Levitt & Nelson, 2010).

The complex and recursive integration between affective and regulatory
processes underpins such multifactorial processes as the sense of self (Feinberg, 2011; Modell, 1993; Northoff, 2013) and the conscious and unconscious
social rules of behavior (Bargh, 2006; Fonagy & Target, 2007). Indeed, the
consistent ways in which we integrate feeling, thinking, and self-regulation
are central to our sense of continuity and coherence (Modell, 1993, Schore,
1994).

Thus, when the brain circuits that mediate any of these processes are affected by brain injury or disease, the outcome can be very painful for the
survivor and their loved ones. When there are disturbances in the generation of emotion and drives, or the cognitive and regulatory processes, one
can lose one's sense of self or have it fundamentally altered or become a
different person in the eyes of loved ones. This is why clinical neuropsychoanalysis is important. When someone has a brain lesion that affects some
discrete sensory or motor function – for example, if they become blind or
have a paralyzed limb – this is a difficult and painful situation. However,
their basic sense of self, their fundamental capacity to regulate their actions
or maintain their relationships, is not fundamentally impaired (Kaplan-
Solms & Solms, 2000). They will certainly have feelings about losing that
sensory or motor capacity and require plenty of support to navigate their
new challenges physically, socially, and psychologically (Prigatano, 2011).
But if someone suffers injury in parts of the cortex that mediate the ability to *think*, to *inhibit impulses*, or to distinguish between self and other,
between fantasy and perception – then that person's *mind* and the relationship of his/her mind to other minds become fundamentally altered, and they
need a different kind of support (Coetzer, 2006; Turnbull & Solms, 2004).

Since neuropsychoanalysis offers an appreciation of a dynamic inner
world, the importance of emotion and fantasy, and the centrality of relationships, we understand that recovery from brain injury involves more
than physical treatment (see, e.g., Coetzer & Balchin, 2014; Kaplan-Solms &
Solms, 2000; Prigatano, 2011; Salas, 2012; Tiberg, 2014; Turnbull & Solms,

2004). Changes in defenses, character structures, new or old fantasies, and more can all be the outcome of brain injury or disease. A neuropsychoanalytic approach, illustrated in the chapters to come, can thus widen the scope of help that can be provided to survivors and their loved ones.

4 An evolutionary context for a neuropsychoanalytic model of the mind and brain

When trying to grasp the brain and mind in the big picture, I have found it very helpful to look at it in the context of evolution (Buckner & Krienen, 2013). Seeing what we have in common with other mammals and what is different in our brains, and thinking about how we are similar and different in our minds, can illuminate the role of various brain regions in psychodynamic processes.

In terms of *structure*, virtually all vertebrate brains have this in common, as shown in Figure 3.1: a brain stem; cerebellum; hypothalamus, thalamus, and basal ganglia; primary sensory and motor cortex; and at least a small amount of association cortex (the kind of cortex that allows for various

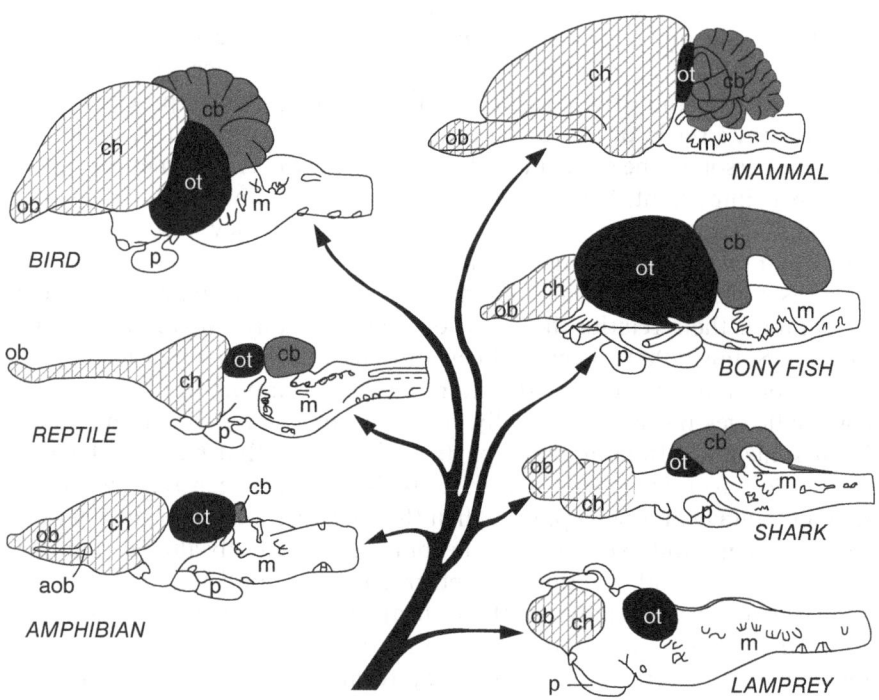

Figure 3.1 Vertebrate brain organization.
Source: From Northcutt, 2002, reprinted with permission.

sensory and motor processes to be integrated). We could say this is the basic "blueprint" for mammalian brains, as all vertebrates have the same brain divisions. Although the relative shapes and positioning of regions differ somewhat from species to species, these differences are variations on a theme, rather than radical departures from each other.

Corresponding with this basic architecture, we can summarize what we have in common in terms of *function* as the following. All mammalian brains have the same infrastructure for primary drives and instincts (Panksepp, 1998). We have the same set of basic needs, species-typical ways to represent those needs, and similar ways of interacting with the environment to meet those needs and ward off dangers. All mammals thus have the capacity to represent the internal body, the external body, and the external world. This is vital for navigating the environment to meet our needs. Finally, all mammals have at least some capacity to inhibit their behavior and to learn in a variety of domains.

The main difference *across* mammalian brains is the amount and proportion of association cortex (Buckner & Krienen, 2013; Krubitzer & Kahn, 2003), as shown in Figure 3.2. Primary association cortex integrates the "raw material" of primary sensory and motor signals into higher order images or motor plans, and multi-model association cortex integrates information and processes from various domains (Mesulam, 2000). Examples of high-level integration include the integration of visual and somatomotor information in the parietal cortex (where we mediate navigating the body and objects in space); visual, auditory, and emotional processes in the temporal lobe (where processes vital to recognition occurs); and cognitive and emotional information and regulatory processes in the anterior prefrontal cortex.

As shown in Figure 3.2, this type of cortex, which integrates various modalities, expands as we go "up" the mammalian evolutionary tree. Humans have significantly more association cortex than nonhuman primates, and this is thought to underlie the major differences between us and them, including language, increased cognitive flexibility, and inhibitory control (Sherwood et al., 2008). Intriguingly, the areas of cortex which are most expanded in humans are also the regions which are most immature at birth and undergo significant development in the first few years of life (Hill et al., 2010). Across species, increased cognitive capacities and inhibitory control are associated with larger brains and/or increased neocortex (MacLean et al., 2014; Sherwood et al., 2008; Stevens, 2014).

Significantly for psychodynamic processes, multimodal association cortex is critical for several major domains of mental life:

- Inhibition (ventromedial and dorso-lateral pre-frontal cortex (vmPFC, dlPFC)
- Generation of imagery (lateral temporal lobe, inferior parietal lobe)
- Computation of relative value (orbito-frontal cortex (OFC), anterior insula)

Common Plan of Organization in Mammals

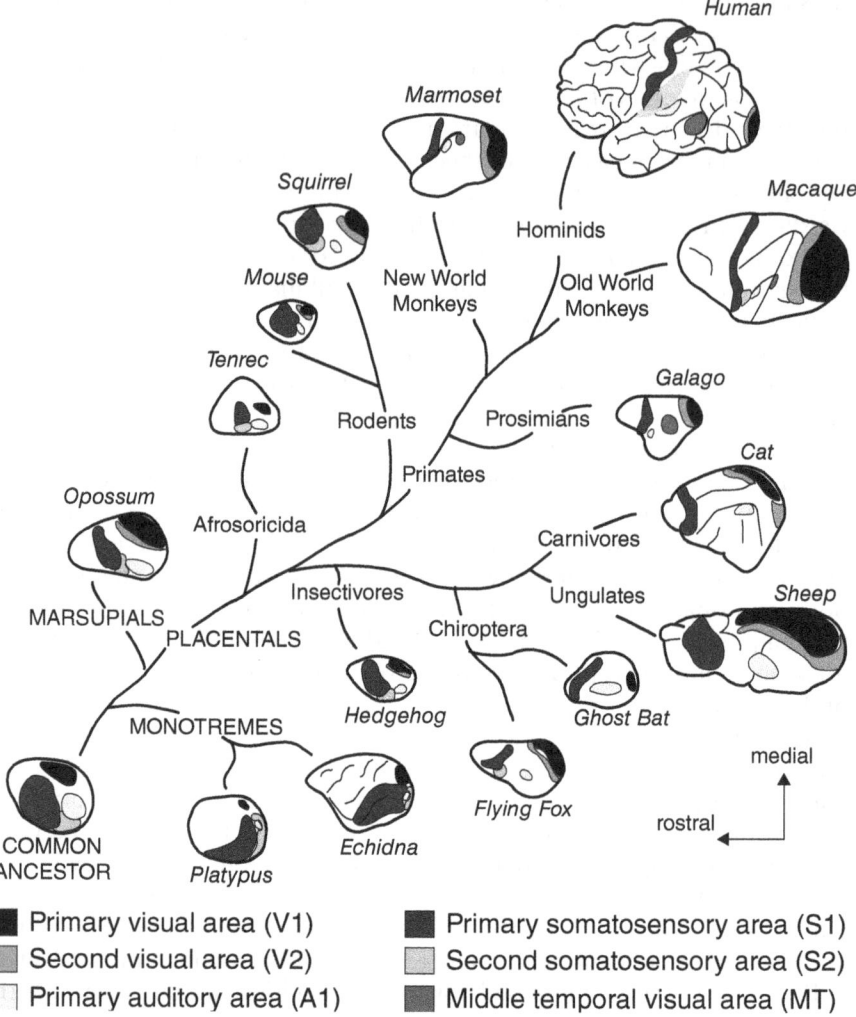

Primary visual area (V1)

Second visual area (V2)

Primary auditory area (A1)

Primary somatosensory area (S1)

Second somatosensory area (S2)

Middle temporal visual area (MT)

Figure 3.2 Expansion of association cortex.
Source: From Buckner & Krienen, 2013, reprinted with permission.

Thus, I suggest that appreciating the dramatic expansion of the association cortex in humans sheds light on the particular strengths and vulnerabilities that humans have. I find that this illuminates the problems I encounter in clinical work and puzzles I encounter when learning about the brain. I find myself imagining what a person can do compared to a rat (which has a fairly small amount of association cortex) and a chimpanzee (which has substantially larger association cortex, but still smaller than a human's). Rats have a wide repertoire of capacities. They can learn a variety of cues and contexts that indicate a reward or punishment and acquire instrumental behavior to gain rewards or avoid punishments (Mackintosh, 1974; Rescorla, 1969). They can also change their behavior as reward contingencies change (Gallagher et al., 1999). Rats appear to engage in "vicarious trial and error," representing the possible outcomes of the end of a maze that it's not currently perceiving, accompanied by corresponding patterns of hippocampal activity (Redish, 2016). Rats exhibit some form of proto-empathy and will work to release a fellow rat from distress (Rice & Gainer, 1962). Compared to rats, great apes show additional capacities. In addition to all of the things rats can do, great apes (like chimps and gorillas) show a range of advanced cognitive capacities, including an ability to manipulate symbols and engage in deception (de Waal, 1992). Evidence suggests that great apes also have theory of mind (Krupenye et al., 2016). A lovely illustration of the capacity of a chimpanzee to take the perspective of another is an anecdote Frans de Waal (2006) shares, in which a chimp on a walk with a group of humans points out a poisonous mushroom to a visitor who has never been to her sanctuary, apparently knowing which of the humans did not yet know about it.

What is harder to explore is whether rats or great apes engage in anything like the volume of imagining that we do. Humans are constantly remembering specific events and imagining the future (Andrews-Hanna et al., 2010). These processes – which can be labeled variously as imagery, imagination, daydreaming, fantasy, "stimulus-independent thought," autobiographical memory, mental time travel, and simulation – are primarily mediated by association cortex, particularly three key hubs grouped into the "default mode network" (DMN; inferior parietal lobe, anterior medial cortex, and posterior medial cortex) (Buckner et al., 2008; Raichle et al., 2001). And certainly humans are capable of inhibiting impulses and reactions to a much greater extent than other animals. We regulate our behavior based on a complex integration of imagining outcomes, imagining others' perspectives, responding to a wide variety of cues, and inhibiting or initiating accordingly.

Thus, it is likely that processes in association cortex – which mediate the lion's share of what we have learned, what we predict, and what we fantasize – are prime candidates for the target of psychoanalytic therapy (Cozolino, 2010). The multimodal areas mediate integrative processes across different domains (including perception, memory, value, and planning), compared to the modality-specific functions of unimodal cortex. Thus, lesions in primary sensory or motor areas lead to discrete and predictable changes, whereas damage to multimodal association cortex leads to more complicated results, which can affect multiple areas of behavior and subjective experience (Mesulam, 2000). In other words, the subjective and/or socioemotional disturbances that follow when multimodal association cortex is affected by brain injury or disease are often more pervasive, and more unpredictable, compared to discrete sensory or motor cortex. The chapters to follow will offer numerous illustrations of this.

To recap, we can divide the brain into an instinctual, emotional subcortical "core," and an inhibitory, learning-influenced, representational/symbolic cortical "mantle" or "canopy."[1] Although expressed in neuroscience terms, I trust that a *psychoanalytic* reader can hear that this division fundamentally correlates with the psychoanalytic division of *id* and *ego/superego* (Solms, 2013).

5 The instinctual/emotional core

As we move into elaborating a correlation between brain circuits and intrapsychic agencies, let's look first at the affective/instinctual core. The oldest, deepest, and most central regions of the brain are involved with embodied, instinctual, affective, motivational, drive-related, and emotional processes (Kringelbach & Berridge, 2009; Panksepp, 1998; Pfaff et al., 2008; Roy et al., 2012; Siegel, 2005). These regions include the brain stem, hypothalamus, and ventral portions of the thalamus and basal ganglia. As mentioned earlier, all mammals have these in common. Circuits in these regions mediate the autonomic and motoric patterns of activity that underlie our homeostatic drives, our basic emotions, and our learned motivational and emotional reactions. In other words, brain stem and subcortical circuits mediate the needs, desires, wishes, and fears that arise from our biological imperative to survive and reproduce – drives and emotions that are evolutionarily given, do not need to be learned, and fundamentally energize and guide all behavior.

A key player, the hypothalamus, receives and sends signals involved with maintaining physiological parameters, promoting individual survival, and facilitating procreation. The hypothalamus registers the needs of the body through hormones, peptides, and other chemical messengers in the blood that indicate the need for food and water, thermoregulation, readiness for sex, and more. When stimulated by other brain circuits, the hypothalamus then triggers specific patterns of motor and autonomic activities to meet the needs (Swanson, 2000). These patterns thus largely correspond to Freud's concept of "instincts" (Solms & Zellner, 2012a). Indeed, the hypothalamus is divided into nuclei which, when activated, trigger all the core instinctual behaviors needed for survival and procreation: eating, copulating, maternal care, defensiveness, and others (Swanson, 2000). The hypothalamus is thus a key node for the "homeostatic" affects like hunger and thirst, and primary emotions like anger (Siegel, 2005).

Much remains to be explored about the brain circuitry mediating emotional behavior, as well as uncertainty about the number of basic emotions (e.g., Ekman, 1992; Wager et al., 2015). However, the evidence summarized by Panksepp (1998, 2011) for discrete circuitry and behavior for seven basic emotion command systems is a solid basis for proceeding with psychoanalytic correlations. As Panksepp suggested, these emotion systems are essentially similar across mammals – similar chemistries, triggers, and patterns of motor and autonomic activation. Based on these similarities, Panksepp argued that it's reasonable to presume that we also have a similar subjective experience, although we may never know that for sure.

Here, I will briefly summarize the systems for the purpose of neuropsychoanalytic correlation. If interested, readers can see Panksepp and Biven (2012) or Panksepp (2011) for more details. First and foremost, the SEEKING system mediates appetitive, foraging behavior – going out into the world to encounter anything that meets needs (and will therefore generate pleasure). This system arises from the top of the brain stem (in the ventral tegmental area [VTA]) and courses through the medial forebrain bundle into the forebrain, synapsing on the ventral striatum, amygdala, and hippocampus on the way. The hypothalamus is a critical sensitizer of the SEEKING circuit. When the SEEKING system is active, we have the psychic energy to exert effort (motivation), and we expect positive things to happen. Because these approach behaviors are central to the activation of this system, Panksepp emphasized the "seeking" aspect. The sustained levels of dopamine associated with foraging and exploration, and the transient increase in dopamine following the consumption of rewards, facilitate learning about cues and environments. In this regard, the activation of expectation and effortful behavior have also been labeled "wanting" by Berridge (2009), which includes the way that cues acquire "incentive salience" when they have been associated with the experience of reward. Thus, the SEEKING system energizes exploratory behavior, increasing our encounters with objects that satisfy needs or present dangers, and also neurochemically facilitates learning about the objects, cues, and environments which satisfy needs or present dangers. However, the SEEKING system does not have a pre-wired notion of the object that is looking for, or non-specific. In psychoanalytic terms, it can be said that this system is "objectless," thus requiring to interact with other systems that attach a value (e.g., reward or punishment) to encountered objects and generate representations of these interactions, thus allowing to learn from experience (Solms & Turnbull, 2002; Solms & Zellner, 2012a).

Panksepp argued that the SEEKING system forms the foundation for the three primary emotion systems that support pro-social behavior: LUST (sexuality), CARE (parental nurturance) (Numan & Insel, 2003), and PLAY (joyful social practicing) (Burgdorf & Panksepp, 2006; Siviy & Panksepp, 2011). These systems are called "pro-social" because they rely on others and ensure positive bonds. First, to have sex, we need another. Second, if there are offspring following sex, they need to be taken care of in order to survive. And third, as offspring develop, they need to practice things they will do as adults. When young animals (including humans) are safe, they will engage in creative, exploratory, "as-if" behavior, which is accompanied by high positive affect and results in positive neurochemical changes in the brain (Burgdorf & Panksepp, 2006). These three systems are mediated by chemicals such as opioids and dopamine, which are associated with strong positive affect (warm, relaxed pleasure with opioids, or excited, appetitive expectation, with dopamine), as well as specific hormones such as estrogen and oxytocin.

We also come "pre-wired" with three systems that produce negative affect, which prepare us to deal with particular challenges. RAGE energizes us to confront threats, competition, or injustice (Siegel, 2005). FEAR causes us to freeze or run away from danger that threatens bodily harm (LeDoux, 2003). PANIC/GRIEF is triggered when we are left alone (Eisenberger, 2012; Panksepp & Abbott, 1990). Since being left alone makes a young mammal or bird vulnerable to future harm (in contrast to FEAR), we are spurred first to protest (to get the caregiver's attention and bring them back), and second to quiet down and save energy until they return (or mourn a loss and move on to new objects). Psychoanalytically educated readers will recognize this last system as a central feature of attachment as described by Bowlby, with the response to loss being the arc from protest to despair (Bowlby, 1973).

Although the basic emotion systems are not learned, in and of themselves, they do play a central role in learning. When emotions are activated, a variety of peptides and neurotransmitters are released, including, in various combinations, dopamine, norepinephrine, acetylcholine, opioids, and stress hormones such as cortisol. These neurochemicals, together with particular patterns of neural activity with emotional arousal, facilitate learning, including emotional memory (mediated by processes in the amygdala and orbitofrontal cortex) (see, e.g., LeDoux, 2003), episodic memory (facilitated by the hippocampus) (Phelps, 2004), and procedural memory (mediated by the striatum) (Gruber & McDonald, 2012; Nicola, 2010). In other words, while we do not have to learn *how* to express our basic emotions or the *essence* of what triggers them, we also have the capacity to acquire a vast number of *new* associations – to learn about new objects and situations that can trigger those basic emotions. This allows mammals to be highly adaptable to a wide range of environments, as we can learn about new rewards and dangers that evolution did not specifically "program" in us.

6 A neuropsychoanalytic link: the affective/instinctual core and the id

So far, I have reviewed some of the central functions of the affective/instinctual core of the brain – the circuits in brain stem, hypothalamus, and related subcortical structures which mediate instinctual motivated behaviors and primary emotions. Based on this evidence, Solms (2013) has argued that these subcortical circuits "do the same intellectual work" as the id: the SEEKING system and the other homeostatic and emotion systems are designed to preserve the well-being of the individual and promote pro-creation. As Freud (1933) described it, the id is

> filled with energy reaching it from the instincts [drives], but it has no organization, produces no collective will, but only a striving to bring about the satisfaction of the instinctual needs subject to the observance of the pleasure principle. The logical laws of thought do not apply in the id, and this is true above all of the law of contradiction. Contrary impulses exist side by side, without cancelling each other out or diminishing each other: at the most they may converge to form compromises under the dominating economic pressure towards the discharge of energy.
>
> (pp. 73–74)

Given the evidence summarized by Panksepp and others that our homeostatic drives and primary emotions have an aim that is associated with an affect – for example, reducing the unpleasure of hunger by eating, the pain of loneliness through companionship, the terror of a predator's approach by finding safety, and so on – it appears that Freud's assertion that the pleasure principle is fundamental to the structure of the mind is born out in the core "architecture" of our brains. At a subjective level, I believe we have all experienced conscious moments where the "id obey[ing] the inexorable pleasure principle," as Freud (1940) put it, breaks through – for example, when we have felt the pressure of a desire or need so strong that it overrules all other considerations. Furthermore, with this linkage of id functions with the subcortical circuits mediating emotion and instincts, it finally made sense to me that Freud labeled this part of the mind the "it" part of ourselves. We all get angry or sad, and we all are "condemned" to having fundamental needs that can't be subverted and must be satiated in order to survive, and which thus fundamentally guide ("drive") our behavior.

Emotions also can seem "timeless" – under the sway of a strong emotion or craving, it feels like the only thing that truly exists or matters in this moment. In everyday life, our mood colors how we think, perceive, and behave. Our emotional state is intrinsically intertwined with our cognition and even our sense of self. The intrinsic fabric of our emotions becomes clearer when they are strongly activated. In the depths of heartbreak, sadness is all there is, and it's hard to imagine ever feeling better. In the grip of strong rage, the desire to punish or destroy can be overwhelming, erasing any memory of this person being kind or loving in the past. In the throes of an addictive compulsion, the pressure to take the drug or engage in the behavior fully takes the reins, even while our wimpy cognition protests that there will be hell to pay later. As Kaplan-Solms and Solms detailed in *Clinical Studies*, and chapters in this book (see chapter 7 by K. Tiberg), these features of the id can be surprisingly visible in patients with damage or disease in areas that normally regulate id functions.

In addition, the fact that emotional and motivational behavior is, first and foremost, not learned corresponds with Freud's assertion of the "heritability" of the id (Solms, 2013) – these are "pre-wired" responses to survival-related events, like approaching rewards and getting away from danger. As Freud put it,

> The experiences of the ego seem at first to be lost for inheritance; but, when they have been repeated often enough and with sufficient strength in many individuals in successive generations, they transform themselves, so to say, into experiences of the id, the impressions of which are preserved by heredity. Thus in the id, which is capable of being inherited, are harboured residues of the existences of countless egos.
>
> (Freud, 1923, p. 38)

This is not as mystical as it may sound; we have indeed inherited "programs" for dealing with the things that our ancestors encountered, the tendency to do the things that allowed them to survive and stay away from the things that would have killed them.

In addition, Freud's idea that drives have "sources" in the body may correspond to activity at the level of the hypothalamus and periaqueductal gray (PAG) (as well as other brain stem nuclei like the parabrachial nucleus), which play a central role in monitoring the needs of the body. When deficits are detected, certain circuits are sensitized to emit movement towards objects in the environment that might satisfy those needs, based on cues acquired through previous experiences of need satisfaction. In other words, the same circuits that respond to messages about the body's needs *also* energize a basic SEEKING tendency, underlying the ability and wiliness to do work to achieve goals. This is consistent with Freud's idea of drives as the demand made upon the mind for work in connection with the body (Freud, 1915; Solms, 2013).

7 The regulatory/inhibitory/symbolic "canopy" and the ego

Having reviewed the instinctual/affective core, which we share with all mammals, we can now turn to the regulatory overlay, which ultimately underlies what makes us distinct from other creatures, particularly in our creativity and our neuroses.

As discussed above, the basic emotions are not learned. We are born with fairly hard-wired emotional instincts, and then learn a lot about things in the world that trigger those emotions. In addition, we are born with circuitry (that matures well after birth) that allows us to regulate and inhibit those emotional responses. However, the rules and contexts in which we regulate ourselves *is* learned. All of these regulatory and inhibitory processes are fundamentally mediated by the cortex. There is wide consensus in neuroscience that the dorsolateral prefrontal cortex (DLPFC) is largely involved with voluntary regulation of behavior and attention (Fuster, 1997; Mesulam, 2000). In contrast, the ventromedial prefrontal cortex (VMPFC) mediates involuntary regulation of emotional response – "gut feelings" about what we should and shouldn't do (Ochsner & Gross, 2005; Roy et al., 2012), in connection with anterior insula (Craig, 2009). Frontoparietal circuits are involved with working memory, critical for staying on task and considering our options before acting (Vincent et al., 2008). Imagining or simulating scenarios recruits a wide range of sensory cortex and, as mentioned earlier, fundamentally involves three cortical areas together called the "default mode network" (inferior parietal lobe, anterior medial cortex, and posterior medial cortex) (Buckner et al., 2008; Raichle et al., 2001).

All of these capacities – to engage in reality testing; to plan, inhibit, and otherwise regulate our behavior; to think before we act – fall under the umbrella of "ego functions" (Freud, 1979; Hartmann, 1968). Therefore, we can, with a broad brush, associate virtually all cortical activity with ego functions (Kaplan-Solms & Solms, 2000; Solms, 2013). According to Freud, the ego is

> that portion of the id which was modified by the proximity and influence of the external world, which is adapted for the reception of stimuli and as a protective shield against stimuli... it has taken on the task of representing the external world to the id – fortunately for the id, which could not escape destruction if, in its blind efforts for the satisfaction of its instincts, it disregarded that supreme external power. In accomplishing this function, the ego must observe the external world, must lay down an accurate picture of it in the memory-traces of its perceptions, and by its exercise of the function of "reality-testing" must put aside whatever in this picture of the external world is an addition derived from internal sources of excitation.
>
> (1933, pp. 75–76)

In Freud's thinking, the foundation of the ego is the mapping of the body and the external world: "The ego is first and foremost a bodily ego; it is not merely a surface entity, but is itself the projection of a surface" (1923, p. 26). This likely corresponds, at least in part, to the cortical circuits which can represent objects in the external world, and thus mediate between what the body needs and what is actually happening in the world, in order to navigate it successfully. However, beyond the concrete mapping of the body, many of the ego functions involved in "reality-testing" are more abstract and involve the capacity for thinking that emerges in conjunction with the ability to inhibit impulses:

> The ego controls the approaches to motility under the id's orders; but between a need and an action it has interposed a postponement in the form of the activity of thought, during which it makes use of the

mnemic residues of experience. In that way it has dethroned the pleasure principle which dominates the course of events in the id without any restriction and has replaced it by the reality principle, which promises more certainty and greater success.

(Freud, 1933, pp. 75–76)

In other words, if we couldn't help trying to meet our needs no matter what is happening in the external world, we wouldn't survive very long. We'd run into trouble right away. It's no good running to the water hole when thirsty if there's a cheetah sitting at the water's edge; grabbing someone to have sex, regardless of how they feel; and stealing food out of our neighbor's hands the moment we get hungry. We wouldn't last long enough to pass our genes on. It's far more adaptive if, once fear has stopped you in your tracks, you can weigh the current variables and imagine ways out of your dilemma. You can determine that the cheetah is actually far enough away that you can manage a sip of water before she could get you; you could make a plan with your tribe to distract the cheetah and take turns drinking.

Thus, a critical role of the ego is *thinking* – and if thinking is affected by brain injury or disease, this can be much more troublesome (for the patient and loved ones) than the more "discrete" outcomes of concrete impairment, as tragic as those losses can be (Kaplan-Solms & Solms, 2000). Because ego functions are quite diverse, and brain injury or disease can target areas throughout the cortex, as well as the connections between areas, the impact of injury can affect ego functions in a wide variety of ways. There can be disturbances in the concrete representation of the body or senses, such as paralysis, blindness, or phantom limbs; difficulty in directing attention or initiating voluntary behavior; impairment in suppressing or inhibiting reflexive or inappropriate responses; deficits in short-term or long-term memory; difficulties expressing or understanding language; and much more.

8 The link between the emotional/involuntary and the cognitive/regulatory: the superego

Thus far, I have been laying out a simple, two-part model, with two distinct anatomical and functional divisions: emotion and instinct, on the one hand; cognition and regulation, on the other. However, the picture is more complex, because not all regulatory processes are "cognitive." In particular, some of the oldest parts of association cortex – the ventromedial and orbitofrontal cortex, anterior cingulate, and anterior insula – straddle the emotional/cognitive divide sketched above. These ancient cortical areas are tightly integrated with the hypothalamic and brain stem structures that mediate instinctual, emotional, and motivational processes (Mesulam, 2000). Cognitive neuroscience has documented how these areas are involved with emotional learning, internalizing social rules, judging affective meaning, and selecting behavior based on the likelihood of reward or punishment (Damasio, 2010; Roy et al., 2012).

Bidirectional, reciprocal connections allow for subcortical emotional processes to strongly influence cortical areas and to influence them in turn. In other words, it is important that there are both "bottom-up" and "top-down" influences (Solms & Zellner, 2012b) – emotional experiences strongly guide learning, as much as, if not more than, cognitively mediated rules can put the brakes on emotional processes (Panksepp, 1998).

Thus, the ventral and anterior cortices are the most "in charge" of regulating the subcortically mediated emotional processes (Ochsner & Gross, 2005, Roy et al., 2012). Because of this bidirectional influence, these regions of association cortex are candidates for the circuits which correspond to Freud's notion of the *superego*. This is the psychic agency overseeing the "shoulds" and "shouldn'ts" of life – what we shouldn't do, for fear of punishment or embarrassment; what we feel compelled or obligated to do, because it just feels right to do so or wrong not to do it. As Freud posited,

> The part which is later taken on by the super-ego is played to begin with by an external power, by parental authority. Parental influence governs the child by offering proofs of love and by threatening punishments which are signs to the child of loss of love and are bound to be feared on their own account. This realistic anxiety is the precursor of the later moral anxiety. So long as it is dominant there is no need to talk of a super-ego and of a conscience. [S]ubsequently ... the external restraint is internalized and the super-ego takes the place of the parental agency and observes, directs and threatens the ego in exactly the same way as earlier the parents did with the child.
>
> (1933, p. 62)

Consistent with this, ventromedial cortical circuits are strongly influenced by early experience, "sculpted" by early social and emotional experiences of reward and punishment (Schore, 1994). As the anterior cingulate is considered the "apex" of the separation distress/GRIEF system (Panksepp, 1998), as well as a key node for monitoring outcomes and switching strategies (Etkin et al., 2006), it is a likely node for mediating the powerful social learning that children take in, based on the approval or disapproval of parents. Indeed, patients suffering disease or injury in these areas often present the most difficulties for their loved ones, as their capacity to regulate their affect and behavior can be severely impaired. Before closing this section, it is important to mention that there is also small literature discussing the "cognitive" aspects of the superego, in particular its simulatory future-oriented (Hopkins, 2012) and verbal-representational nature (Salas, 2016; Salas & Yuen, 2016). This less-attended aspect of the superego has been stressed by classic psychoanalytic authors as well (Bion, 1992; Grotstein, 2004).

9 Recap of the big picture

The sketch in this chapter is extremely abbreviated and has left out a tremendous amount of detail and nuance. But my intention is to offer a simplified correlation between brain circuits and Freud's psychic agencies, to help give context to the rich and complex discussions to follow in the rest of this volume. In this simple sketch, we can say in broad brushstrokes that the *id* is correlated with instinctual/motivational/affective circuits that are primarily subcortical; the *ego* is correlated with cortical circuits mediating reality-perceiving, inhibitory, symbolic, and/or cognitive processes; and the *superego* is tentatively correlated, at minimum, with VMPFCs which mediate the value-laden, primitive, emotional rule-based guidance of behavior (Solms & Zellner, 2012c). In slightly more elaborated terms, we can say that

- The *id* is the "wanting and needing" part of the mind. It is constituted by the need for survival and reproduction. It operates according to the pleasure principle, in the here and now. Key candidate brain circuits include the brain stem, hypothalamus, ventral striatum, and amygdala. These parts of the brain are where we humans have the most in common with our fellow mammals; they are the most "given" by our evolutionary heritage.
- The *ego* is the "execution and regulation" part of the mind. It represents and navigates the external world and negotiates the impulses of the id, based on the ability to inhibit behavior and the capacity to learn and predict. It operates according to the reality principle, creating a space between impulse and action, in which multiple representations of options, and weighing of outcomes, can take place. Ego functions are mediated by primary sensorimotor cortex and virtually all of the neocortex.
- The *superego* is the "should" part of the mind, which weighs in on what the ego regulates and how to regulate it. It is built from identifications with, and internalizations of, prohibitions from the parents and guides the behavior based on social rules. It is likely correlated at minimum with the most ancient parts of the association cortex, including orbitofrontal cortex (OFC) and VMPFC, parahippocampal cortex, and anterior insula. These brain areas are most tightly integrated with the brain stem and ventral basal ganglia. Therefore, they are the cortical regions, on the one hand, that are most deeply informed by the experience of pain and pleasure and, on the other hand, that most efficiently and automatically regulate those body-related subcortical circuits.

For those relatively new to the neuroscience mentioned here, it may be helpful if I put this in experience-near, clinically relevant terms. We are first and foremost *feeling* creatures, trying to meet our needs, maximizing pleasure and minimizing unpleasure. If we feel relatively safe and our basic needs are met, we will engage in pro-social behaviors, based on the four positive affect systems: exploration, play, caring for others, and engaging in sexual activity. If we are threatened, we can react using the three negative affect systems: when challenged by an obstacle, or if our young ones are threatened, we can be defensive; if confronted by danger, we can freeze or run away; if we suffer a loss, we can strive for reunion or grieve and let go. All of these affect systems can be grouped under id functions.

As we go about the world trying to meet our needs and engaging in social life, ego functions allow us to navigate the environment and predict events with ever greater precision. We accumulate knowledge and memories. We learn rules and procedures, predictions that are shaped by the rewards and punishments we have experienced. If things are good enough in our early development, we should have a healthy capacity to inhibit our impulses, delay action, think, and fantasize, using these abilities in the service of maximizing our pleasure and building positive social relationships.

However, if we grow up in families or cultures which have some degree of dysfunction or pathology, some of the rules we live by may get in the way of effectively responding to opportunities and dangers in the world. We may have learned that certain ways of acting, thinking, or feeling are dangerous and should be avoided. We may inhibit ourselves unnecessarily, or predict inaccurately, and then we end up neurotic and suffering. We may have insufficient brakes on our impulses and reactions, and cause suffering for ourselves and others. Psychodynamic treatment and other psychological modalities, as well as addressing socioeconomic conditions that contribute to suffering, are necessary to help us out of the problems created by problematic ego and superego functioning.

If we are unlucky and suffer brain injury or disease, numerous circuits mediating various id, ego, or superego functions may be affected. In these cases, our abilities to regulate ourselves and navigate the world, our relationships or our own subjective experience of selfhood can be distorted or completely derailed. Hopefully the neuropsychoanalytic explorations in this book and elsewhere can help us understand ourselves in our own "derailments" and help others with theirs.

10 Dynamic interactions

While this chapter has focused on segregating various divisions of the brain in order to correlate with Freud's agencies of the mind, we do not want to overstate the distinctions, because in fact the brain is highly interconnected. Indeed, Freud himself said that "one must not take the difference between ego and id in too hard-and-fast a sense, nor forget that the ego is a specially differentiated part of the id" (1923, p. 38).

Neighboring local areas influence each other; most circuits of the brain are incorporated into one or more networks; and large-scale brain networks are dynamically influencing each other in every moment (Fox et al., 2005; van den

Heuvel & Sporns, 2013; Yeo et al., 2011). This degree of dynamic integration and relationship between circuits resonates profoundly with the psychoanalytic perspective of dynamic interaction between agencies; between past, present, and future; between internal fantasy and perception; between wish and fear, impulse and defense; between fast-acting intersubjective processes; and more (Zellner, 2012). Thus, as we think about id/ego/superego dynamics, or emotional/cognitive interactions, or subcortical–cortical connectivity, it's critical to appreciate how interrelated, and reciprocally connected, they are. Each subdivision affects the others. The relationships are inherently dynamic and multidirectional. Indeed, there is such a high level of connectivity and interpenetration that, notwithstanding the simple model sketched in this chapter, these levels of the mind are actually hard to dissociate in lived experience. Overall, the body of affective and cognitive neuroscience ultimately support a psychodynamic picture of a mind and brain in which emotion and cognition, memory and value, past and present, and self and other are all interrelated.

Certainly, in terms of the interactions between the major subdivisions sketched out in this chapter, there is a highly integrated interaction in both directions, as Panksepp and Solms (Panksepp, 2011; Solms & Panksepp, 2012) have emphasized. First, Panksepp (2011) succinctly summarized dynamic interactions, shown in Figure 3.3, when describing the defining characteristics of the emotion command systems:

> They all have a few (1) intrinsic inputs, which behaviorists called Unconditional Stimuli (UCSs); (2) various instinctual behavioral and bodily, especially autonomic-visceral, outputs, which behaviorists called Unconditional Responses (UCRs); (3) the input of various other stimuli into higher brain regions – potential conditional stimuli (CSs) – if they predict rewards and punishments, is controlled by emotional systems

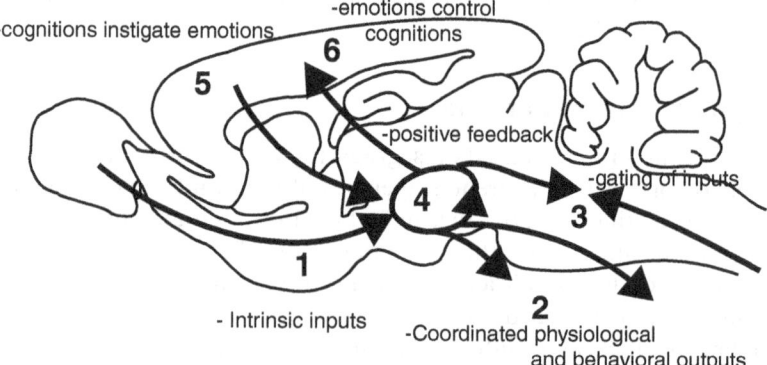

Figure 3.3 Defining characteristics of basic instinctual emotional systems (Panksepp, 2011).

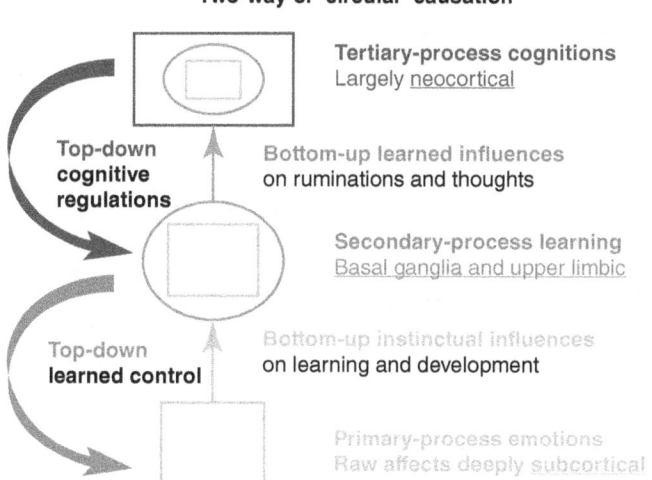

Two-way or 'circular' causation

Tertiary-process cognitions
Largely neocortical

Top-down **cognitive regulations**

Bottom-up learned influences
on ruminations and thoughts

Secondary-process learning
Basal ganglia and upper limbic

Top-down **learned control**

Bottom-up instinctual influences
on learning and development

Primary-process emotions
Raw affects deeply subcortical

Figure 3.4 Nested hierarchies of circular emotional control and regulation within the brain (Panksepp & Solms, 2011).

(yielding what some people call "incentive salience"); (4) emotions out-last the stimuli that activated the systems, whether external (UCSs) or internal ruminations, such as those that arise from, (5) higher cortical areas, especially in the frontal cortex activating or inhibiting emotions, and (6) emotional systems clearly have the power to control and modify higher brain functions – the affective feeling of an emotion largely pro-duced by an internal brain process summarized by attribute 4.

(Panksepp, 2011, p. 1798)

11   Conclusions

As a final offering in this chapter, I think nothing more eloquently expresses the dynamic interactions between different levels of the brain and their re-lationship to central psychodynamic processes, as shown in Figure 3.4 from Panksepp and Solms (2011). Some of the components of that beautifully par-simonious flowchart has been fleshed out in the information surveyed in this chapter, and much more will come in the following chapters.

Much more could have been said in this chapter, of course; we have only covered the most minimum ground. I hope this overview has prepared you for the rich discussions to come in the next chapters and support your en-gagement in this neuropsychoanalytic dialogue. Neuroscience and psycho-analysis are each vast universes in themselves; to bring them together is at times a daunting project. But the neuropsychoanalytic project is filled with discovery, enlightenment, and more "aha" moments than you can count.

Note

1   This is how Jaak Panksepp often referred to the cortex; this architectural term seems appropriate to me, since it drapes over, but does not fully encapsulate, the subcortical structures and brain stem.

References

Andrews-Hanna, J. R., Reidler, J. S., Huang, C., & Buckner, R. L. (2010). Evidence for the default network's role in spontaneous cognition. *Journal of Neurophysiology*, *104*(1), 322–335. http://doi.org/10.1152/jn.00830.2009

Bargh, J. A. (2006). *Social Psychology and the Unconscious: The Automaticity of Higher Mental Processes*. New York: Psychology Press.

Berridge, K. C. (2009). Wanting and liking: Observations from the neuroscience and psychology laboratory. *Inquiry*, *52*(4), 378–398. http://doi.org/10.1111/j.0963-7214.2004.00288.x

Bion, W. R. (1992). *Cogitations*. London: Karnac Books.

Blass, R. B., & Carmeli, Z. (2007). The case against neuropsychoanalysis. On fallacies underlying psychoanalysis' latest scientific trend and its negative impact on psychoanalytic discourse. *The International Journal of Psycho-Analysis*, *88*(Pt 1), 19–40.

Boag, S. (2014). Ego, drives, and the dynamics of internal objects. *Frontiers in Psychology*, *5*, 666. http://doi.org/10.3389/fpsyg.2014.00666

Bowlby, J. (1973). *Attachment and loss, vol. II: Separation*. London: Basic Books.

Buckner, R. L., Andrews-Hanna, J. R., & Schacter, D. L. (2008). The brain's default network: Anatomy, function, and relevance to disease. *Annals of the New York Academy of Sciences*, *1124*, 1–38.

Buckner, R. L., & Krienen, F. M. (2013). The evolution of distributed association networks in the human brain. *Trends in Cognitive Sciences*, *17*(12), 648–665. http://doi.org/10.1016/j.tics.2013.09.017

Burgdorf, J., & Panksepp, J. (2006). The neurobiology of positive emotions. *Neuroscience and Biobehavioral Reviews*, *30*(2), 173–187. http://doi.org/10.1016/j.neubiorev.2005.06.001

Carhart-Harris, R. L., & Friston, K. J. (2010). The default-mode, ego-functions and free-energy: A neurobiological account of Freudian ideas. *Brain: A Journal of Neurology*, *133*(Pt 4), 1265–1283. http://doi.org/10.1093/brain/awq010

Carhart-Harris, R. L., Mayberg, H. S., Malizia, A. L., & Nutt, D. (2008). Mourning and melancholia revisited: Correspondences between principles of Freudian metapsychology and empirical findings in neuropsychiatry. *Annals of General Psychiatry*, *7*(1), 9. http://doi.org/10.1186/1744-859X-7-9

Champagne, F. A. (2008). Epigenetic mechanisms and the transgenerational effects of maternal care. *Frontiers in Neuroendocrinology*, *29*(3), 386–397. http://doi.org/10.1016/j.yfrne.2008.03.003

Coetzer, R. (2006). *Traumatic Brain Injury Rehabilitation: A Psychotherapeutic Approach to Loss and Grief*. New York: Nova Biomedical Books.

Coetzer, R., & Balchin, R. (2014). *Working with Brain Injury: A Primer for Psychologists Working in Under-Resourced Settings*. East Sussex: Psychology Press.

Cozolino, L. (2010). *The Neuroscience of Psychotherapy: Healing the Social Brain* (Norton Series on Interpersonal Neurobiology). W.W. Norton & Company: New York.

Craig, A. D. B. (2009). How do you feel – now? The anterior insula and human awareness. *Nature Reviews Neuroscience*, *10*(1), 59–70.

Damasio, A. (2010). *Self Comes to Mind: Constructing the Conscious Brain*. New York: Pantheon Books.

De Waal, F. (1992). Intentional deception in primates. *Evolutionary Anthroplogy*, *1*(3), 86–92.

De Waal, F. (2006). *Our Inner Ape*. New York: The Berkeley Publishing Group.

Dehaene, S. (2014). *Consciousness and the Brain: Deciphering How the Brain Codes Our Thoughts*. New York: Penguin Books.

Eagle, M. (2011). *From Classical to Contemporary Psychoanalysis: A Critique and Integration*. New York: Routledge.

Eisenberger, N. I. (2012). The pain of social disconnection: Examining the shared neural underpinnings of physical and social pain. *Nature Reviews Neuroscience*, *13*(6), 421.

Ekman, P. (1992). An argument for basic emotions. *Cognition and Emotion*, *6*, 169–200.

Etkin, A., Egner, T., Peraza, D., Kandel, E., & Hirsch, J. (2006) Resolving emotional conflict: a role for the rostral anterior cingulate cortex in modulating activity in the amygdala. *Neuron*, *51*, 871–882.

Feinberg, T. E. (2011). The nested neural hierarchy and the self. *Consciousness and Cognition*, *20*(1), 4–15. http://doi.org/10.1016/j.concog.2010.09.016

Fonagy, P., & Target, M. (2007). The rooting of the mind in the body: New links between attachment theory and psychoanalytic thought. *Journal of the American Psychoanalytic Association*, *55*(2), 411–456.

Fox, M. D., Snyder, A. Z., Vincent, J. L., Corbetta, M., Van Essen, D. C., & Raichle, M. E. (2005). The human brain is intrinsically organized into dynamic, anticorrelated functional networks. *Proceedings of the National Academy of Sciences of the United States of America*, *102*(27), 9673–9678. http://doi.org/10.1073/pnas.0504136102

Fox, S. E., Levitt, P., & Nelson, C. A. (2010). How the timing and quality of early experiences influence the development of brain architecture. *Child Development*, *81*(1), 28–40. http://doi.org/10.1111/j.1467-8624.2009.01380.x

Freud, A. (1979). *The Writings of Anna Freud, Volume II, 1936: The Ego and the Mechanisms of Defense*. London: International Universities Press.

Freud, S. (1915). Instincts and their vicissitudes. *Standard Edition*, *14*, 117–140.

Freud, S. (1923). The Ego and the Id. *The Standard Edition of the Complete Psychological Works of Sigmund Freud, Volume XIX (1923–1925): The Ego and the Id and Other Works*, 1–66.

Freud, S. (1933). New Introductory Lectures on Psycho-Analysis. *The Standard Edition of the Complete Psychological Works of Sigmund Freud, Volume XXII (1932–1936): New Introductory Lectures on Psycho- Analysis and Other Works*, 1–182.

Freud, S. (1940). An outline of psychoanalysis. *Standard Edition*, *23*, 144–207.

Friston, K. (2010). The free-energy principle: a unified brain theory? *Nature Reviews Neuroscience*, *11*(2), 127–138. http://doi.org/10.1038/nrn2787

Fuster, J. M. (1997). *The Prefrontal Cortex: Anatomy, Physiology, and Neuropsychology of the Frontal Lobe*. London: Lippincott Williams and Wilkins.

Gallagher, M., McMahan, R. W., & Schoenbaum, G. (1999). Orbitofrontal cortex and representation of incentive value in associative learning. *The Journal of Neuroscience*, *19*(15), 6610–6614.

Grotstein, J. S. (2004). Notes on the superego. *Psychoanalytic Inquiry, 24*(2), 257–270.

Gruber, A. J., & McDonald, R. J. (2012). Context, emotion, and the strategic pursuit of goals: Interactions among multiple brain systems controlling motivated behavior. *Frontiers in Behavioral Neuroscience, 6*, 50.

Hartmann, H. (1968). *Ego Psychology and the Problem of Adaption*. New York: International Universities Press.

Hassin, R. R., Uleman, J. S., & Bargh, J. A. (2006). *The New Unconscious*. Oxford: Oxford University Press.

Hasson, U., Ghazanfar, A. A., Galantucci, B., Garrod, S., & Keysers, C. (2012). Brain-to-brain coupling: A mechanism for creating and sharing a social world. *Trends in Cognitive Sciences, 16*(2), 114–121.

Hill, J., Inder, T., Neil, J., Dierker, D., Harwell, J., & Van Essen, D. (2010). Similar patterns of cortical expansion during human development and evolution. *Proceedings of the National Academy of Sciences of the United States of America, 107*(29), 13135–13140. http://doi.org/10.1073/pnas.1001229107

Hopkins, J. (2012). Psychoanalysis, representation, and neuroscience: The Freudian unconscious and the Bayesian brain. In A. Fotopoulou, D. Pfaff, & M. Conway (Eds.), *From the Couch to the Lab: Trends in Psychodynamic Neuroscience* (pp. 231–265). New York: Oxford University Press.

Ishai A (2010). Seeing faces and objects with the "mind's eye". *Archives Italiennes de Biologie, 148*, 1–9.

Kaplan-Solms, K., & Solms, M. (2000). *Clinical Studies in Neuro-Psychoanalysis*. London: Karnac.

Kosslyn, S. M., Ganis, G., & Thompson, W. L. (2001). Neural foundations of imagery. *Nature Reviews Neuroscience, 2*(9), 635–642. http://doi.org/10.1038/35090055

Kringelbach, M. L., & Berridge, K. C. (2009). Towards a functional neuroanatomy of pleasure and happiness. *Trends in Cognitive Sciences, 13*(11), 479–487. http://doi.org/10.1016/j.tics.2009.08.006

Krubitzer, L., & Kahn, D. M. (2003). Nature versus nurture revisited: An old idea with a new twist. *Progress in Neurobiology, 70*(1), 33–52.

Krupenye, C., Kano, F., Hirata, S., Call, J., & Tomasello, M. (2016). Great apes anticipate that other individuals will act according to false beliefs. *Science (New York, NY), 354*(6308), 110–114. http://doi.org/10.1126/science.aaf8110

LeDoux, J. (2003). The emotional brain, fear, and the amygdala. *Cellular and Molecular Neurobiology, 23*(4–5), 727–738.

Mackintosh, N. J. (1974). *The Psychology of Animal Learning*. London: Academic Press.

MacLean, E. L., Hare, B., Nunn, C. L., Addessi, E., Amici, F., Anderson, R. C., ... & Boogert, N. J. (2014). The evolution of self-control. *Proceedings of the National Academy of Sciences, 111*(20), E2140–E2148.

Makari, G. (2008). *Revolution in Mind: The Creation of Psychoanalysis*. New York: Harper Books.

Meaney, M. J. (2001). Maternal care, gene expression, and the transmission of individual differences in stress reactivity across generations. *Annual Review of Neuroscience, 24*, 1161–1192.

Mesulam, M. M. (2000). *Principles of Behavioral and Cognitive Neurology*. Oxford: Oxford University Press.

Modell, A. M. (1993). *The Private Self*. Cambridge, MA: Harvard University Press.

Nicola, S. M. (2010). The flexible approach hypothesis: Unification of effort and cue-responding hypotheses for the role of nucleus accumbens dopamine in the activation of reward-seeking behavior. *Journal of Neuroscience, 30*, 16585–16600.

Northcutt, R. G. (2002). Understanding vertebrate brain evolution. *Integrative and Comparative Biology, 42*(4), 743–756. https://doi.org/10.1093/icb/42.4.743

Northoff, G. (2013). Brain and self - A neurophilosophical account. *Child and Adolescent Psychiatry and Mental Health, 7*(1), 28. http://doi.org/10.1186/1753-2000-7-28

Northoff, G., Bermpohl, F., Schoeneich, F., & Boeker, H. (2007). How does our brain constitute defense mechanisms? First-person neuroscience and psychoanalysis. *Psychotherapy and Psychosomatics, 76*(3), 141–153. http://doi.org/10.1159/000099841

Numan, M., & Insel, T. R. (2003). *The Neurobiology of Parental Behavior.* New York: Springer.

Ochsner, K. N., & Gross, J. J. (2005). The cognitive control of emotion. *Trends in Cognitive Science, 9*, 242–249.

Pally, R. (2007). The predicting brain: Unconscious repetition, conscious reflection and therapeutic change. *The International Journal of Psycho-Analysis, 88*(Pt 4), 861–881.

Pally, R. (2010). The brain's shared circuits of interpersonal understanding: Implications for psychoanalysis and psychodynamic psychotherapy. *The Journal of the American Academy of Psychoanalysis and Dynamic Psychiatry, 38*(3), 381–411.

Panksepp, J. (1998). The periconscious substrates of consciousness: Affective states and the evolutionary origins of the SELF. *Journal of consciousness studies, 5*(5–6), 566–582.

Panksepp, J. (2011). The basic emotional circuits of mammalian brains: Do animals have affective lives? *Neuroscience and Biobehavioral Reviews, 35*(9), 1791–1804. http://doi.org/10.1016/j.neubiorev.2011.08.003

Panksepp, J., & Abbott, B. B. (1990). Modulation of separation distress by α-MSH. *Peptides, 11*(4), 647–653.

Panksepp, J., & Biven, L. (2012). *The Archeology of Mind: Neuroevolutionary Origins of Human Emotions.* New York: W.W. Norton & Company.

Panksepp, J., & Solms, M. (2011). What is neuropsychoanalysis? Clinically relevant studies of the minded brain. *Trends in Cognitive Sciences*, 1–3. http://doi.org/10.1016/j.tics.2011.11.005

Pfaff, D., Ribeiro, A., Matthews, J., & Kow, L.-M. (2008). Concepts and mechanisms of generalized central nervous system arousal. *Annals of the New York Academy of Sciences, 1129*, 11–25. http://doi.org/10.1196/annals.1417.019

Phelps, E. A. (2004). Human emotion and memory: interactions of the amygdala and hippocampal complex. *Current Opinion in Neurobiology, 14*(2), 198–202.

Pine, F. (1990). *Drive, Ego, Object, and Self: A Synthesis for Clinical Work.* New York: Basic Books.

Prigatano, G. P. (2011). The importance of the patient's subjective experience in stroke rehabilitation. *Topics in Stroke Rehabilitation, 18*(1), 30–34. http://doi.org/10.1310/tsr1801-30

Raichle, M. E., MacLeod, A. M., Snyder, A. Z., Powers, W. J., Gusnard, D. A., & Shulman, G. L. (2001). A default mode of brain function. *Proceedings of the National Academy Science of the Untied States America, 98*, 676–682.

Redish, A. D. (2016). Vicarious trial and error. *Nature Reviews Neuroscience, 17*(3), 147–159. http://doi.org/10.1038/nrn.2015.30

Rescorla, R. A. (1969). Pavlovian conditioned inhibition. *Psychological Bulletin, 72*, 77–94.

Rice, G. E., & Gainer, P. (1962). "Altruism" in the albino rat. *Journal of Comparative and Physiological Psychology, 55*(1), 123.

Rizzolatti, G., Alberto Semi, A., & Fabbri-Destro, M. (2013). Linking psycho-analysis with neuroscience: The concept of ego. *Neuropsychologia*. http://doi.org/10.1016/j.neuropsychologia.2013.10.003

Roffman, J. L., & Gerber, A. J. (2009). Neural models of psychodynamic concepts and treatments: Implications for psychodynamic psychotherapy. *Trends in Cognitive* Neuroscience, *9*(5), 305–338. http://doi.org/10.1016/j.tics.2005.03.010

Roy, M., Shohamy, D., & Wager, T. D. (2012). Ventromedial prefrontal-subcortical systems and the generation of affective meaning. *Trends in Cognitive Sciences, 16*(3), 147–156. http://doi.org/10.1016/j.tics.2012.01.005

Salas, C. E. (2012). Surviving catastrophic reaction after brain injury: The use of self-regulation and self-other regulation. *Neuropsychoanalysis, 14*(1), 77–92.

Salas, C. E. (2016). Revisiting the left convexity hypothesis: Changes in the mental apparatus after left dorso-medial prefrontal damage Response to commentaries. *Neuropsychoanalysis, 18*(2), 125–131.

Salas, C. E., & Yuen, K. S. (2016). Revisiting the left convexity hypothesis: Changes in the mental apparatus after left dorso-medial prefrontal damage. *Neuropsychoanalysis, 18*(2), 85–100.

Schore, A. N. (1994). *Affect Regulation and the Origin of the Self: The Neurobiology of Emotional Development*. Hillsdale, NJ: Lawrence Erlbaum.

Sherwood, C. C., Subiaul, F., & Zawidzki, T. W. (2008). A natural history of the human mind: Tracing evolutionary changes in brain and cognition. *Journal of Anatomy, 212*(4), 426–454. http://doi.org/10.1111/j.1469-7580.2008.00868.x

Siegel, A., (2005). *The Neurobiology of Aggression and Rage*. Boca Raton, FL: CRC Press.

Siviy, S. M., & Panksepp, J. (2011). In search of the neurobiological substrates for social playfulness in mammalian brains. *Neuroscience and Biobehavioral Reviews, 35*(9), 1821–1830. http://doi.org/10.1016/j.neubiorev.2011.03.006

Solms, M. (2013). The conscious id. *Neuropsychoanalysis, 15*(1), 5–19. http://doi.org/10.1080/15294145.2013.10773711

Solms, M., & Panksepp, J. (2012). The "Id" knows more than the 'ego' admits: Neuropsychoanalytic and primal consciousness perspectives on the interface between affective and cognitive neuroscience. *Brain Sciences, 2*(2), 147–175. http://doi.org/10.3390/brainsci2020147

Solms, M., & Turnbull, O. (2002). *The Brain and the Inner World: An Introduction to the Neuroscience of Subjective Experience*. New York: Karnac Books.

Solms, M., & Zellner, M. R. (2012a). Freudian drive theory and contemporary neuroscience. In A. Fotopoulou, D. W. Pfaff, & M. A. Conway (Eds.), *Trends in Neuropsychoanalysis: Psychology, Psychoanalysis and Cognitive Neuroscience in Dialogue*. Oxford: Oxford University Press.

Solms, M., & Zellner, M. R. (2012b). Emotion in Freudian metapsychology and contemporary psychoanalysis. In A. Fotopoulou, D. W. Pfaff, & M. A. Conway (Eds.), *Trends in Neuropsychoanalysis: Psychology, Psychoanalysis and Cognitive Neuroscience in Dialogue*. Oxford: Oxford University Press.

Solms, M., & Zellner, M. R. (2012c). The Freudian unconscious and evidence from cognitive and affective neuroscience. In A. Fotopoulou, D. W. Pfaff, & M. A. Conway (Eds.), *Trends in Neuropsychoanalysis: Psychology, Psychoanalysis and Cognitive Neuroscience in Dialogue*. Oxford University Press.

Stevens, J. R. (2014). Evolutionary pressures on primate intertemporal choice. *Proceedings Biological Sciences / the Royal Society*, *281*(1786), 20140499. http://doi.org/10.1037/a0031869

Suomi, S. J. (2011). Risk, resilience, and gene-environment interplay in primates. *Journal of the Canadian Academy of Child and Adolescent Psychiatry = Journal De l'Académie Canadienne De Psychiatrie De L'Enfant Et De L'adolescent*, *20*(4), 289–297.

Swanson, L. W. (2000). Cerebral hemisphere regulation of motivated behavior. *Brain Research*, *886*(1–2), 113–164.

Tiberg, K. (2014). Confabulating in the transference. *Neuropsychoanalysis*, *16*(1), 57–67. http://doi.org/10.1080/15294145.2014.898410

Turnbull, O. H., Solms, M. (2004). Depth psychological consequences of brain damage. In J. Panksepp (Ed.), *A Textbook of Biological Psychiatry* (pp. 571–596). New York: John Wiley & Sons.

Turnbull, O. H., & Solms, M. (2007). Awareness, desire, and false beliefs: Freud in the light of modern neuropsychology. *Cortex*, *43*(8), 1083–1090.

Uhlhaas, P. J., & Singer, W. (2011). The development of neural synchrony and large-scale cortical networks during adolescence: Relevance for the pathophysiology of schizophrenia and neurodevelopmental hypothesis. *Schizophrenia Bulletin*, *37*, 514–523.

van den Heuvel, M. P., & Sporns, O. (2013). Network hubs in the human brain. *Trends in Cognitive Sciences*, *17*(12), 683–696.

Vincent, J. L., Kahn, I., Snyder, A. Z., Raichle, M. E., Buckner, R. L. (2008). Evidence for a frontoparietal control system revealed by intrinsic functional connectivity. *Journal of Neurophysiology*, 100, 3328–3342.

Wager, T. D., Kang, J., Johnson, T. D., Nichols, T. E., Satpute, A. B., & Barrett, L. F. (2015). A Bayesian model of category-specific emotional brain responses. *PLoS Computational Biology*, *11*(4), e1004066. http://doi.org/10.1371/journal.pcbi.1004066

Watt, D. F. (1990). Higher cortical functions and the ego: Explorations of the boundary between behavioral neurology, neuropsychology, and psychoanalysis. *Psychoanalytic Psychology*, *7*(4), 487.

Watt, D. F., & Panksepp, J. (2009). Depression: An evolutionarily conserved mechanism to terminate separation distress? A review of aminergic, peptidergic, and neural network perspectives. *Neuropsychoanalysis*, *11*(1), 7–51.

Yeo, B. T. T., Krienen, F. M., Sepulcre, J., Sabuncu, M. R., Lashkari, D., Hollinshead, M., et al. (2011). The organization of the human cerebral cortex estimated by intrinsic functional connectivity. *Journal of Neurophysiology*, *106*(3), 1125–1165. http://doi.org/10.1152/jn.00338.2011

Zellner, M. R. (2012). Toward a materialist metapsychology: Major operating principles of the brain provide a blueprint for a fundamentally psychodynamic infrastructure. *The Psychoanalytic Review*, *99*(4), 563–588.

Chapter 4

Relational neuropsychoanalysis

Giles Yeates and Christian Salas

I Introduction

In the first decade following the publication of *Clinical Studies in Neuropsy-choanalysis* (CSNP; Kaplan-Solms & Solms, 2000), a polemical exchange of perspectives was widely evident in psychoanalytic circles, and within this many would have viewed the construct of *relational neuropsychoanalysis* as a contradiction. An interest for the neuro-anatomical basis of complex psychological processes was viewed as profoundly incompatible with relational psychoanalytic ideas, which emphasised the relevance of the space between people in the constitution of subjectivity. This tension paralleled similar debates that occurred at the same time outside psychoanalysis, for example, between social constructionists and experimental neuropsychologists (Abrams, 2004).

However, during the same 10–15 years there have been two concurrent developments in related fields that have supported the emergence of a relational view in neuropsychoanalysis. Firstly, the social neuroscience revolution, which offered an enormous corpus of evidence regarding the interactional nature of human communicative processes that connect two or more brains, such as emotion recognition and regulation, attachment and mentalizing, or emotional resonance and empathy (e.g., Frith & Wolpert, 2004). Studies from this field provided the possibility to explore the brain in health and pathology from a relational point of view and with novel experimental methodologies that allowed capturing the interpersonal dynamics of these processes.

Secondly, the clinical consideration of neuro-disability (developmental, acquired and progressive) gradually moved towards a relational conceptualisation emphasising the interpersonal and social impact of these conditions. Such paradigm shift allowed clinicians to pay attention to how neurological pathologies not only changed the individual mind but, more importantly, the interpersonal processes by which patients and relatives connect to each other. A growing number of studies described how relatives (e.g., partners, parents, children, siblings, friends) routinely presented to services and articulated their distress regarding changes in the relationship and connection between them and the person with a neurological condition. Even though, in the surface, relative's complaints focused on the patient, for example, his/her changed personality, such transformation inevitably referred to an experience of alienation and the concurrent disruptions of their own self-experience due to this altered connection. Given this level of distress affecting multiple people around one survivor, the previous prioritisation by neuropsychologists on certain modules of neurocognitive function in the individual patient had to necessarily shift to meet these concerns. In addition, clinicians themselves who work over a long period of time with the same service users have also described the impact on their subjective experience, and the therapeutic relationship, arising from prolonged contact with another where a neurological lesion is present (e.g., Lewis, 1999).

So, the clinician making theory–practice links, and the researcher focused on the social dimension of neuro-disability, have both increasingly required theoretical bridging constructs to explain how neurological lesions of different etiologies/locations can not only alter patient–relative communication processes but also impact the minds of others interconnected within the intersubjective field around a patient, including the clinician themselves. From this applied position, in 2017, the polemical exchange in psychoanalytic circles following the publication of CSNP in 2000 seems outdated and unhelpful. What is required is a guiding account incorporating the pathology of the neurological and material level from a relational dimension, a perspective that is sensitive to the qualities of affect, subjectivity and communication, and also considering the wider influences of social contextual processes. So, where to start looking for such a scheme or for important published elements to build this framework if it is insufficiently developed at this point in time?

In this chapter, we present an overview of such sources, starting from the relational seeds to be found in CSNP itself. We then take the main developments over the last century from the progressively relational turn in psychoanalysis and intersect these with the social neuroscience knowledge base, to arrive at a proposal for a contemporary relational neuropsychoanalysis. We will then road-test it with reference to the core interpersonal challenges confronting those with neurological conditions, their loved ones and the clinicians supporting them.

2 Historical elements of a contemporary relational neuropsychoanalysis

2.1 Psychodynamic theory

Freud's original works have both been retrospectively positioned as irreconcilably individualist and containing the embryonic elements that nourished the subsequent relational turn in the field (Frosh, 1987). It is true that the

Freudian classical writings, and the views of neo-Freudians since, position the mind of the analysand as the isolated subject of the analyst's inquiry, with the events of the therapist's mind during the therapeutic process considered but treated with caution. However, Freud's concepts included the first description of the representation of others being incorporated and influencing the mind of the patient (e.g., the introjection of a loved object to maintain in *Mourning and Melancholia*), the articulation of intrapsychic conflict with real interpersonal conflicts and the 'carrying over' of feelings, desires and modes of relating between patient and therapist (*transference-countertransference*).

It was these elements that Melanie Klein used to forge her important developments in psychoanalytic theory. She took Freud's account of projection and introjection from *Mourning and Melancholia* (1917) and incorporated significant new constructs arising from her novel infant observation and child analysis to develop a rich account of the two-way traffic and contortions of multiple minds and the unconscious communication that exists between them (both the developmental dimension in the past and the interactional dimension in the present). Her specific introduction of the projective identification concept (Klein, 1952), as an intrapsychic mechanism, provided a new lens to understand how the organisation of one person's mind (ego-boundaries) is intertwined with, and at times disruptive to, another. Later post-Kleinian authors developed this concept further by stressing the communicative and regulatory nature of projective identification in the patient–therapist interaction (the therapist as a *container*, Money-Kyrle, 1956; Bion, 1959, 1962; Money-Kyrle, 1956). Thus, object relations theorists progressively placed the psychodynamic lens on the space between people and the communication between minds, and parts of minds, within a psychological transaction. These ideas have formed a core corpus that has permeated applied fields beyond traditional psychoanalysis, such as couples/family psychotherapy (e.g., Balfour, 2012), Mentalization-Based Therapy (MBT; e.g., Bateman & Fonagy, 2012) and Dynamic Interpersonal Therapy (Lemma, Target & Fonagy, 2011).

A main limitation of these ideas was that they still privileged the encapsulated minds of each interactional agent while elaborating the unconscious communication between both. Two postclassical psychoanalytic movements have adopted a theoretical stance that focuses on the interaction between minds. The *intersubjective* approach (Atwood & Stolorow, 1984) seeks to understand phenomena that emerge within the psychological field constituted by the intersection of the patient and analyst's subjectivities, and it focuses on the interplay between the differently organised subjective worlds of patient and analyst whom constitutes an indissoluble psychological system (p. 34). The *relational* approach emphasises the role of real and imagined relationships in the configuration of human motivations. As noted by Mitchell (1988),

> we are not a conglomeration of physical urges, but a being shaped by and inevitably embedded within a matrix of relationships with other people, struggling both to maintain our ties to others and to differentiate

ourselves from them (...) In this view, the basic unit of analysis is not the individual as a separate entity whose desires clashes with external reality, but an interactional field within which the individual arises and struggles to make contact to articulate himself (...) The mind is composed of relational configurations.

(p. 3)

2.2 Neuropsychoanalytic theory

The trends in evolved psychodynamic theory above can also be usefully mapped on to developments in neuropsychoanalysis itself. The so-called *depth neuropsychology* in CSNP was strongly based on a classical Freudian metapsychology (Turnbull & Solms, 2004, Fotopoulou, Pfaff & Conway, 2012). But Freud's interpersonal embryonic seeds were inspiringly present in the original book in several ways. Firstly, Kaplan Solms and Solms (KS-S) systematically observed and explored the affective and representational impact that relating to patients, with lesions in diverse brain areas, had in the therapist's mind and behaviour. In other words, how it felt working with a patient who was unable to express his thoughts in words (Broca's aphasia) or acknowledge the functional loss of a paralyzed limb (anosognosia and anosodiaphoria). For us, novel clinicians working in the neurorehabilitation field, such a categorised consideration was extremely novel, since traditional training rarely considered this phenomenon as an object of clinical enquiry or a source of information. Secondly, Freudian ideas on introjective and projective mechanisms were innovatively applied by KS-S to understand the relational corollaries of different lesions, and corresponding neuropsychological impairments, and the specific requirements of the psychotherapist as a result. Memorable offerings of such kind include the explicit statement that the therapist (and significant others) will often need to act as an auxiliary ego that scaffolds impaired abilities in order to optimise patient's functioning. This idea resonates with Luria's emphasis on the need to consider the *inter-mental* space when designing rehabilitation interventions (Luria, 1963).

However, it was perhaps the chapter on lesions to the right peri-sylvian convexity that made the most significant pioneering steps towards a truly relational neuropsychoanalysis. Here, KS-S proposed a theoretical link between the classic right hemisphere syndrome (attentional, visuo-spatial and constructional disorders) and pathognomonic interpersonal problems. The latter were evident too in the transferential–countertransferential patterns within the therapeutic relationship, such as oscillating idealisation and denigration of the therapist, who came to represent hated aspects of the external world that could not be omnipotently controlled by the patient. The authors used Freud's (1914) formulation of narcissism to propose an underlying pathological disruption to intersubjectivity in these patients, characterised by the collapse of the brain's represented peri-personal space and a corresponding regression to ego-centric, part-object ways of relating. In other words, the right hemisphere syndrome not only altered the construction of *real* objects and space, but, more importantly, it severely compromised the constitution of *internal* objects and the relationship of the self with those objects and their virtual minds.

Subsequent neuropsychoanalytic authors working from a relational frame have both valued these initial pioneering offerings and argued for further steps taken towards an interpersonal focus in neuropsychoanalytic formulations of common neuro-rehabilitation topics, such as amnesia (Moore, Salas, Dockree & Turnbull, 2017), awareness of disability (Clarici & Giuliani, 2008; Morin et al., 2005; Yeates, Henwood, Gracey & Evans, 2007), executive function (Yeates et al., 2008), confabulation (Fotopoulou, Solms & Turnbull, 2003; Tiberg, 2014) and emotion dysregulation (Salas, 2012; Salas & Castro, 2014; Salas et al., 2014). The reader should consult the variety of ideas and clinical formulations presented in this current volume as a contemporary picture of this diverse evolution of neuropsychoanalytic thought. These authors have applied ideas from the historical figures of the relational trends in psychoanalysis mentioned above to take these new steps and have commonly placed additional emphasis on the minds and influences of significant others in the maintenance of interpersonal difficulties over time as a core element of neuro-disability.

There is another strand of literature, not directly linked to Freud's work, that has strongly influenced relational views in neuro-rehabilitation and neuropsychoanalysis as well. Kohut's Self-Psychology (Kohut, 1977), for example, proposes that a person's sense of well-being and self-cohesion builds on the many interactions that the person had with his/her caretakers. Kohut's ideas have been foundational in the development of the intersubjective and relational psychoanalytic movement. In Kohut's view, caretakers act as *self-objects* by initially sustaining the child's self-cohesion through the support of physiological and psychological needs (Wolf, 1988). In adulthood, people continue to need self-objects, using friends, family and activities to accomplish such purpose. The idea of self-objects has been used in neurorehabilitation, particularly in order to understand the experience of self-fragmentation and the interpersonal mechanisms used to recover from such states (Klonoff, Lage & Chiapello, 1993; Salas, 2012). It has also been used to consider the diverse forms of transferences that can unfold in the patient-therapist relationship, in order to maintain self-cohesion: mirroring, idealising and twinship (Klonoff & Lage, 1991; Lewis, 1999).

2.3 Social neuroscience

We will not attempt to review the breadth of contemporary social neuroscience constructs here (for reviews see Cacioppo et al., 2002; Harmon-Jones & Winkielman, 2007). Rather, we will comment on basic assumptions from this knowledge base that can be used to substantiate a relational neuropsychoanalysis project. It is argued here that the most important concept from social neuroscience is the idea of a 'shared manifold' (Gallese, 2001; Gallese, Keysers & Rizzolatti, 2004). This idea refers to a field of mind that emerges from the functioning of two or more brains in interaction. This common tapestry of mind and communication has different emergent qualities, dependent on which social cognition neuro-anatomical systems are activated in the brains involved in the social encounter. The interaction of one system (e.g., the medial frontal-temporal sulcus-temporal pole mentalizing system, see below) interacts with that same neuro-anatomical system of the other person. According to Gallese (2003), "it is through this shared manifold that it is possible to recognize other human beings as being similar to us. It is just because of this shared manifold that intersubjective communication and attribution of intentionality become possible" (p. 171). This common tapestry has been described by neuroscientists as an 'intersubjective field' through which the social minds of those linked in interaction are constituted and communicated. In using the methodologies of both functional neuroimaging – to show the contribution of certain systems to this shared manifold – and neuropathology/neuropsychology – to link anatomy to specific forms of dysfunction to social communicative processes – a degree of specificity has been arrived at by social neuroscientists.

A picture has emerged across studies of different types of intersubjective fields of communication, emerging from the activation of specific systems in the brains of social agents. One kind has been described by Gallese, Keysers and Rizzolatti (2004) as *perspectival intersubjective space* and defined as a relational framing of theory of mind/mentalising concepts in the traditional psychology and cognitive neuropsychology fields. This emerges from the activation of medial frontal cortices, temporal poles and superior temporal sulci, and creates a communicative field where social agents can be orientated to divergences between each other's experiences, that is, to compare and contrast perspectives, intentions and points of view, either in the present or in an anticipated future mental state. Many researchers (e.g., Frith & Frith, 2003) have characterised this process as largely effortful and deliberated, where information about a person's external behavior is linked to the context in which it occurs to infer an underlying representation of agency and intention. Other investigators have used different methodologies and metaphors to show how a representation of another's intentions can be more automatically and reflexively elicited by certain cues, such as the facial expression around the eyes of another (Baron-Cohen, 1999). These findings have been linked to certain philosophical traditions that emphasise the automatic relational nature of communication and the representation of intentions, notably the work of Merleau-Ponty (1978): "It is as if the other person's intentions inhabited my body and mine his".

A second form of shared manifold between social agents has been described by Gallese (2010) as *we-centric intersubjective space*, a reciprocal field of neuro-social contact defined by the communication and processing of sameness/shared experience. Here, information processing has been described as characteristically fast, automatic and embodied. The reader is invited to recall a time that they inadvertently walked to a room where two other people in the room have just had an argument. You may not have explicitly known what has just taken place prior to your arrival. However, you feel uncomfortable at the bodily level, in your skin, experiencing awkwardness and discomfort. These feelings may motivate you differentially to tend and facilitate some reconciliation between the other parties, or alternatively propel your quick exit from the situation to relieve your discomfort. These qualities of social experience emerge from a we-centric intersubjective space. It has been proposed that this field emerges from the interaction of those neural systems that contain an overlap of self- and other social and body processing, that is, systems containing neurons that fire when an individual is performing a motor or sensory process with a social meaning, and also fire when an individual sees or hears another encountering the same stimuli and/or performing the same action. This property was initially discovered in cells within the inferior parietal and frontal cortices related to hand actions by Rizzolatti and colleagues (1996) in their now seminal work on 'mirror neurons'. Subsequent researchers have demonstrated simultaneous self/other firing for eyes and mouth movements and the self-perception/other observation of the experience of neutral tactile stimulation, pain (Singer et al., 2004), disgust (e.g., Calder et al., 2000) anger and anxiety (Adolphs, Tranel, Damasio & Damasio, 1994; Goldman & Sripada, 2005). This system recruits somatosensory cortices, anterior cingulate and insula cortices and amygdala. While neuro-anatomically diverse, these areas and abilities share the core tasks of integrating internal bodily and external stimuli within social interactions. Importantly for a relational neuropsychoanalysis, there is empirical evidence to support the unconscious nature of we-centric space communication. Scandinavian neuroscientists (Sonnby-Borgenström, 2008) have studied the automatic facial mimicry that occurs when a person views a human face expressing one of the core emotions. These investigators demonstrated that when these facial stimuli are presented so rapidly that participants have no conscious experience of seeing anything, their facial muscles still mimic the emotion expressed in the subliminal stimulus.

This shared manifold has been shown to also be an important element for decision-making, problem-solving and the regulation of behaviour, when this occurs in socially ambiguous contexts. The work of Antonio Damasio and colleagues (e.g., 1994, 1999) exemplifies repeating findings across groups and paradigms that our social behavior towards others is potently elicited by bodily cues in the expressions of others (evidenced in autonomic arousal as measured through galvanic skin response and cardiac activity) and is guided by our own interoceptive and visceral processes in a fast intuitive, feeling-led way, rather than a rational, cognitive, deductive fashion.

Putting this all together, what assumptions does this social neuroscience literature allow us to make as foundations for a relational depth neuropsychology? Firstly, much of our mind, mental processes and subjective experience, as emergent through neural activity, is inherently relational, formed through the neural activity of multiple brains and via a relational field between people. Secondly, and approaching this from another perspective, our social and interpersonal processes have a neural dimension. We agree with critical social and social constructionist perspectives that emphasise how relational and social contextual processes shape and form mental and psychological phenomena, thereby rejecting a reductionist-cognitivist inputs and outputs account. However, our neuro-focus holds that any material disruption to the neural basis (through developmental difference, acquired lesions or degenerative pathology) will be expressed through and alter these relational and socially constructive processes. Thirdly, in returning to the subjective level (importantly and uniquely for a relational neuropsychoanalytic perspective), this alteration would be experienced by all of those connected within a relational exchange and intersubjective space. One person's insula lesion will be a directly influence on other's perturbed sense of difference or alienation in his/her intimate connection with the neurological patient, with a corresponding disruption to his/her sense of self (e.g., Feigelson, 1993), that is, a tear in the intersubjective fabric between people that results in a corresponding disruption to mind for all those interconnected.

Finally, given the unconscious-automatic dimension to many of these socio-emotional communicative processes when they are working optimally, it is likely that the pathological disruption to these same functions will have unconscious influences on a given social exchange. These influences may overdetermine misalignments between people during socio-emotional communication, and accompanying subjective experiences of alienation, intrusion and disturbance in experiences of self and other for everyone within a social transaction. This hypothesis is congruent with the findings on progressive social isolation and rejection of people with neurological conditions.

2.4 Arriving at a relational clinical neuropsychoanalysis

These four assumptions emergent from social neuroscience, when connected with complementary theoretical elements from the aforementioned progressively relational turn in psychoanalysis, can provide a foundation for a relational psychoanalytic perspective to be applied in clinical neuro-rehabilitation. This point of convergence can be characterised by a prioritisation of the relational/intersubjective dimension as *the field* in which the many deficits and disabilities generated by neuropathology manifest. Any clinician considering this perspective should pay attention – during assessment and treatment – to how a patient negotiates the minds and social communication of others, his/her subjective experience of the relational encounter, and the experience of others in relation to the patient himself/herself. A relational clinical neuropsychoanalytic perspective would encourage to develop therapeutic settings that consider individual, couple, family and group interventions, in addition to informing community neuro-rehabilitative initiatives. Importantly, the minds of the treating therapists, and the process of the clinical team as a whole, would not be considered immune or independent from the relational impact of an identified patient's neuropathology. As such, this would be a constant invitation to reflect about the relationship patterns that emerge during the therapeutic encounter. In other words, to consider how psycho-historical elements from the patient and therapists influence each other's mental states, as well as how the neuropathological profile of the patient shapes such interaction. In view of the impossibility to be immune to the patient and patient's family influence, rehabilitation teams should systematically develop self-care practices as part of their everyday work. Both conscious and unconscious levels of enquiry would be part of all that has been mentioned above. As we move on to summarise the recent focus on relationships within the wider clinical neuropsychological rehabilitation, the potential relevance and contribution of these characteristics of a relational clinical neuropsychoanalysis become clear.

3 The relational turn in neuropsychological rehabilitation

The mapping of the impact of different neurological conditions has progressively broadened in scope over the past three decades. Patients' performance on standardised medical and neuropsychological tests has been complemented by a strong consideration of ecologically valid real-world functional outcomes at the individual level (e.g., personal, domestic, vocational and community independence). The emotional and subjective-existential dimension of patient's experience, while always having been a focus of inquiry for clinicians, became a priority for research and clinical service remit in the late 1990s and early 2000s. A common observation of early studies on this topic was the presence of important levels of distress in those connected to patients with neurological conditions. Furthermore, it was also noted that emotional distress tended to increase over time and, in many cases, was associated with a breakdown in significant relationships (e.g., high divorce and separation rates, Thomsen, 1974) or a deterioration of the social network (Elsass & Kinsella, 1987; Hilari & Northcott, 2017; Northcott, Hirani & Hilari, 2017). Couples and families have always presented their shared relational distress following the onset of a neurological condition to professionals in rehabilitation services, yet have received mixed levels of understanding and systematic support in response.

Empirical research during the past 20 years has highlighted the extent and significance of relationship changes around a lesion or pathology in one person's brain. Studies in both acquired and progressive conditions have demonstrated the presence of clinical levels of distress – anxiety, depression, psychological trauma, anger, adjustment disorders – in romantic partners (e.g., Perlesz et al., 2000), ageing parents (Kreutzer, Gervasio & Camplair, 1994), child relatives of a parent with a neurological condition (Daisley & Webster, 2008), siblings (Willer et al., 1990), friends (Salas et al., 2016) and wider community relations (Elsass & Kinsella, 1987). Interestingly, it has been noted in vocational rehabilitation that changes in social interaction between brain injury survivors and work colleagues were more predictive of employment status/outcome than the survivor's ability to perform the core job competencies (Watt & Penn, 2000). Importantly for this discussion, it is the survivor's social cognition difficulties rather than generic illness adjustment factors that have predicted these interpersonal outcomes. For example, survivor's emotion recognition difficulties have shown to be related to couples' relationship outcome (Blonder et al., 2012), and survivor's mentalising ability and executive difficulties have predicted the appraisal of work social behaviours by vocational informants (Yeates et al., 2016). Inversely, a couple of studies have shown that relative's well-being appears to predict patient's well-being and even rehabilitation outcome (e.g., Carnwath & Johnson, 1987; Sander et al., 2002).

As noted above, the relationship between patient and rehabilitation clinicians is not immune to the interpersonal challenges associated with neurological conditions – this is, of course, unsurprising to psychoanalytic-minded readers. Lisa Lewis (1999) and Mary Pepping (1993), using a psychodynamic framework, drew attention to the different qualities of transference and counter-transference patterns that could emerge between patient and rehabilitation professionals (e.g., idealisation and denigration of the therapist with the clinician's corresponding over-confidence or doubt in his/her ability; collusion in denial of deficits). On a more recent study, Schonberger, Yeates and Hobbs (in press) found that certain social cognition difficulties in brain injury survivors predicted therapist's ratings of their therapeutic working alliance with the service user. Recent interest in the factors that influence the strength of working alliance between patients and rehabilitation teams (Stagg, Douglas & Iacono, 2017) could benefit from this relational perspective.

This emerging picture of widespread and significant interpersonal challenges in many different forms of relationship around the person with neurological conditions has stimulated new innovations in clinical neuropsychological services to prioritise and intervene directly on the relational level, such as group milieu therapies (e.g., Ben-Yishay & Diller, 2011; Gracey, Evans & Malley, 2009; Klonoff, 1997, 2005; Prigatano, 1999), family interventions (e.g., Bowen, Yeates & Palmer, 2010; Evans-Roberts, Weatherhead & Vaughan, 2014; Norup, 2018), couples therapy interventions (Yeates et al., 2013) and the creation of informal therapeutic settings that promote the social encounter (e.g., Miller, 1992; Salas, 2020; Vickers, 2010).

Many of these approaches have acknowledged the need to account for the direct influence of social neuropsychological deficits on both presenting problems and necessary adaptations to therapeutic responses. At the same time, the embryonic literature on social cognition rehabilitation interventions has been criticised for its neglect of both survivor emotional processes and working with live relationships in the room (Yeates, 2014). Given the current evidence for both negative interpersonal outcomes associated with neurological conditions and the acceptance in the professional community of the need to work on such issues in innovative ways, the time is indeed right for interventions informed by an applied relational clinical neuropsychoanalysis to feature in neuro-rehabilitation services.

4 Case example of relational clinical neuropsychoanalytical interventions

We draw to an end of this chapter by an example of the aforementioned ideas and assumptions in practice. To summarise, when informed by the range of ideas and influences shared above, these interventions can be commonly characterised by primarily working on the level of relationships. Those significant to the patient are discerned and any changes to the connection between patient and these people are assessed with the corresponding impact on the patient's subjective experience. The presence of relevant neuropsychological deficits is systematically assessed and incorporated into an emerging formulation, which draws much upon ideas from the progressive relational turn in the psychoanalytic literature, as from social neuroscience and broader neuropsychological literature. The therapist's experience and responses, no matter how unusual or how hard to articulate, are significant sources of information at all times.

Arthur (age 32) was referred by his General Practitioner (GP) to the community neuro-rehabilitation service where one of the authors (GY) works, in order to receive ongoing psychological support to manage the distress he routinely experienced when dealing with others. He reported a history of problematic schooling and early failed attempts to maintain successful employment. His narratives, plus some of his school attainment records, were consistent with a diagnosis of high-functioning Asperger's syndrome, although he never formally received a diagnosis. When he was in his mid-20s, a glioma affecting both right frontal and temporal cortices was diagnosed, and this tumour was surgically removed. He underwent a full neuropsychological assessment with us eight years post-surgery, and this investigation highlighted difficulties in executive functioning, specifically cognitive flexibility – responding to changing patterns of information and implementing multi-part plans in response to multiple goals, attentional switching and mentalizing of others' intentions, plus related aspects of social inference (but he did have intact emotion recognition abilities). The assessment also highlighted a piecemeal perceptual processing style consistent with an autistic spectrum neuropsychological profile (Happé, 1997).

The therapist had an unusual and very strong experience upon entering the waiting room to meet Arthur for the first time. Looking down at the file as he entered the waiting room, the therapist was startled by hearing inside his head: "you piece of shit" (the therapist had never experienced anything like this before). The therapist looked up and scanned the busy waiting room, and eventually made eye contact with a large man staring back in a very contemptuous and dismissive manner. It was Arthur. He was invited in to the consulting room, and he narrated his story of how he was engaged with multiple conflicts with public organisations – the police, the county council and his landlord. He was very distressed as he described a repeating and historical pattern with such organisations: he would contact them to make a complaint about some aspect of the service that was being provided, but the telephone call would quickly deteriorate into conflict when he inevitably felt the representative of the organisation was not *trying* to understand his point of view and *deliberately* lying to him and making judgements about him. This was more likely to occur when dealing with call centres, a lack of a nominated point of contact and representatives reading from customer service scripts. Arthur would become angry and frustrated, and the member of staff would feel abused and threatened, cancelling the call. Over time the organisation would restrict Arthur's ability to contact them.

When some organisations did provide a point of contact, Arthur would follow a pattern of being initially weary of them, then following any positive initial experiences would place the person on a pedestal of perfection, only to be followed by a mistake on the member of staff's part leading to significant distress for Arthur, with a *certainty* that this was a deliberate, malevolent act, reflecting a broader conspiracy on the part of the organisation. In this paranoid state of mind, Arthur would sometimes seek out individual staff members via online social networks and launch vindictive personal campaigns against them. Arthur had frequent arguments with his neighbours (he lives alone) and described many historical relationships where he felt powerless against an unjust, cruel powerful figure of authority (he did not identify any overt episodes of physical or sexual abuse, or profound neglect during any point in his life).

A series of fortnightly clinical neuropsychology sessions were initially agreed. These contained a central psychotherapy element with additional liaison roles for the therapist with the other organisations in Arthur's life and whom he felt were the source of his distress. The therapist has been seeing Arthur for nine years now, with session frequency changing between monthly and fortnightly gaps depending on the challenges faced by Arthur. The very modest aim, given Arthur's profound interpersonal difficulties and tendency to eventually disengage with any collaborative professional relationship, is to maintain an engagement with Arthur and use a formulation of his interpersonal patterns and subjective experience to help him manage his responses to others, to guide liaison with other services, to maintain the safety of the therapeutic relationship for both Arthur and the therapist (alongside the therapist's extensive use of supervision) and to ultimately keep him out of the criminal justice system.

We present here some reflections on the intersubjective field as experienced by the therapist and shared in dialogue with Arthur. These elements were subsequently used to generate a formulation that would become a pivotal resource in the liaison with other services and attempts to guide the interactional patterns with these groups away from the historical end points of conflict. The therapist was initially overwhelmed with feelings of intimidation when in the company of Arthur, feeling like walking on eggshells or trying to blindly negotiate a field of hidden landmines. When trying to reach out to Arthur and offer a view that was meant to clarify or empathise, this would quickly become a trigger for Arthur to become frustrated and angry at times, feeling that once again he was being misunderstood by a professional. He would often return to subsequent sessions having ruminated during the interceding week about a comment or non-verbal gesture on the therapist's part, confirming his suspicion that the therapist's intentions towards him may secretly be malevolent, as with all the others, and would more likely come to be so the longer the therapist worked with him ("when you find out what I'm really like you'll won't be able to manage me"). The marching of time would only bring us towards both the inevitable end point of relationship rupture, disconnection and rejection, and the inevitable end point of conflict and cruelty between us.

The therapist's own process felt like a roller coaster: trying to provide a perfect comprehensive response to Arthur's needs, which was more likely to be met by criticism from Arthur and in turn a privately angry response by the therapist ("how ungrateful..."), which ran the danger of evolving into sadistic and/or dismissive feelings towards Arthur. In parallel to this, it became discernible as the therapist developed a liaison role with some of the aforementioned organisations that towards the end of an increasingly conflictual relationship with Arthur, individual members of staff would act in unambiguously sadistic and/or dismissive ways towards him, beyond the limits of acceptable professional practice.

MBT (Bateman & Fonagy, 2012) informed the main core of the intervention, guiding the therapist to support the mentalisation between both he and Arthur at all times. The intervention began with an early warning to Arthur that being another human being, the therapist would inevitably let him down the way all the others have done, and that they both would need to expect this and have a survival plan in place. Arthur's representations of others' intentionality were highlighted and formulated early on, helping him to become more aware of how he chose to keep himself safe when he encountered that 'kind of mind' in another. The relationship with the therapist was the main testing ground for this work, where Arthur would be encouraged and validated to share moments where he became unclear about the therapist's internal world, and the therapist would explore the distress these moments would cause him. Following the principles of MBT, the therapist would try and maintain clarity and honesty about his intentions and perspectives throughout, to avoid further escalation of anxiety on Arthur's part that would further reduce his ability to mentalise. This approach allowed Arthur, at times, to move away from certainty of another's malevolence to tolerating the 'not knowing' of another person's inner world when they act in a way that surprised him (moving away from a 'psychic equivalence' mode in MBT terms). However, this progress was easily reversed when a trigger (the therapist's actions not being clearly enough indicative that he was 'on Arthur's side') was too big, and the work would have to start back at square one, rebuilding foundations to get to a place where the transference/intersubjective field processes could be jointly considered by both Arthur and the therapist once again.

At the same time, the therapist used a Kleinian framework to recognise the visceral turmoil of projective identificatory processes and the pull these would have on him. Rather than acting on these, the therapist would use these as stimuli to wonder in session (when it felt safe to do so and not overwhelm Arthur) if Arthur was suddenly feeling unsafe and to discern together the occurrence of any interpersonal trigger. The therapist and Arthur created a shared language (and a visual formulation) together of these 'unsafe' moments for both he and the person upon which he was relying. This formulation would then be used in abbreviated form to inform other key points of contact in organisations of such moments before they occurred and to invite them to use the therapist's help to negotiate these turbulent waters. Family sessions also benefited from this understanding.

Bringing to bear the theoretical ideas explored above, the core assumption held by the therapist/clinical neuropsychologist is that the damaged neuro-anatomical networks in Arthur's brain subserving socio-emotional processing influence a shared transaction of mind with others. This transaction is experienced subjectively by others as a very powerful disruption to self when in the company of Arthur, undermining their ability to mentalise, attune to emotion and respond accordingly. These disruptions to self-other organisations were experienced as violent attacks and elicit early infantile anxieties for both Arthur and those temporarily connected with him (before these processes become too unbearable and force disconnection and rejection, repudiation of these feelings and him). Of course, these factors have manifested through a wider context of Arthur's experiences of psychological trauma and the effects of such on his relations with others. However, this relational clinical neuropsychoanalytic perspective maintains a spotlight on the underlying interpersonal vulnerability affecting all past, current and future contact with others, as a function of neuro-anatomical difference.

These ideas have allowed the creation and maintenance of a useful theoretical lens that links altered neuropathology with the immediacy of the interpersonal experience with Arthur. Furthermore, it has created a road map to guide the work in a way that has seen the maintenance of Arthur's engagement over nine years, while other organisations have been dismissed by him. In addition, such relational formulation has helped the therapist in maintaining his own mental health and usefulness in the face of very strong conscious and unconscious interpersonal processes, thus contributing to treatment adherence and helping the patient to remain outside of the criminal justice system for nearly a decade.

5 Conclusions

We have described how the interpersonal elements evident in Kaplan-Solms and Solms's (2000) classic work have matured during the past 20 years gaining the attention of many clinical neuropsychologist working with brain-injured populations. Such process has benefited as well by the evolution of relational strands in psychoanalytic theory, which have underscored the need to consider psychological development, psychopathology and therapeutics from an interpersonal angle. In addition, the emerging field of social neuroscience has also contributed to understand the neural architecture and neuropsychological mechanisms that support socio-emotional functions in human interaction. We believe that a relational neuropsychoanalytic approach can not only have a theoretical value but, most importantly, contribute to individual case formulations as well as informing the work of rehabilitation services and rehabilitation teams with brain-injured patients. This is particularly relevant at this historical moment in neurorehabilitation, where the relational impact of disability has become increasingly a focus of assessment and intervention.

The elements of the proposed configuration of theory and practice have been selected from the rich heritage of the progressively relational turn in psychoanalysis, social neuroscience and clinical neuro-rehabilitation research. This has been by no means a definitive selection of theoretical components, and alternative proposals are welcomed. However, we would request that future contributions to a relational neuropsychoanalysis are not subjected to reductionist positioning that would de-emphasise the relational field between people as the domain in which clinical phenomena are encountered, made sense of, and supported.

References

Abrams, D. (2004). Chair of the research board's report. *The Psychologist*, May, 260.

Adolphs, R., Tranel, D., Damasio, H., & Damasio, A. R. (1994). Impaired recognition of emotion in facial expressions following bilateral damage to the human amygdala. *Nature*, *372*, 669–672.

Anderson, S. W., Bechara, A., Damasio, H., Tranel, D., & Damasio, A. R. (1999). Impairment of social and moral behavior related to early damage in human prefrontal cortex. *Nature Neuroscience, 2*(11), 1032–1037.

Atwood, G. E., & Stolorow, R. D. (1984). *Structures of subjectivity: Explorations in psychoanalytic phenomenology and contextualism.* London: Routledge.

Balfour, A. (2012). *How couples relationships shape our world.* London: Routledge.

Baron-Cohen, S. (1999). *The evolution of a theory of mind.* In M. C. Corballis & S. E. G. Lea (Eds.) *The descent of mind: Psychological perspectives on hominid evolution* (pp. 261–277). Oxford University Press.

Bateman, A. W., & Fonagy, P. (Eds.). (2012). *Handbook of mentalizing in mental health practice.* Washington, DC: American Psychiatric Pub.

Ben-Yishay, Y., & Diller, L. (2011). *Handbook of holistic neuropsychological rehabilitation: outpatient rehabilitation of traumatic brain injury.* New York: Oxford University Press.

Bion, W. R. (1959). Attacks on linking. *International Journal of Psychoanalysis, 40,* 308–315.

Bion, W. R. (1962). *Learning from experience.* London: Routledge.

Blonder, L. X., Pettigrew, L. C., & Kryscio, R. J. (2012). Emotion recognition and marital satisfaction in stroke. *Journal of Clinical and Experimental Neuropsychology, 34*(6), 634–642.

Bowen, C., Yeates, G., & Palmer, S. (2010). *A relational approach to rehabilitation: Thinking about relationships after brain injury.* London: Karnac Books.

Cacioppo, J. T., Berntson, G., Adolphs, R., Carter, S., Davidson, R., McClintock, M., McEwen, B., Meaney, M., Schacter, D., Sternberg, E., Suomi, S., & Taylor, S. (2002) *Foundations in social neuroscience.* Cambridge, MA: The MIT Press.

Calder, A. J., Keane, J., Manes, F., Antoun, N., & Young, A. W. (2000). Impaired recognition and experience of disgust following brain injury. *Nature Neuroscience, 3,* 1077–1078.

Carnwath, T. C. M., & Johnson, D. A. W. (1987). Psychiatric morbidity among spouses of patients with stroke. *British Medical Journal, 294,* 409–411.

Clarici, A., & Giuliani, R. (2008). Growing up with a brain-damaged mother: Anosognosia by proxy?. *Neuropsychoanalysis, 10*(1), 59–79.

Daisley, A., & Webster, G. (2008). Familial brain injury: Impact on and interventions with children. In A. Tyerman & N. King (Eds.), *Psychological approaches to rehabilitation after traumatic brain injury* (pp. 475–509). Oxford: Blackwell.

Elsass, L., & Kinsella, G. (1987). Social interaction following severe closed head injury. *Psychological Medicine, 17*(1), 67–78.

Evans-Roberts, C., Weatherhead, S., & Vaughan, F. (2014). Working with families following brain injury. *Revista Chilena de Neuropsicología, 9*(1), 21–30.

Feigelson, C. (1993). Personality death, object loss, and the uncanny. *The International Journal of Psycho-Analysis, 74*(2), 331.

Fotopoulou, A., Pfaff, D., & Conway, M. A. (Eds.). (2012). *From the couch to the lab: Trends in psychodynamic neuroscience.* New York: Oxford University Press.

Fotopoulou, A., Solms, M., & Turnbull, O. (2003). Wishful reality distortions in confabulation: A case report. *Neuropsychologia, 42*(6), 727–744.

Freud, S. (1914). *On narcissism.* Standard edition of the works of Signmund Freud, 24.

Freud, S. (1917). *Mourning and melancholia.* Standard edition of the works of Sigmund Freud, 14.

Frith, U., & Frith, C. D. (2003). Development and neurophysiology of mentalizing. *Philosophical Transactions of the Royal Society of London. Series B: Biological Sciences, 358*(1431), 459–473.

Frith, C. D., & Wolpert, D. (2004). *The neuroscience of social interaction: Decoding, influencing, and imitating the actions of others*. New York: Oxford University Press.

Frosh, S. (1987). *The politics of psychoanalysis: An introduction to freudian and post-freudian theory*. London: Macmillan.

Gallese, V. (2001). The 'shared manifold' hypothesis. From mirror neurons to empathy. *Journal of Consciousness Studies, 8*(5–6), 33–50.

Gallese, V. (2003). The roots of empathy: the shared manifold hypothesis and the neural basis of intersubjectivity. *Psychopathology, 36*(4), 171–180.

Gallese, V. (2010). Embodied simulation and its role in intersubjectivity. In T. Fuchs, H.C. Sattel, P. Henningsen (Eds.) *The embodied self. Dimensions, coherence and disorders* (pp. 78–92). Stuttgart: Schattauer.

Gallese, V., Keysers, C., & Rizzolatti, G. (2004). A unifying view of the basis of social cognition. *Trends in Cognitive Sciences, 8*(9), 396–403.

Goldman, A. I., & Sripada, C. S. (2005). Simulationist models of faced based emotion recognition. *Cognition, 94*, 193–213.

Gracey, F., Evans, J. J., & Malley, D. (2009). Capturing process and outcome in complex rehabilitation interventions: A "Y-shaped" model. *Neuropsychological Rehabilitation, 19*(6), 867–890.

Happé, F. G. E. (1997). Central coherence and theory of mind in autism: Reading homographs in context. *British Journal of Developmental Psychology, 15*, 1–12.

Harmon-Jones, E., & Winkielman, P. (Eds.). (2007). *Social neuroscience: Integrating biological and psychological explanations of social behavior*. New York: Guilford Press.

Hilari, K., & Northcott, S. (2017). "Struggling to stay connected": Comparing the social relationships of healthy older people and people with stroke and aphasia. *Aphasiology, 31*(6), 674–687.

Kaplan-Solms, K., & Solms, M. (2000). *Clinical studies in neuro psychoanalysis*. London: Karnac Books.

Klein, M. (1952). On observing the behaviour of young infants. In *Developments in psychoanalysis* (pp. 237–270). New York, London.

Klonoff, P. S. (1997). Individual and group psychotherapy in milieu-oriented neurorehabilitation. *Applied Neuropsychology, 4*(2), 107–118.

Klonoff, P. S. (2005). The art and science of milieu-oriented neurorehabilitation. *Barrow Quarterly, 21*(2), 14–21.

Klonoff, P. S., & Lage, G. A. (1991). Narcissistic injury in patients with traumatic brain injury. *The Journal of Head Trauma Rehabilitation, 6*(4), 11–21.

Klonoff, P. S., Lage, G. A., & Chiapello, D. A. (1993). Varieties of the catastrophic reaction to brain injury: A self psychology perspective. *Bulletin of the Menninger Clinic, 57*(2), 227.

Kohut, H. (1977). *The restoration of the self*. Madison, WI: International Universities Press Inc.

Kreutzer, J. S., Gervasio, A. H., & Camplair, P. S. (1994). Primary caregivers' psychological status and family functioning after traumatic brain injury. *Brain Injury, 8*, 197–210.

Lemma, A., Target, M., & Fonagy, P. (2011). *Brief dynamic interpersonal therapy: A clinician's guide*. London: Oxford University Press.

Lewis, L. (1999). Transference and countertransference in psychotherapy with adults having traumatic brain injury. In K. Langer, L. Laatsch & L. Lewis (Eds.) *Psychotherapeutic interventions for adults with brain injury or stroke: A clinician's treatment resource* (pp. 113–130). Madison: Psychological Press.

Luria, A. R. (1963 [1948]). *Restoration of function after brain injury* (B. Haigh, Trans.). Oxford: Pergamon Press.

Merleau-Ponty, M. (1978). *Phenomenology of perception*. London: Routledge & Kegan Paul.

Miller, L. (1992). When the best help is self-help: or, everything you always wanted to know about brain injury support groups. *Journal of Cognitive Rehabilitation, 10*(6), 14–17.

Mitchell, S. A. (1988). *Relational concepts in psychoanalysis*. Cambridge: Harvard University Press.

Money-Kyrle, R. E. (1956). Normal counter-transference and some of its derivations. *The International Journal of Psycho-Analysis, 37*, 360.

Moore, P. A., Salas, C. E., Dockree, S., & Turnbull, O. H. (2017). Observations on working psychoanalytically with a profoundly amnesic patient. *Frontiers in Psychology, 8*, 1418.

Morin, C., Thibierge, S., Bruguière, P., Pradat-Diehl, P., & Mazevet, D. (2005). "Daughter-somatoparaphrenia" in women with right-hemisphere syndrome: A psychoanalytic perspective on neurological body knowledge disorders. *Neuropsychoanalysis, 7*(2), 171–184.

Northcott, S., Hirani, S. P., & Hilari, K. (2017). A typology to explain changing social networks post stroke. *The Gerontologist, 58*(3), 500–511.

Norup, A. (2018) Family matters in neurorehabilitation: why, when, who and how? *Revista Iberoamericana de Neuropsicologia, 1*(1), 17–31.

Pepping, M. (1993). Transference and countertransference issues in brain injury rehabilitation: implications for staff training. In C. Durgin, N. Schmidt and J. Fryer (Eds.), *Staff development and clinical intervention in brain injury rehabilitation* (pp. 87–103). Maryland: Aspen Publication.

Perlesz, A., Kinsella, G., & Crowe, S. (2000). Psychological distress and family satisfaction following traumatic brain injury: Injured individuals and their primary, secondary, and tertiary carers. *Journal of Head Trauma Rehabilitation, 15*, 909–929.

Prigatano, G. P. (1999). *Principles of neuropsychological rehabilitation*. New York: Oxford University Press.

Rizzolatti, G., Fadiga, L., Galles, G., & Fogassi, L. (1996). Premotor cortex and the recognition of motor actions. *Cognitive Brain Research, 3*, 131–141.

Salas, C. E. (2012). Surviving catastrophic reaction after brain injury: The use of self-regulation and self-other regulation. *Neuropsychoanalysis, 14*(1), 77–92.

Salas, C., Casassus, M., Rowlands, L., & Pimm, S. (2020). Developing a model of long-term social rehabilitation after traumatic brain injury: The case of the head forward centre. *Disability and rehabilitation*, 1–12.

Salas, C. E., & Castro, O. (2014). Mente desorganizada y reaccion catastrofica: regulacion emocional intrinseca y extrinseca en sobrevivientes de lesion cerebral adquirida. *Revista Chilena de Neuropsicología, 9*(1), 38–45.

Salas, C. E., Radovic, D., Yuen, K. S., Yeates, G. N., Castro, O., & Turnbull, O. H. (2014). "Opening an emotional dimension in me": Changes in emotional reactivity and emotion regulation in a case of executive impairment after left fronto-parietal damage. *Bulletin of the Menninger Clinic, 78*(4), 301–334.

Sander, A., Caroselli, J., High, W., Becker, C., Neese, L., & Scheibel, R. (2002). Relationship of family functioning to progress in a post-acute rehabilitation programme following traumatic brain injury. *Brain Injury, 16,* 649–657.

Schonberger, M., Yeates, G. N., & Hobbs, P. (in press). Associations between therapeutic working alliance and social cognition in neuro-rehabilitation. *Neuropsychological Rehabilitation.*

Singer, T., Seymour, B., O'Doherty, J., Kaube, H., Dolan, R., & Frith, C. D. (2004). Empathy for pain involves the affective but not sensory components of pain. *Science, 303,* 1157–1162.

Sonnby-Borgenström, M. (2008). Imitation responses and verbally reported emotional contagion from spontaneous, uncionscious to emotionally-regulated, conscious information-processing levels. *Neuropsychoanalysis, 10*(1), 81–85.

Stagg, K., Douglas, J., & Iacono, T. (2017). A scoping review of the working alliance in acquired brain injury rehabilitation. *Disability and Rehabilitation, 41*(4), 489–497.

Thomsen, I. V. (1974). The patient with severe head injury and his family. *Scandinavian Journal of Rehabilitation Medicine, 6,* 180–183.

Tiberg, K. (2014). Confabulating in the transference. *Neuropsychoanalysis, 16*(1), 57–67.

Turnbull, O. H., & Solms, M. (2004). Depth psychological consequences of brain damage. In J. Panksepp (Ed.) *Textbook of biological psychiatry* (pp. 571–595). New Jersey: Wiley & Sons.

Vickers, C. P. (2010). Social networks after the onset of aphasia: The impact of aphasia group attendance. *Aphasiology, 24*(6–8), 902–913.

Watt, N., & Penn, C. (2000). Predictors and indicators of return to work following traumatic brain injury in South Africa: Findings from a preliminary experimental database. *South African Journal of Psychology, 30,* 27–37.

Willer, B., Allen, K., Durnan, M. C., & Ferry, A. (1990). Problems and coping strategies of mothers, siblings and young adult males with traumatic brain injury. *Canadian Journal of Rehabilitation, 3,* 167–173.

Wolf, E. (1988). *Treating the self.* New York: Guilford Press.

Yeates, G. N. (2014). Social cognition interventions in neuro-rehabilitation: An overview. *Advances in Clinical Neuroscience & Rehabilitation, 14*(2), 12–13.

Yeates, G., Edwards, A., Murray, C., Creamer, N., & Mahadevan, M. (2013). The use of Emotionally-focused Couples Therapy (EFT) for survivors of acquired brain injury with social cognition and executive functioning impairments, and their partners: A case series analysis. *Neuro-Disability and Psychotherapy, 1*(2), 151–197.

Yeates, G., Hamill, M., Sutton, L., Psaila, K., Gracey, F., Mohamed, S., & O'Dell, J. (2008). Dysexecutive problems and interpersonal relating following frontal brain injury: Reformulation and compensation in cognitive analytic therapy (CAT). *Neuropsychoanalysis, 10*(1), 43–58.

Yeates, G., Henwood, K., Gracey, F., & Evans, J. (2007). Awareness of disability after acquired brain injury and the family context. *Neuropsychological Rehabilitation, 17*(2), 151–173.

Yeates, G. N., Rowberry, M., Dunne, S., Goshawk, M., Mahadevan, M., Tyerman, R., Salter, M., Hillier, M., Berry, A., & Tyerman, A. (2016). Social cognition and executive functioning predictors of others' appraisal of interpersonal behaviour in the workplace following acquired brain injury. *Neurorehabilitation, 38*(3), 299–310.

Chapter 5

Lacanian neuropsychoanalysis

On the role of language motor dynamics for language processing and for mental constitution

Ariane Bazan, Gertrudis Van de Vijver and Diana Caine

In the first volume of *Clinical Neuropsychoanalysis*, Kaplan-Solms and Solms (2001) compare a patient with a Broca-type aphasia, Mr. J, and one with a Wernicke-type aphasia, Mrs. K. Broadly speaking, the authors find that Mr. J's 'ego functioning' is 'normal', i.e. that he can reappraise and adjust to changed realities, even if he has enormous difficulties expressing himself verbally, while Mrs. K's speech production is fluent but she often 'goes blank' mentally, being unable both to understand non-idiomatic speech and to bring her own speech intentions into execution. The authors conclude that (1) "The motor aspect of the word, then, and therefore the motor component of the speech apparatus – Broca's area – (...) is little more than an output channel for the ego's complex workings; its role in verbal *thinking* is superfluous." (p. 89; their italics) and (2) "the auditory-component of word presentation does participate in some way in the executive functioning of the ego." (p. 114). In what follows we will spell out how, to the contrary, in our view the motor component of the speech apparatus is actually constitutive of access to symbolic language (and hence of ego-functioning), while the auditory component is no more than an auxiliary for this access. Having done so, we provide an alternative explanation for Mrs. K's mental failures and Mr. J's mental robustness, in terms of dorsal and ventral language pathways, and of secondary and primary processing, in place of the traditional framework of Broca's and Wernicke's aphasias.

The Lacanian viewpoint on psychoanalysis serves as the main background for this chapter. This implies basically two things in this context. Firstly, in line with Lacan, its focus is first and foremost on the signifier in its constitutive relation to the subject. The Lacanian signifier is a phonemic form, the determination of which depends on its relation with other phonemic forms. Even if we will not mobilize this concept directly in the present chapter, the Lacanian background further implies that the subject, then, is "what is represented by a signifier for another signifier". This means that the subject is an effect of the interplay between signifiers. Secondly, a Lacanian viewpoint also questions the possibility and the validity of a metalanguage: as a signifier cannot signify itself, a subject cannot signify itself either. A detour via the other, via language and via the Other is needed. This detour via the Other and the signifier as an articulate motor pattern are central to the present chapter.

I   The motor component of speech is constitutive for the understanding of language

I.I   Word forms have autonomous mental (and clinical) effects

In *On Aphasia*, Freud (1891) presents his well-known 'word presentation/thing presentation' model (see Figure 5.1). Mental representations are formed through the perceptual and motor experiences we have of things in the world: this is the object presentation level. A word, however, is no less an object, inasmuch as it is encoded through its own perceptual and motor characteristics – namely, through its sound image and its articulatory program. This material substrate is the word presentation according to Freud. The linguistic reference function of language is constituted by the connections between the word- and object presentation levels. Using the structural linguistics of de Saussure, Lacan (1957) formalizes Freud's concept of word presentation into the concept of signifier, which is the form of the word, given by the motor (articulatory) and acoustic properties of its phonology. Crucially, the signifier is not to be understood as just another attribute of

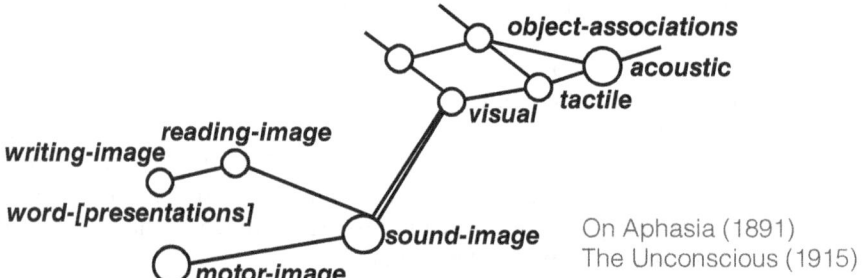

PSYCHOLOGICAL DIAGRAM OF A WORD-PRESENTATION

Figure 5.1 Freud (1891, pp. 77–78): "The word, then, is a complicated concept built up from various impressions, i.e., it corresponds to an intricate process of associations entered into by elements of visual, acoustic and kinaesthetic origins. However, the word acquires its significance through its association with the "idea (concept) of the object" (*Objektvorstellung* or object presentation), at least if we restrict our considerations to nouns. The idea, or concept, of the object is itself another complex of associations composed of the most varied visual, auditory, tactile, kinesthetic, and other impressions."

the thing presentation at the same level as the visual, auditory and other characteristics of the thing. The signifier is, in the first place, consistent with Freud's model, in itself a thing, which only secondarily acquires its linguistic dimension in relation to something it may denote.

Lacan (1957) subverts de Saussure's classical model of structural linguistics by proposing that the operator that organizes mental life is not "the signified" (the meaning of the word), but rather the signifier. In so doing, Lacan formalizes Freud's intuition from *On Aphasia* that word forms are relatively independent of their meaning and produce mental effects of their own. This is obvious throughout Freud's entire oeuvre. In the famous forgetting of the word 'Signorelli', Freud (1901) recalls that he intentionally pushed away the signifier or word presentation 'Herr', because it was the beginning of a phrase with a scabrous theme, involving sexuality and death. However, Freud has pushed away 'Herr' so efficiently that the inhibition spilled over to the associates of the word, including its Italian translation 'signor'. Subsequently, Freud can't find the word 'Signorelli', which is related to 'Herr' not on a (direct) semantic basis (which would involve the idea of a painter) but on a phonological basis – 'signor' being (no more than) the first two syllables of 'Signorelli'. Instead of 'Signorelli', one of the substitutes that pop up in Freud's mind is 'Boltraffio', the name of another Italian painter. At that point he realizes that he had recently received the news that a patient, for whom he had made a big effort, had killed himself in Trafoi for reasons of sexual dysfunction. Freud elegantly demonstrates how the repressed theme 'death and sexuality' makes displacements along phonemic (Herr/Signor[1] – traffio/Trafoi) to produce mental symptoms; these elements are Lacan's signifiers.

1.2 Humans have a mental lexicon, independent of semantics and phonological in structure

The models of Freud and Lacan have found corroboration in the neurobiological observation that the mental representation of word forms is relatively independent of semantic representations. Hannah Damasio and colleagues (1996) combined neuropsychological data and brain imaging to show that language has specific, organized circuitry in the left basotemporal lobe, organized along lexical principles distinct from the distributed bilateral hemispheric fields encoding object properties. This relative independence shows itself most strikingly in the dissociation between stroke aphasic patients who lose the ability to name pictured objects without losing knowledge of their meaning and patients with progressive fluent aphasia (semantic dementia) who lose meaning but retain access to the word forms (Suárez-González et al., 2014). In other words, there is a word level, the lexical level, which is as such materially present in the brain and which is to be distinguished from the object level or the semantic fields.[2]

A common characteristic of Freud's word presentation, Lacan's signifier and Damasio's lexical unit is that they are phonologically encoded. Lacan (1957, p. 120) explicitly refers to motor articulation in defining phonemes: "Now the structure of the signifier is, as it is commonly said of language itself, that it should be *articulated*. This means that (...) these elements, one of the decisive discoveries of linguistics, are *phonemes*." (our italics).

In other words, Lacan's signifier is first and foremost a *motor* structure.[3] Importantly, psycho- and neurolinguistic studies have well established now that there is no such thing as a purely acoustic registration of language (see also Hickok, 2014). For instance, attempts to map the minimal spectrographic acoustic elements that would permit the classification of phones unambiguously to particular classes of phonemes have been inconclusive (for review, see Cutler & Clifton, 1999). Liberman, Cooper, Shankweiler and Studdert-Kennedy (1967) and Liberman and Mattingly (1985) have therefore proposed the 'motor theory of speech perception', which supposes that the listener does not try to trace the information needed to recompose the acoustic record, but rather the information that would permit the reconstruction of the articulatory *motor intention* of the speaker. Upon hearing the other speak, a subject activates its own articulatory apparatus and by means of mirror neurons tries to find the articulatory movements which, were he himself to execute them, would lead to the same perceptual result (Rizzolatti & Arbib, 1998). The McGurk[4] effect (1976) shows how much we rely on visual lip-reading cues, which inform the listener about the movement made by the speaker, not about the sound uttered, to enable *hearing* the identity of the uttered sound.

Chomsky and Halle (1968) also define phonemes in terms of articulatory feature clusters. Actually, the very essence of what makes a sound a linguistic sound is its being articulated. For example, the phonemes /r/ and /l/ have neighboring acoustic characteristics, and it is possible to artificially produce sounds which vary in a continuous way between /r/ and /l/. If language were first and foremost sound, we would be able to hear these variations, but research shows that people do not hear a gradual change: for a whole variation of /r/ acoustic sounds, we judge they are the result of the /r/ articulatory movement, i.e. we *hear* /r/, until when the acoustic parameters come too close to /l/, and then we judge they are the result of the /l/ articulatory movement, i.e. we *hear* /l/. Speech perception, therefore, is categorical (Liberman, 1970). Neurolinguistic data have confirmed the implication of Broca's area in listening (e.g. Ojemann, 1979, 1983, 1991; Price et al., 1996).

There are also many indications that Freud considered the articulatory motor aspects as constitutive for language. Based on his observation of 'echolalia', Freud (1891/1978, pp. 91–92; our italics) defended the idea that

> understanding of spoken words is probably not to be regarded as simple transmission from the acoustic elements to the object association;

it rather seems that in listening to speech with understanding, the function of verbal association is stimulated from the acoustic elements at the same time, so that we more or less *repeat to ourselves the word heard, thus supporting our understanding with the help of kinaesthetic impressions.*

Earlier in the same study (1891/1978, pp. 73–74), he had proposed that "we learn to speak by associating a 'word sound image' with an 'impression of word innervation'" and "by endeavoring to equate the sound image produced by ourselves as much as possible to the one which had served as the stimulus for *the act of innervation of our speech muscles*".

Here Freud introduces an enigmatic new element, namely, that of 'the impression' of 'the language innervation'. It is highly improbable that this is the proprioceptive feedback of the articulation, which he clearly refers to as the 'kinaesthetic word image' (p. 73). An alternative interpretation is that of the 'efference copy' which feeds back to the neocortex whenever an efferent motor command leaves the motor cortex (see Figure 5.2). The modern efference copy or so-called internal models are derived from von Helmholtz (1878/1971, p. 123) who first proposed the idea of a direct sensation of the motor command: "The impulse to move, which we initiate through the innervation of our motor nerves, is immediately perceptible." This idea reappeared in motor physiology as the 'corollary discharge' by von Holst (1954) and Sperry (1950). More recently it has become reintegrated as the efference copy model (Blakemore, Wolpert & Frith, 1998; Jeannerod, 1997, 2001; Wolpert, 1997).

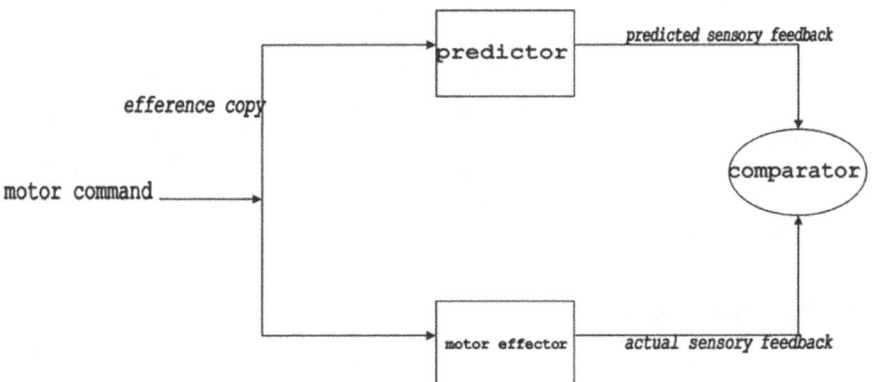

Figure 5.2 The efference copy model (Blakemore, Wolpert & Frith, 1998; Georgieff & Jeannerod, 1998; Sperry, 1950; van Holst, 1954).

Freud adhered to the views of the late 19th-century physiologist, von Helmholtz. The historical, neuroanatomical, and even semantic closeness of Freud's concept of 'indications of reality' and the modern sensorimotor concept of 'efference copies', then, is remarkable (see Bazan, 2007a, 2007b, for a detailed discussion). The efference copies inform the neocortex that a motor command has been sent out, while the proprioceptive feedback informs the neocortex that a motor command has been executed. According to Freud, phonemic access is gained whenever a motor innervation impression reaches some level of identity with a perceptual acoustic image in line with what was laboriously learned through association during infancy. Precisely this was recently proposed by the neurolinguist Gregory Hickok (2014) who specifies:

> In motor control terms, [the] phonological level is the 'internal model', which is divided into two representational components, a motorphonological component (the internal model of the motor effector) and an auditoryphonological component (where the auditory consequences of actions are coded).

We thus conclude that there is a high coherence between psychoanalytical clinical and neuroscience empirical observations.

2 The ventral and dorsal language pathways

To explain the cases of Mr. J and Mrs. K, it is important to reappraise language dynamics, not so much in terms of the contrast between Wernicke's and Broca's aphasias, but rather between ventral and dorsal language pathways. There is now consensus that just as there are dorsal versus ventral pathways for visual, visuomotor, and auditory processing, so this distinction applies also to language processing (Hickok & Poeppel, 2000, 2004, 2007; Rauschecker & Scott, 2009; Saur et al., 2008; see Figure 5.3). In each of these domains, spatial stimulus processing and sensorimotor integration – the so-called *where* stream – are subserved by a dorsal pathway, whereas stimulus perception and recognition – the so-called *what* stream – are transmitted via a ventral pathway. The language model assumes that the ventral stream is largely bilaterally organized and that the dorsal stream is strongly left-hemisphere dominant.

2.1 The ventral pathway

The ventral pathway connects the frontal and temporal cortices ventrally and subserves "phonology-to-meaning" mapping (Hickok & Poeppel, 2004, 2007; Rauschecker & Scott, 2009), i.e. processing speech signals for comprehension, sometimes described as "the relation between phonological words

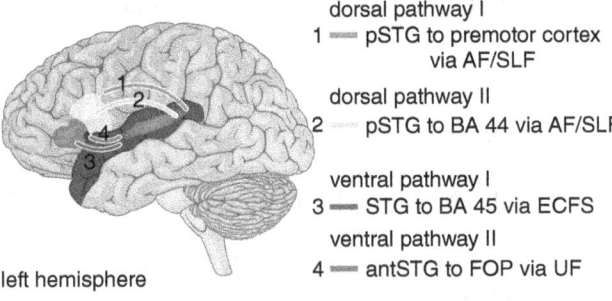

dorsal pathway I
1 ═══ pSTG to premotor cortex
      via AF/SLF

dorsal pathway II
2 ─── pSTG to BA 44 via AF/SLF

ventral pathway I
3 ━━ STG to BA 45 via ECFS

ventral pathway II
4 ━━ antSTG to FOP via UF

left hemisphere

Figure 5.3 Schematic view of two dorsal and two ventral language pathways. Ventral pathway I, the ECFS, also named the inferior fronto-occipital fascicle, connects BA 45 and BA 47 (the ventrolateral prefrontal cortex) and the temporal cortex. Ventral pathway II, the UF, connects the FOP and the anterior temporal STG/superior temporal sulcus (STS). Dorsal pathway I connects STG to *the dorsal* PMC (BA 6) via the AF and the SLF. Dorsal pathway II connects the STG (Wernicke's area) to BA 44, i.e. the posterior portion of Broca's area, via the AF/SLF.

and conceptual representations" (Hickok & Poeppel, 2000, 2004, 2007; Rauschecker & Scott, 2009; Wernicke, 1874/1977). First, *the extreme capsule fiber system* (ECFS) connects BA 45 and BA 47 to the superior temporal gyrus (STG), the middle temporal gyrus (MTG) and the occipital cortex (Saur et al., 2008, 2010; Sarubbo, Benedictis, Maldonado, Basso & Duffau, 2013; Turken & Dronkers, 2011). This fiber system is seen as the major pathway supporting semantic processes (Saur et al., 2008) and is activated during auditory comprehension. Second, *the uncinate fascicle* (UF) connects the frontal operculum (FOP) and orbitofrontal cortex to the anterior STG. Friederici et al. (2006) suggest that this route may be involved in the building up of local phrases through which adjacent elements are combined syntactically. Interestingly, the UF is also considered a limbic pathway mainly connecting the amygdala and hippocampus in the medial temporal region with the prefrontal lobe (Schmahmann et al., 2009). Thus, the ventral pathway, with its subcomponents, supports elementary semantic processes and local phrase building processes.

2.2 The dorsal pathway

The dorsal pathway was initially described as emanating from the planum temporale in the posterior superior temporal region running through the *inferior parietal lobule to the dorsal premotor cortex* (PMC; BA 6): this pathway is involved in establishing the relation between speech gestures and the sounds they produce (Hickok & Poeppel, 2000, 2004, 2007; Raus-checker & Scott, 2009). It has a sensorimotor mapping function (Saur et al., 2008; through the efference copy system, see further), and functionally, it is involved in speech repetition, i.e. in the production and articulation of perceived speech sounds (Hickok & Poeppel, 2000, 2007). A second major dorsal fiber tract terminates in *BA 44* and connects this area directly *with the posterior temporal cortex* (Wernicke's area). One proposed function for this arcuate fascicle (AF)/superior longitudinal fascicle (SLF) to BA 44 route is that it is particularly involved in processing syntactically complex sentences (Friederici, 2015). Interestingly, this fiber bundle is not myelinized in newborns (Perani et al., 2011).

2.3 Ventral and dorsal syntax

Note that, for syntactic processes, a differentiation is made between local phrase structure, which recruits a ventral fiber tract, and the structure of hierarchical syntactic dependencies in grammar sequences, which involve a dorsal pathway (Friederici, 2015). Concerning local phrase structure, Saur and colleagues (2008) proposes the following:

> an iterative exchange with the prefrontal cortex, which is involved in executive aspects of semantic processing (Bookheimer, 2002) – e.g., controlled semantic retrieval (Thompson-Schill, D'Esposito, Aguirre & Farah, 1997), semantically based analysis of grammatical structures (Dapretto & Bookheimer, 1999), and application of cognitive rules (Musso et al., 2003).

This is complementary to Friederici (2015; see also Friederici et al., 2006; Grodzinsky & Friederici, 2006) who proposes that processing of simple grammatical structures (e.g. computing local phrase structures) was found to involve the ventral pathway connecting the anterior STG and the FOP.[5] The dorsal pathway (AF/SLF), however, is needed for the processing of sentences with hierarchical syntax (Brauer, Anwander & Friederici, 2011; Wilson et al., 2011). Thus, both the ventral and the dorsal pathway are involved in syntactic processes, albeit in different ways (Griffiths, Marslen-Wilson, Stamatakis & Tyler, 2013).

2.4 The primary and secondary modes of language processing

We have argued before that there is a parallel between ventral processing and primary process mentation, and between dorsal processing and secondary process mentation, respectively (Bazan, 2007a, 2007b; Bazan & Snodgrass, 2012).

2.4.1 Primary and secondary language processes

The primary process (Freud, 1895, 1900) is essentially an associative functioning modus that connects representations on the basis of their (superficial) attributes. It is typically described in psychoanalytic literature as being the mental mode characteristic of the unconscious, but it is present in *any* mental life, since it is the modus that furnishes positive content elements. However, the proliferation of associations is much more unconstrained in unconscious mental life, while it is mostly very much constrained by secondary processes in conscious mental life. Secondary processes are both the fact, in and of itself, of the constraining of primary processes and its result. These processes essentially draw their ability for inhibition from the aimed-for end result of the action (which is the only way to counteract strong associative links); for this reason, secondary processes take into account both the intentionality of the subject and the environment. Secondary processes, therefore, are said to follow the reality principle: their support base is at the end point of the arrow. Primary processes, in contrast, follow the pleasure principle: their support base is at the start point of the arrow.

2.4.2 Primary versus ventral and secondary versus dorsal processing

In the previous work (Bazan, 2006, 2007a, 2007b, 2012), we have argued that the associative proliferation of content elements of the primary process is subserved by the ventral pathway, which allows for identification and solving of the "What?" question. In this perspective, it is interesting that the UF is connected to the hippocampus: we might speculate that whenever primary process associates are disinhibited, the search for other meanings involves this memory structure. However, there are neither spatial nor temporal coordinates in this pathway; these are provided by the dorsal "Where?" pathway, which involves a construction of reality on the basis of external perceptual information as well as of the intentionality of the subject in his or her environment on the basis of interoceptive information. This processing of both the intention of the subject and the context is also the mental mode of the secondary process. In addition, only the dorsal pathway has the means to exert inhibitory influences, thanks to the efference copies dynamics. If, as we have argued before, there is equivalence between the efference copy and Freud's 'indications of reality' (see also below), and if only the secondary process has access to the 'indications of reality' (Freud

1950/1966, p. 325), this further confirms a logical coherence between the secondary process and the dorsal pathway.

2.4.3 Primary versus ventral and secondary versus dorsal language processing

Speculatively, we propose that what happens at the level of the ventral route, described as the resolution of 'local syntactic phrases through which adjacent elements are combined syntactically' (Friederici, 2015, p. 184), is the local restriction of possible interpretations of a given phonological 'chunk'[6] (a group of phonemes, a word or a phrase). This, we propose, happens by means of what we previously called 'lexical labels' (Bazan, 2007a, 2007b) – be these labels of a grammatical nature (subject versus verb versus object, substantive versus pronoun, etc.) or of a more strictly lexical nature (person versus man-made object, etc.; see Damasio et al., 1996). For example, the phrase "Mary pours ...." anticipates a 'substantive' with the property of being 'liquid'.[7] Whatever the word will be that completes this phrase, the search for it will be narrowed down by the preorientation given by these lexical labels 'substantive' and 'liquid'.

We propose now to see the dynamic tension as follows: the ventral pathway is always (structurally) ready to proliferate with possible candidates for language chunks; this is the primary processing of language. It is then the involvement of prefrontal structures (Broca) – strictly speaking a dorsal structure – which cuts short this proliferating search. This, then, is one level of the secondary processing of language corresponding with the 'ventral' syntactic pathway, which operates the selection of the contextual meaning by means of lexical labels, but needs involvement of the dorsal Broca area to be able to do so.

However, local phrase structure resolution is not always enough: when the phrases are complicated, or – we speculate – when their structure is novel or surprising and unanticipated, it might be necessary to refer back to the intention of the speaker. These processes, then, would involve the posterior STG and BA 44/45 (Grozinsky & Friederici, 2006), areas connected via the dorsal pathway (Friederici et al., 2006). The role of the dorsal syntactic pathway, we speculate, would be to reactualize the original linguistic grasp we were trying to deploy upon the world (or which we attribute to another) or, in other words, to reactualize the linguistic action intention. This would need to be the case when the intended utterance cannot sufficiently rely upon idiomatic – i.e. automatic, thoughtless, ready-made – phrase components. This aspect might also be important in understanding language, when the local phrase information is not sufficient to decide between competing interpretations.[8] Again, this would correspond to secondary process mentation, though maybe of a much more fundamental kind than the 'ventral' secondary process, with its aim to resolve local syntax: this kind of secondary process would reactualize the aimed-for end result as the target for the action of the subject in the world, i.e. his or her (unconscious) intentionality. The dorsal syntactic pathway also involves prefrontal brain structures (BA 44/45); therefore, its mode of operation is also thought to be through inhibition. However, it might be less the kind involving the inhibition of competing meaning candidates, but rather the kind of cutting that would be at the service of creative recomposition: indeed, the dorsal pathway would go in search of novel handles to grasp by cutting short the existing ones and thereby eliminating competition in favor of the ones that are sometimes only very poorly invested, i.e. very weakly present in mind. It thereby is the kind of cutting that is thought to have a revelatory power. Speculatively, we propose that these syntactic operations are strategically crucial for the access to, and the making of, symbolic language.

3 The linguistic and paternal metaphors: constituting the mental

In 1957, inspired by the work of Jacobson, Lacan introduces both the formula of the linguistic metaphor and that of the paternal metaphor. The metaphors truly formalize the logical dynamics of how primary and secondary processes interact for targeted action. If we keep in mind that the secondary process has the asset of holding on to the wished-for end configuration and the primary process has the asset of a wide range of handles to direct action, then the formula of the metaphor shows how the secondary process is able to open the primary process valve in an attuned, controlled, measured way so as to pick up from its associative stream the one handle that is best targeted for the wished-for end configuration. What is thereby dug up is the metaphorized result, an original subjective creation.

3.1 The linguistic metaphor: grasping language

3.1.1 Mental dynamics of the linguistic metaphor

Metaphorization is an operation whereby a current (associative) meaning of a signifier is put into an unusual lexical position which then enforces the reading of the signifier (Bazan, 2007a, pp. 47–62): in essence, then, it is secondary processes getting hold of primary process language associativity. For example, the phrase "did you see her walking hand in hand with [this wardrobe]?" grammatically speaking anticipates a substantive, and lexically speaking a person (Bazan, 2007a: 58). When the word 'wardrobe' appears, which is commonly (i.e. associatively) known as a piece of furniture, this lexical determination (furniture) is ripped from the signifier. New ones, predetermined by the other signifiers in the sentence – namely, substantive and person – are imposed on it. This is an operation by which new meaning arises: here 'wardrobe' comes to signify 'a burly man'. Lacan (1955–1956: p. 218; italics added) says: "Metaphor presupposes that a meaning is the dominant datum and that it deflects,[9] commands, the use of the signifier to such an extent that *the entire species of pre-established, I should say lexical, connections comes undone.*" Adding: "And yet it's clear that the use of a language is only susceptible to meaning once (...) the meaning has ripped the signifier from its lexical connections." He thereby gives the formula of the metaphor[10]:

$$\frac{S}{\$'} \cdot \frac{\$'}{x} \to S \cdot \frac{1}{s}$$

with S = signifier 1, $'$ = signifier 2, x = an unknown signification, and s = the emerging signified, induced by the metaphor.

Concretely,

$$\frac{\text{a person}}{\text{wardrobe}} \cdot \frac{\text{wardrobe}}{\text{(big, large)}} \longrightarrow \text{a person.} \frac{1}{\text{burly}}$$

In other words, for a metaphor "pin a signifier to a signifier and see what that produces. But, in this case, something new is always produced which is sometimes as unexpected as a chemical reaction, namely the emergence of a new signification" (Lacan, 1957, p. 141).

Note that it is only at the end of the metaphor operation that it becomes possible to pinpoint, in hindsight, which of the attributes of the object will have 'delivered' the excitations that were discharged – e.g. here, 'burly' pinpoints 'big, large' in the wardrobe, and the wardrobe reveals 'burly' in the person indicated. It is the symbolic structure of language and, specifically, the metaphor, which endows humans with a structurally open potential to endlessly reveal new aspects of reality.[11]

3.1.2 Physiology of the metaphor

As indicated earlier, only the motor – i.e. dorsal – dynamics have the means for targeted inhibition through the efference copy-attenuation principle. Indeed, Hickock (2014, p. 8) reminds us that motor control models

assume a kind of cancelling operation as the basis for comparing motor predictions with overt sensory feedback, with the motor prediction implemented as an inhibitory signal. If the prediction (−) and the overt sensory input (+) cancel, then this indicates an accurate prediction. Prediction error, then, is sensory activation that is not cancelled.

Even if this mechanism may seem merely technical, we have argued elsewhere (Bazan, 2012) that its role may be properly constitutive. Following Hickok (2014, p. 7[12]), we would like to venture a comparison between the movement of language and grasping: if the dorsal pathway has pre-calculated the right grasp towards the thing-to-grasp, then there is no prediction error, and further processing of the thing-to-grasp is efficiently stopped. In language terms, if the word-to-be-said or to-be-understood was sufficiently predetermined by the surrounding signifiers, that is, if that word (or that chunk) was already adequately predefined by the sum of the lexical labels gathered by the sentence so far, then there is no prediction error, and further (associative) processing of the word is efficiently stopped. However, if, once arrived at the spot where the word has to be grasped, the lexical labels are unusual or surprising – as in the example of person-wardrobe – then there is a prediction error. Consequently, the further associative (semantic) processing is not stopped, and primary process-mode associations are disinhibited in a continued search for identity: this is a good thing, because another way, besides the usual one, has to be found amidst the freed associations to grasp the word anew. The handle 'person' obliges us to look beyond furniture associations for those associative meanings of wardrobe, which could also apply to a person. Here, the associations found are 'big, large'. We see, now, how metaphorization crucially depends on the dorsal route-mediated motor organization of language. The motor aspect of language is by no means "little more than an output channel" (Kaplan-Solms & Solms, 2001, p. 89).

3.2 The paternal metaphor: grasping intentions

The metaphor, as we have just discussed, is an instantiation of a more basic, constitutive metaphor, which Lacan (1957, p. 456) calls the "Name-of-the-Father", the character and function of which we will now outline.

3.2.1 From drives to discharge

When thrown into life, a newborn is subjected to a chaos of inner body excitations for which, in order to survive, it will be important to find ways to discharge. The first other, often the mother, is a recipient of these excitations, but she unavoidably also induces them in the child. This is expressed in the second term of the father-metaphor 'Mother's Desire/Signified to the Subject': what has to be processed are the excitations, signified to the child by the coming and going of the mother, inducing a first distinction between more or less excitation (see Figure 5.4). But since outbursts of excitations are also induced in the child through the interaction with the mother, the

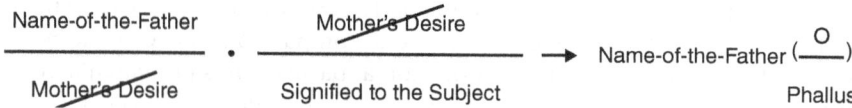

Figure 5.4 Schematic representation of the Name-of-the-Father metaphor. See text for explanation.

mother cannot offer an effective means of discharge to the child. Without such means, the child cannot acquire a perspective on or a limit to these excitatory outbursts.

But the child and the mother are not alone. A second other – who is the actual other – interferes between the child and the first (m)other, on the condition that there is also desire between this first and second other. Indeed, only on that account the desire of the mother is also eliciting excitation in the father, an excitation, however, to which he will in some way respond, for which he has, in some way, however partially, the means of discharge. These means of discharge fall under the term the 'Name-of-the-Father', according to Lacan the constitutive and fundamental metaphor.

The father will name, i.e. give words to the desiring interactions between the mother and himself. This is expressed in the first term of the father-metaphor 'Name-of-the-Father/Mother's Desire'. Crucially, any naming or acting operation induces another type of temporality: while the coming and going of excitations is diffuse, any naming cuts a precise – even if completely arbitrary – parcel of time out of a diffuse continuity. Thereby, the 'Name-of-the-Father' introduces a so-called *coupure*, a cut, which structures the desiring interactions between the first and the second other. What is important is that mother and father, first and second other, are *logical* positions, which do not even have to be equated to unitary physical persons as such. The logic is one whereby a primary caregiver of the child has also desire for another person, who will respond to this desire with language interventions, structuring the interaction.

The metaphor now is a transitivity operated by the child: if the child assumes that the desire of the mother, to which the father responds, is in some ways comparable to the desire induced in him by the mother, then the reactions given by the father may enable the child to grasp his own excitations in the same move. The child has no direct access to the way the mother's desire works on the father: the naming by the father, the imposition of a signifier, is an external operation. However, insofar as the naming has allowed the child to hypothesize that what it refers to is related to what he himself experiences in relation to the mother's desire, then the naming in and by itself gives the child a means to attach the diffuse excitations he or she experiences to a phoneme structure. The Name-of-the-Father metaphor is accomplished. The Name-of-the-Father might thus be described as the device by which the drive derivatives are linked to the language discharge system (the motor component), the apparatus on the basis of which inner body excitations are transposed into outer body dischargeable forms.

3.2.2 ...to the emergence of something new

What, then, is the relation between the paternal and the linguistic metaphor? The second term in our prosaic earlier example was 'wardrobe/(big large)': an object (a mother or a wardrobe) induces experiential excitations, which refer to the characteristics (attributes or affordances) of the object; these excitations are initially chaotic, i.e. unnamed. In the same way that 'the Name-of-the-Father' indicates to the subject how to grasp 'the desire of the mother', the first signifier S1 of the metaphor formula indicates how to grasp the experiential excitation, induced by the second signifier S2 – for example, 'a person' indicates how to grasp 'wardrobe'. This means precisely that S1 provides the lexical constraints to which the semantics of S2 should be submitted: in the case of the wardrobe, S1 dictates that S2 should be taken as the qualification of a person. If the semantics of 'wardrobe' is to be submitted to 'qualification of a person', then 'burly' is generated, thereby revealing in hindsight that wardrobe has induced excitations also by its large, broad dimensions. The lexical constraints are thereby equivalent to the structuring constraints imposed by the naming of the father to the excitations induced by the desire of the mother. Both types of constraints impose the regularities to which the experience has to be submitted, thereby introducing the subject to the dimension of the law.

However, the logic of the two metaphors – far from being mere discharge devices – shows how the need for discharge transforms into the generation of a new form and, more precisely, how the condition for the generation of this new form is the interplay with two 'others'. This is to say, it is only by there being two others, that we can be sure there is at least one. Indeed, if discharge is played out between the subject and a single other, then any change will be mirrored in the back-and-forth movement between the child and the first other. As a consequence, there will be neither real discharge nor the emergence of something new. The paternal metaphor intends to show how the subject, when not exhaustively taken by the interplay with a first other, uses the desiring interplay between this other and a second other, to intentionally derange and interfere in this interplay: by doing so, something unforeseen emerges (e.g. a parental response), something which properly manifests the subject, in his difference, i.e. in his singularity. The parental response here is not a simple mirroring but minimally the sign of an effect, and even often of a surprise. The child thereby himself or herself is taken by surprise that his or her movement had an unexpected effect of making a difference, i.e. of creating an 'event'. This will be the incentive for him or her to repeat and experiment with interfering and 'disturbing'. Metaphorization, far from being an all-or-nothing operation, thus, is an open-ended dynamic.

The advantage of the Name-of-the-Father metaphor over simpler drive-to-intention-translation models is that it succeeds in capturing various dimensions of this transformation simultaneously: (1) the dimension, close to a biological approach, of transforming diffuse excitation into dischargeable outer body motor forms; (2) the linguistic dimension whereby it is the arbitrary naming of the Father which thrusts this transformation; (3) the oedipal dimension with a constitutive role of the desiring interaction between the first and the second other for the subjectivation of the child; and (4) the sexual dimension introduced by the sexual differentiation of the parents which, through the way this differentiation is appraised by the child, is thought to leave a mark on his or her so-called fundamental phantasy. We will for now not develop this last dimension.

4 Reappraisal of the cases of Mrs. K and Mr. J

4.1 Mrs. K

Mrs. K suffered "an acute left fronto-parietal subdural hematoma (with slight midline shift) and a left temporo-parietal intracerebral hemorrhage – a substantial hemorrhagic lesion in the mid-temporal area, extending posteriorly to include the supramarginal gyrus" (p. 92), which resulted in "fluent 'empty speech' (i.e. a stream of connected discourse that lacks substantives) with abundant verbal paraphasias (i.e. misuse of words)", a Wernicke's aphasia which "had resolved (...) into what Luria (1947) called 'acoustic-mnestic aphasia'", with as essential feature, "an inability to retain audioverbal material in working memory (i.e. in consciousness)" (p. 93). Although her speech was fluent, she had marked problems with understanding and meaningful expression, from which Kaplan-Solms and Solms (2001) conclude that the 'acoustic aspect' is central to the word presentation and a fortiori to the mental apparatus. We will come back to that acoustic aspect, but for now we propose that Mrs. K's frontoparietal and temporoparietal lesions have more crucially affected the dorsal syntactic pathways than Mr. J's, principally affecting her secondary process functioning. We propose that since it is the constraining inference of the secondary process which enables metaphorization, this leads to *a fundamental metaphorization defect in Mrs. K*. Indeed, in Mrs. K both the metaphorization principle giving access to language beyond its idiomatic use, the linguistic metaphor, and, more fundamentally, the principle by which drive excitations are grasped into action intentions, the paternal metaphor, seem to be harmed.

4.1.1 Mrs. K's linguistic metaphor

Take for example the following confusion: The therapist said that she appeared a moment earlier to have lost track of herself and the world. Mrs. K misunderstood this, and thought that she [the therapist] was speaking about international travel. The therapist explained that by 'world' she was referring to Mrs. K's experience of what was going on around her.[13] Then Mrs. K said, "Oh yes, I am in bits and pieces. I am in bits and pieces through my mind" (Kaplan-Solms & Solms, 2001, p. 101). The context of "losing track of herself and the world" should have enabled her to constrain the associative meaning of the word 'world' which would have stopped the association with 'international travel'. Inasmuch as the term 'world' was not taken up into an active metaphorization operation, it was released from secondary process constraints regaining primary process object status, where it *metonymically* gave rise to the association of 'international travel'.

"On a subsequent occasion", Kaplan-Solms and Solms (2001, p. 105) recount, Mrs. K

> said that she was going to visit some friends of hers in another ward of the hospital, only to realize later that these were friends who had lived in her residential hotel – they were not living in this hospital. This reduplicative error was especially interesting, because it seemed to concretize an aphasic error that she frequently made: she confused the words 'hospital' and 'hotel'.

This example again shows that when metaphorization, a secondary process, fails, words revert to a primary process mode. In this instance, 'hotel' (which etymologically comes from 'hostel') metonymically becomes 'hospital'. What is interesting here is that the primary process metonymy guides the actions (and even action intentions) of the patient (language commands the doing, and not the reverse); that is, when the secondary process fails, our drive-guided, intentional grip on what we are doing is lost in favor of a primary process mode of language over which we do not have control.

Thus, we would argue, Mrs. K's defective metaphorization underlies her inability to attach meaning to language, especially when it comes to non-idiomatic language, implying that either the associative meaning is not the contextual one, or that there is no associative meaning at all: "but here is another example of how silly I've become! You know, I just *can't* understand what you're saying. I know it's English, but I don't know what it *means*. What do you *mean*?" (Kaplan-Solms and Solms, 2001, p. 99).

4.1.2 Mrs. K's paternal metaphor

Kaplan-Solms and Solms (2001) indicate that the patient complains about an "inability to think" (p. 94) and "I know what I want to say but I can't find the words; they just aren't there. And then, before I can find the words, the *thought* is gone. I just can't *think* anymore." (p. 104; their italics). The authors add:

> She was far from being truly unable to think. Rather, we would like to suggest, she suffered from an inability to a*ttach words to her thoughts*, resulting in an inability to *bring her thoughts to consciousness* (and to *keep* them there).
>
> (2001, p. 108; their Italics)

By this line of reasoning, then, thoughts are supposed to exist 'as such', merely awaiting language to get expressed. What we propose, in contrast, regarding Mrs. K is that what is 'broken' is not a passive attachment of thoughts to words but, the very process of metaphorization itself, the sub-jectification of language – that is, not only the linguistic metaphor but more-over the paternal metaphor, the fundamental function of language which allows for drive excitations to find discharge into (phonemic) motor pro-grams: "often I can't even remember what I was trying to say, and then I just drop the whole thing and forget about it." (Kaplan-Solms & Solms, 2001, p. 101). As noted above, the metaphoric function is not simply a matter of discharge but also the device by which new forms emerge, which truly are the mark of a subject that has interfered, cut, and selected in human linguis-tic exchange, and that thereby manifests its singularity as a subject. This, then, might be a more formal, logical way to grasp what Kaplan-Solms and Solms (2001, p. 113) indicate by saying that "her ego operations were being undermined".

4.2 Mr. J

Mr. J suffered an "infarction of the left inferior frontal and anterior tempo-ral lobes of the brain, and the involvement of the underlying white matter" (p. 75), which resulted in "a severe, non-fluent aphasia", which

> conformed to the classical syndrome of Broca's aphasia. Mr J's spon-taneous speech was sparse, severely telegraphic, and agrammatical. His repetition (...) was only slightly superior to his spontaneous output. (...) Comprehension was essentially preserved (...) the main feature of Mr. J's clinical presentation (...) [was] the striking integrity of this ego functioning. He was fully aware of the difficulties that he was having in communicating, and he spared no effort in overcoming these difficulties. (...) The content of his communications, too, revealed, the same intact-ness of his ego functions. (...) this high degree of ego integrity in a case of severe Broca's aphasia was indeed remarkable. This fact provides us with a first important clue as to the role that this region of the brain

plays in the deep psychological organization of the mental apparatus in general. Whatever this role, it certainly cannot be too central to what the ego does on the whole.

(p. 76)

In light of the previous, it is indeed amazing how little Mr. J is affected by the lesion.

To help us out here, we go back to Hickok (2014) who reminds us that it has been shown before how well speech perception can be accomplished with a damaged, deactivated, or undeveloped motor speech system (Bishop et al., 1990; Eimas, Siqueland, Jusczyk & Vigorito, 1971; Hickok, Costanzo, Capasso & Miceli, 2011; Hickok et al., 2008; Kuhl & Miller, 1975; Rogalsky, Love, Driscoll, Anderson & Hickok, 2011). However, as Hickok (2014, p. 10) adds, even with a damaged dorsal route, a "modulatory contribution of the motor system to speech perception remains a possibility", provided that what crucially is preserved is that *"activation of motor speech units generate[s] a forward prediction for their corresponding auditory speech units"* (Hickok, Houde, et al., 2011; our italics), i.e. the generation of the efference copies of the articulatory motor commands.

Returning to the question of the 'acoustic aspect' of language, we propose that what is important is not the perceptual, acoustic aspect as such of language but rather, as we have argued here, *the contribution of the motor dynamics to the understanding of language*. Hickok and colleagues' prescription is that the minimal function needed from the motor pathway is the generation of a forward prediction: indeed, as we have seen, the contribution of these efference copies is constitutive precisely, if paradoxically, for the hearing of language (see 1.2 and the McGurk effect), which explains the apparent importance of the acoustics. These efference copies might also be crucially involved in prefrontal working memory (Jacobs & Silvanto, 2015). For example, Kaplan-Solms and Solms (2001, pp. 107, 93) qualify Wernicke's aphasia as a "loss of memory for words", i.e. "an inability to retain audioverbal material in working memory (i.e. in consciousness) (...) she kept forgetting what it was that she was intending to say".

Moreover, the efference copy dynamics are also what is at the heart of the secondary process: it is through these efference copies, or indications of reality, that the constraining effect upon the primary process (and, by extension, the metaphor function), is realized. In other words, as long as the efference copy generation is preserved dorsally, the metaphorization – and thus, speculatively, what Kaplan-Solms and Solms call the 'ego-functions' – is preserved, even if the pathway to execute articulation, further downstream, is damaged (such as in the case, probably, of Mr. J). Moreover, since efference copies are not implied in motor execution as such, the reverse is also true: if this efference copy-generation mechanism is damaged or disturbed, the metaphorization – or what would be called the 'ego-functions' – is jeopardized, even if the execution of articulation is preserved (such as, probably, in Mrs. K). So, in sum, we speculate that Mr. J's capacity for metaphorization was kept intact, due to the intact functioning of the efference copy-generation mechanism, with, however, the impossibility to come to the motoric expression of this intact functioning. This could explain the fact that Mr. J witnesses to an intact situatedness in space and time, due to the correct dorsal inhibitory functioning of language. Mrs. K, on the other hand, suffers precisely this: the absence of a properly functioning metaphorization, leading to an incapacity to find herself 'in the world' and 'in time'.

4.3 The mental is not the physiological

The linear equation of Mrs. K's and Mr. J's symptoms to their deficits, broadly speaking a Wernicke's and a Broca's aphasia, had resulted in what we might qualify as 'overly general propositions' – such as, e.g. a 'normal ego-functioning'. Instead, what we have proposed is first and foremost an understanding of the mental logics of language in and by itself, developed through the mechanics of the linguistic and the paternal metaphor. This has resulted in proposing a single line of interpretation of Mrs. K's symptoms, in terms of a metaphorization deficit, which is at once able to explain all her various difficulties – not only her understanding of language but also her functioning in the primary process mode, her self-function difficulties, her working memory problems, her inability to think, etc. Moreover, it leads us to interpret Ms. J's case in terms of an inability to motorically express an otherwise correctly functioning metaphorization function. This explains the capacity of Mr. J to comprehend his subjective situatedness in space and time, being meanwhile in the inability to have the motoric linguistic expression correspond with this experience.

What we wish to underscore, then, at the end of this exercise, is that the most proximal interpretation lines for 'disorders of the mental, of the psyche' is *a mental interpretation line.* Indeed, we venture that metaphorization might have instantiated somewhat differently in the anatomy or in the physiology of the brain, depending on the subject, and thus predict that, whatever the precise locations of the lesions, if the metaphorization function is attained, we will find symptoms which are logically similar – and the other way around, whatever the brain deficits, if the metaphorization function is not damaged, essential linguistic mechanisms constitutive for mental functioning will be preserved. In other words, what we propose epistemologically is that from the brain to the symptoms the connexion is not linear, but articulates over the mental: the mental principle – here the metaphorization function – could well succeed in explaining the symptoms better than the physiological. This gives weight to the idea that the mental is an autonomous organization level, not reducible to the brain dynamics.

Moreover, in the spirit of Hickok's suggestion, we would conjecture more generally that an attained brain function common to all subjects with met-aphorization deficits would involve the the function of generating forward predictions for the activation of motor speech units. This function, then, is the crucial contribution of the dorsal pathway to the language dynamics. It would, of course, be relevant to attempt to substantiate this hypothesis on the basis of more clinical cases, However, what has been revealed in the present exercise through the careful clinical analyses of the speech and un-derstanding of these singular cases supports that the heuristic revelatory direction for the neuropsychoanalytical endeavor is from the mental to the brain, far more than from the brain to the mental.

Notes

1 One might object that Herr/Signor is a semantic, not a phonological, bridge structure. However, it must be remembered that what Freud pushed away was 'Herr' in the meaning of 'Sir'. By doing so, he pushes away all the primary pro-cess associates to 'Herr' – some of which are phonological, some of which se-mantic. One of the semantic associates, undergoing inhibition, is 'Sir', but it is by a phonological association with 'Signorelli' that the symptom arises, namely, the forgetting of the painter's name. This shows that even the semantic bridge associations are not secondary but primary processes. But the existence of this associative 'mindless' dynamic is revealed by the phonological, not the semantic associates (as for semantic associations, one can always propose that they are the result of secondary 'mindful' dynamics).

2 Words, therefore, even if they are no less objects than other objects, are still a particular kind of objects: besides having (motor and perceptual) character-istics of their own, they are also constituted by the fact of referring to other objects – those other objects being themselves either words or not.

3 Even if many Freudian, and even Lacanian, psychoanalysts still refer to the word presentation, the signifier, as an 'acoustic' element.

4 The McGurk effect is often called 'an illusion'. However, this would imply that the acoustic trace is the 'real trace' and that hearing speech is hearing the acous-tic trace of speech. This, we think, is fundamentally mistaken: when it comes to language, what we hear is structured by the sensorimotor feedback of the recognized speech movements matched with the acoustic information (Hickok, 2014). Therefore, in the McGurk effect, seeing the mouth movements of 'ga ga ga' together with hearing the acoustic trace of 'ba ba ba', results in the effective hearing of 'da da da', and not in its illusion.

5 Therefore, in contrast with Saur, Friederici indicates the ventral unicate fiber bundle as the prime player for this.

6 "sequences of phonemes that form the syllables or words of a language might be efficiently coded as motor chunks, a mental syllabary to use Levelt's term" (Hickock, 2014, p. 5).

7 Savage-Rumbaugh (1986) trained chimpanzees to use the combination of the lexigrams 'give' and 'banana' if they wished a banana and 'pour' and 'juice' if they wished juice. The teaching of these separate combinations was easy, but

when they received the four lexigrams at the same time, they perseverated in making random, including impossible, combinations (e.g. 'give give', 'pour banana'). In order to make a logical use of the lexigrams, the chimpanzees needed extra sessions to *unlearn* the impossible combinations. Deacon (1997, p. 85) interprets these observations by concluding that the unlearning sessions correspond to the acquisition of linguistic rules such as, here, 'a verb asks for a substantive' and 'the object of 'to pour' is liquid'.

8   In this perspective, it should be logical that this route has some connection to brain centers gathering inner body, i.e. drive, information.

9   In this the question remains whether it is the semantics that commands the signifier: in the present text we propose, inversely, that it is the lexical position that commands the semantics.

10   Lacan's first presentation of the signifier can be found in "The agency of the letter in the unconscious or reason since Freud" (Lacan 1977 [1966], pp. 146–178).

11   In the example used by Lacan (1957), Boaz, a major figure in the Book of Ruth in the Bible, is described as *"His sheaf was neither miserly nor spiteful."*, pinpointing not-so-commonly stressed attributes of a 'sheaf', namely, 'opulent, giving, feeding', and thereby revealing the person so qualified (Boaz) as 'generous'.

12   "if you reach for the same cup in the same location repeatedly, you will need to rely less and less on sensory information for achieving a successful reach. In general, there is an inverse relation between familiarity with the action-object pairing and the need for sensory involvement in the action: the more familiar the situation, the less you need sensory guidance (...). The same is true in speech, I suggest. Articulating less familiar words will require more input from the auditory-phonological component of the network than articulating highly familiar words."

13   Here, we feel, the therapist was acutely mindful in picking up something important.

References

Bazan, A. (2006). Primary process language. *Neuro-Psychoanalysis, 2*, 157–159.

Bazan, A. (2007a). *Des fantômes dans la voix. Une hypothèse neuropsychanalytique sur la structure de l'inconscient.* Collection *Voix Psychanalytiques.* Editions Liber, Montréal.

Bazan, A. (2007b). An attempt towards an integrative comparison of psychoanalytical and sensorimotor control to psychoanalytical theories of action. P. Haggard, Y. Rossetti, & M. Kawato (eds.), *Attention and Performance XXII.* New York: Oxford University Press, 319–338.

Bazan, A. (2012). From sensorimotor inhibition to Freudian repression: Insights from psychosis applied to neuroris. *Frontiers in Psychology, 3*, 452.

Bazan, A. & Snodgrass, M. (2012). On unconscious inhibition: Instantiating repression in the brain. In A. Fotopoulou, D. Pfaff, & M. A. Conway (Eds.). *From the couch to the lab: Trends in psychodynamic neuroscience.* Oxford University Press, 307–337.

Bishop, D. V., Brown, B. B. & Robson, J. (1990). The relationship between phoneme discrimination, speech production, and language comprehension in cerebral-palsied individuals. *Journal of Speech and Hearing Research, 33*(2), 210–219.

Blakemore, S. J., Wolpert, D. M. & Frith, C. D. (1998). Central cancellation of self-produced tickle sensation. *Nature Neurosciences, 1*, 635–640.

Bookheimer, S. (2002). Functional MRI of language: New approaches to under-standing the cortical organization of semantic processing. *Annual Review of Neu-roscience, 25*(1), 151–188.

Brauer, J., Anwander, A. & Friederici, A. D. (2011). Neuroanatomical prerequisites for language functions in the maturing brain. *Cerebral Cortex, 21*(2), 459–466.

Chomsky, N. & Halle, M. (1968). *The sound pattern of English*. Cambridge, MA: The MIT Press.

Cutler, A. & Clifton, C. (1999). Comprehending spoken language: A blueprint of the listener. *The Neurocognition of Language*, 123–166.

Damasio, H., Grabowski, T. J., Tranel, D., Hichwa, R. D. & Damasio, A. R. (1996). A neural basis for lexical retrieval. *Nature, 380*, 499–505.

Dapretto, M. & Bookheimer, S. Y. (1999). Form and content: Dissociating syntax and semantics in sentence comprehension. *Neuron, 24*(2), 427–432.

Deacon T. 1997. *The symbolic species: the co-evolution of language and the brain*. New York: W.W. Norton & Co.

Eimas, P. D., Siqueland, E. R., Jusczyk, P. & Vigorito, J. (1971). Speech perception in infants. *Science, 171*(968), 303–306.

Freud, S. (1891/1978). *On aphasia, a critical study* (E. Stengel, translator). New York: Universities Press.

Freud, S. (1895/1966 [1950]). *Project for a scientific psychology* (J. Stratchey, transla-tor). In *Standard Edition I* (281–397/410). London: The Hogarth Press.

Freud, S. (1900/1975). *The interpretation of dreams* (J. Stratchey, translator). In *Standard Edition IV-V*. London: The Hogarth Press.

Freud, S. (1901/1990). *The psychopathology of everyday life* (J. Stratchey, translator). In *Standard Edition VI*. London: The Hogarth Press.

Freud, S. (1950/1966). *Project for a scientific psychology* (J. Stratchey, translator). In *The Standard Edition I* (281–392). London: The Hogarth Press.

Friederici, A. D. (2015). White-matter pathways for speech and language process-ing. *Handbook of Clinical Neurology, 129*(3), 177–186.

Friederici, A. D., Bahlmann, J., Heim, S., Schubotz, R. I. & Anwander, A. (2006). The brain differentiates human and non-human grammars: Functional localiza-tion and structural connectivity. *Proceedings of the National Academy of Sciences of the United States of America, 103*(7), 2458–2463.

Georgieff, N. & Jeannerod, M. (1998). Beyond consciousness of external reality. A "Who" system for consciousness of action and self-consciousness. *Conscious Cognition, 7*, 465–477.

Gonzalez, C. C. & Burke, M. R. (2013). The brain uses efference copy information to optimise spatial memory. *Experimental Brain Research, 224*(2), 189–197.

Griffiths, J. D., Marslen-Wilson, W. D., Stamatakis, E. A. & Tyler, L. K. (2013). Functional organization of the neural language system: Dorsal and ventral path-ways are critical for syntax. *Cerebral Cortex, 23*(1), 139–147.

Grodzinsky, Y. & Friederici, A. D. (2006). Neuroimaging of syntax and syntactic processing. *Current Opinion in Neurobiology, 16*(2), 240–246.

Helmholtz, H. von (1878/1971). The facts of perception. In R. Kahl (ed.), *Selected writings of Hermann von Helmholtz*. Middletown, CT: Wesleyan University Press, 115–185.

Hickok, G. (2014). The architecture of speech production and the role of the pho-neme in speech processing. *Language, Cognition and Neuroscience, 29*(1), 2–20.

Hickok, G., Costanzo, M., Capasso, R. & Miceli, G. (2011). The role of Broca's area in speech perception: Evidence from aphasia revisited. *Brain and Language*, *119*(3), 214–220.

Hickok, G., Houde, J. & Rong, F. (2011). Sensorimotor integration in speech processing: computational basis and neural organization. *Neuron*, *69*(3), 407–422.

Hickok, G., Okada, K., Barr, W., Pa, J., Rogalsky, C., Donnelly, K., ... Grant, A. (2008). Bilateral capacity for speech sound processing in auditory comprehension: Evidence from Wada procedures. *Brain and Language*, *107*(3), 179–184.

Hickok, G. & Poeppel, D. (2000). Towards a functional neuroanatomy of speech perception. *Trends in Cognitive Sciences*, *4*, 131–138.

Hickok, G. & Poeppel, D. (2004). Dorsal and ventral streams: A framework for understanding aspects of the functional anatomy of language. *Cognition*, *92*(1), 67–99.

Hickok, G. & Poeppel, D. (2007). The cortical organization of speech processing. *Nature Reviews Neuroscience*, *8*(5), 393–402.

Jacobs, C. & Silvanto, J. (2015). How is working memory content consciously experienced? The 'conscious copy' model of WM introspection. *Neuroscience & Biobehavioral Reviews*, *55*, 510–519.

Jeannerod, M. (1997). *The cognitive neuroscience of action*. New Jersey: Blackwell Publishing.

Jeannerod, M. (2001). Neural simulation of action: A unifying mechanism for motor cognition. *Neuroimage*, *14*(1), S103–S109.

Kaplan-Solms, K. & Solms, M. (2001). *Clinical studies in neuro-psychoanalysis. Introduction to a depth neuropsychology*. Madison, CT: International Universities Press.

Kuhl, P. K. & Miller, J. D. (1975). Speech perception by the chinchilla: Voiced-voiceless distinction in alveolar plosive consonants. *Science*, *190*, 69–72.

Lacan, J. (1955–1956/1993). *The psychoses, the seminar of Jacques Lacan*. Edited by Jacques-Alain Miller, translated with notes by Russell Grigg, Routledge.

Lacan, J. (1957/1966). *The insistence of the letter in the unconscious* (J. Miel, translator) in J. Ehrmann (ed.), *Yale French Studies*, (36/37), 112–147.

Lacan, J. (1977/1966). *The agency of the letter in the unconscious or reason since Freud, Ecrits: A selection*, trans. Alan Sheridan. London: Tavistock, pp. 146–178.

Liberman, A. M. (1970). The grammars of speech and language. *Cognitive Psychology*, *1*(4), 301–323.

Liberman, A. M., Cooper, F. S., Shankweiler, D. P. & Studdert-Kennedy, M. (1967). Perception of the speech code. *Psychological Review*, *74*, 431–461.

Liberman, A. M. & I. G. Mattingly (1985). The motor theory of speech perception revised. *Cognition*, *21*, 1–36.

Luria, A. R. (1947). *Traumatic aphasia: Its syndromes, psychology and treatment*. The Hague: Mouton.

Musso, M., Moro, A., Glauche, V., Rijntjes, M., Reichenbach, J., Büchel, C. & Weiller, C. (2003). Broca's area and the language instinct. *Nature Neuroscience*, *6*(7), 774–781.

Ojemann, G. A. (1979). Individual variability in cortical localization of language. *Journal of Neurosurgery*, *50*, 164–169.

Ojemann, G. A. (1983). Brain organization of language from the perspective of electrical stimulation mapping. *Behavioral and Brain Sciences*, *2*, 189–230.

Ojemann, G. A. (1991). Cortical organization of language. *Journal of Neuroscience*, *11*, 2281–2287.

Perani, D., Saccuman, M. C., Scifo, P., Anwander, A., Spada, D., Baldoli, C., ... & Friederici, A. D. (2011). Neural language networks at birth. *Proceedings of the National Academy of Sciences*, *108*(38), 16056–16061.

Price, C. J., Wise, R. J. S., Warburton, E. A., Moore, C. J., Howard, D., Patterson, K., ... Friston, K. J. (1996). Hearing and saying: The functional neuro-anatomy of auditory word processing. *Brain: A Journal of Neurology*, *119*(3), 919–931.

Rauschecker, J. P, & Scott, S. K. (2009). Maps and streams in the auditory cortex: Nonhuman primates illuminate human speech processing. *Nature Neuroscience*, *12*(6), 718–724.

Rizzolatti, G. & Arbib, M. A. (1998). Language within our grasp. *Trends in Neurosciences*, *21*, 188–194.

Rogalsky, C., Love, T., Driscoll, D., Anderson, S. W. & Hickok, G. (2011). Are mirror neurons the basis of speech perception? Evidence from five cases with damage to the purported human mirror system. *Neurocase*, *17*(2), 178–187.

Sarubbo, S., De Benedictis, A., Maldonado, I. L., Basso, G. & Duffau, H. (2013). Frontal terminations for the inferior fronto-occipital fascicle: Anatomical dissection, DTI study and functional considerations on a multi-component bundle. *Brain Structure and Function*, *218*(1), 21–37.

Saur, D., Kreher, B. W., Schnell, S., Kümmerer, D., Kellmeyer, P., Vry, M. S., Umarova, R., Musso, M., Glauche, V., Abel, S., Huber, W., Rijntjes, M., Hennig, J. & Weiller, C. (2008). Ventral and dorsal pathways for language. *Proceedings of the National Academy of Sciences*, *105*(46), 18035–18040.

Saur, D., Schelter, B., Schnell, S., Kratochvil, D., Küpper, H., Kellmeyer, P., Kümmerer, D., Klöppel, S., Glauche V., Lange, R., Mader, W., Feess, D., Timmer, J. & Weiller, C. (2010). Combining functional and anatomical connectivity reveals brain networks for auditory language comprehension. *Neuroimage*, *49*(4), 3187–3197.

Savage-Rumbaugh, E. S. (1986). *Ape language: From conditioned response to symbol.* New York: Columbia University Press.

Schmahmann, J. D. Schmahmann, J., & Pandya, D. (2009). *Fiber pathways of the brain*. New York: Oxford University Press.

Sperry, R. W. (1950). Neural basis of the spontaneous optokinetic response produced by visual inversion. *Journal of Comparative and Physiological Psychology*, *43*, 482–489.

Suárez-González, A., Heredia, C. G., Savage, S. A., Gil-Néciga, E., García-Casares, N., Franco-Macías, E., ... Caine, D. (2014). Restoration of conceptual knowledge in a case of semantic dementia. *Neurocase*, *21*(3), 309–321.

Thompson-Schill, S. L., D'Esposito, M., Aguirre, G. K. & Farah, M. J. (1997). Role of left inferior prefrontal cortex in retrieval of semantic knowledge: A reevaluation. *Proceedings of the National Academy of Sciences*, *94*(26), 14792–14797.

Turken, A. U. & Dronkers, N. F. (2011). The neural architecture of the language comprehension network: Converging evidence from lesion and connectivity analyses. *Frontiers in Systeme Neurosciences*, *5*, 1.

van Holst, E. (1954). Relations between the central nervous system and the peripheral organs. *British Journal of Animal Behavior*, *2*, 89–94.

Wernicke, C. (1874/1977). Der aphasische symptomencomplex: Eine psychologische studie auf anatomischer basis. In G. H. Eggert (ed.), *Wernicke's works on aphasia: A sourcebook and review*. The Hague: Mouton, 91–145.

Wilson, S. M., Galantucci, S., Tartaglia, M. C., Rising, K., Patterson, D. K., Henry, M. L., Ogar, J. M., DeLeon, J., Miller, B. L. & Gorno-Tempini, M. L. (2011). Syntactic processing depends on dorsal language tracts. *Neuron, 72*(2), 397–403.

Wolpert, D. M. (1997). Computational approaches to motor control. *Trends in Cognitive Sciences, 1*, 209–216.

Case studies

Chapter 6

A mother and wife, after right-hemisphere stroke

A self psychological perspective

Pamela Klonoff

Psychotherapy has grown in its recognition and utilization in neurore-habilitation for people with brain injuries (Ben-Yishay & Diller, 2011; Klonoff, 2010; Langer, Laatsch & Lewis, 1999; Newby, Coetzer, Daisley & Weatherhead, 2013; Ponsford, 2004; Prigatano et al., 1986; Ruff & Chester, 2014; Wilson, Gracey, Evans & Bateman, 2011). Among these therapies, psychoanalytic approaches have imparted valuable insights into how brain injury can alter the ways in which individuals relate to themselves and others. Self psychology has particularly contributed by describing how brain damage can harm the coherence and continuity of the self. The goal of this case is to exemplify the effectiveness of self psychology concepts in comprehending psychological changes after brain injury. In order to do so, the case of a woman with a right-hemisphere stroke who underwent psychotherapy and holistic rehabilitation is presented.

I Self psychology and selfobject relations

Self psychology, like so many other fields within psychoanalysis, developed as a clinical discipline, without any reference to neurobiology. The field is predicated on the seminal work of Heinz Kohut and explored four facets of psychoanalysis: how relational affective transactions with the social environment spur the development of the self, how experiences are internalized into maturing self-regulating structures, how early deficits in self-structure result in later self-pathologies, and how the therapeutic relationship restores the self (Schore, 2009).

The self is the essence of an individual's psychological being, consisting of sensations, feelings, thoughts, and attitudes toward oneself and the world (Banai, Mikulincer & Shaver, 2005). Self psychology purports that healthy narcissism is a nondefective structural completeness of the self which can sustain its coherence, continuity, and self-esteem (Banai et al., 2005; Kohut, 2009). Kohut posited that the essential task of psychological development and existence is the growth and maintenance of the cohesive functioning self, also with a yearning for connection (Terman, 2014). The selfobject is the necessary precondition for development of a cohesive self (Wolfe, 1989). Selfobjects in the psychic world are objects who are experienced as part of the self, not as separate and independent (see Wolfe, 1989, for a review). Kohut posited that "parents with mature psychological organizations serve as selfobjects which perform critical regulatory functions for the infant, who has an immature, incomplete, psychological organization" (Kohut, 1977; Schore, 2009, pp. 191–192). Of note, the self needs selfobjects throughout the life span and their form changes with maturity (Kohut, 2009; Lage & Nathan, 1991). The neurobiological basis of such selfobjects has never been a reference point for the field, but there are some potential points of contact, of which the clearest might come from the themes of empathy and mirroring.

Through the reciprocal transactions with the selfobject (episodes of empathic "mirroring" or admiration of the individual's qualities and accomplishments), the infant is able to maintain his or her internal homeostatic equilibrium, self-worth, value, and internal self-respect (Baker & Baker, 1987; Banai et al., 2005; Kohut & Wolf, 1978; Schore, 2009). Other forms of selfobjects are "idealizing," in which an external selfobject provides calming, comforting, and protective functions through merging with idealized selfobjects (Baker & Baker, 1987; Banai et al., 2005; Brown, 2010; Kohut, 2009; Kohut & Wolf, 1978) and "twinship" or "alter ego" selfobject needs, defined as a degree of alikeness with other people and feeling bonded with the human community (Baker & Baker, 1987; Brown, 2010; Kohut, 2009). A firm self has three constituents: one pole which fundamental strivings for power and success emanate from, another pole that holds basic idealized goals, and an intermediate area of talents and skills which are activated by a tension arc between ambitions and ideals (Kohut & Wolf, 1978).

Empathic responses from critical selfobjects during formative years are necessary for the development of self-cohesion (i.e., the ability to tolerate stress) (Lage & Nathan 1991). Disorders of the self result from developmental arrests and traumatic failings resulting from parental (and/or their substitutes' shortcomings). There is an underlying lack of self-cohesion, a dearth of confidence in dealing with life's hardships, and vulnerable self-esteem (Baker & Baker, 1987; Banai et al., 2005). In the therapeutic process, the defective self and archaic struggles are reactivated; through the mirroring, idealizing, or twinship/alter ego transferences, the self can be reconstituted (Lage & Nathan, 1991).

2 Right hemisphere function

One further potential link between self psychological concepts and neuropsychology might come from a consideration of the functions of the right cerebral hemisphere (in those with conventional cerebral dominance). Right-hemisphere strokes naturally produce a wide range of common sequelae, often involving primarily cognitive impairment. These include hemianopia, and various forms of neglect; visuoperceptual, visuospatial, and constructional apraxia deficits; visual search difficulties; topographical orientation problems; and contralateral hemiplegia or hemiparesis, spasticity, and other motor challenges (Árnadóttir, 2011; Byars & Heilman, 2015; Capruso, Hamsher & Benton, 2006; Festa, Lazar & Marshall, 2008; Gottesman & Hillis, 2010; Matano, Iosa, Guariglia, Pizzamiglio & Paolucci, 2015; Ten Brink et al., 2016).

In addition to these, and of particular interest in the context of self psychology, right-hemisphere stroke also produces emotional processing and communication disorders: recognizing or categorizing facial emotions, as well as comprehension and expression of emotional prosody (Byars & Heilman, 2015; Festa et al., 2008). The right hemisphere is also implicated in other cognitive activities on the emotion–cognition boundary, including attending to relevant stimuli, as well as deciding when to initiate, persist, and complete actions (Byars & Heilman, 2015). Perhaps as a result of these many impairments, such neurological patients can present with a range of "psychiatric-like" symptoms. Thus, patients with right-hemisphere stroke can exhibit depression, which potentially negatively impacts attention, visual perception, working memory, episodic verbal memory and semantic memory, auditory and written language, constructional apraxia, and impairments in verbal fluency (Oliveira et al., 2015).

A related set of issues arise from the fact that damage affecting the frontal lobes have long been implicated in executive system dysfunction, producing cognitive, communication, mood, and behavioral challenges (Gottesman & Hillis, 2010; see Klonoff, 2014, for a review). Executive functions are also considered part of metacognition, defined as "thinking about thinking" (see Purdy, 2014, for a review). Metacognitive beliefs are dynamic, in that they are created and updated based on new experiences and circumstances, including consideration of patients' own personal task failures and successes (Levine et al., 2011; Purdy, 2014). Interestingly, right hemisphere damage has also been correlated with an "updater" failure, an inability to construct, utilize, or update representational models. This translates to a reduced capacity to alter mental models through detection of novel stimuli that do not fit with the current conceptualization and subsequently shift to a new representation (Stöttinger et al., 2014). These deficits have a deleterious effect on recovery and outcomes (Gillen, 2011; Matano et al., 2015; Ownsworth & Shum, 2008) and are clearly relevant to a self psychology perspective.

How might this rather abstract list of neuropsychological impairments map onto the real-life experiences of a stroke survivor?

3 Sara's background history

Sara was a "stay-at-home" mom who also homeschooled two of her four children, ages 2, 4, 6, and 8. Her husband, Tim, is (and was) a fire fighter. At age 29, she suffered a large right middle cerebral artery infarct including the insula. She presented with left-sided weakness, left facial droop, slurred speech, behavioral change, nausea, and vomiting. Sara was 13 weeks pregnant with her fifth child (named Amaziah: God will strengthen). A medical workup revealed a protein S deficiency. Sara was discharged to inpatient rehabilitation three days later and then home after 16 days. Upon discharge, the physician suggested to Tim that he buy a hospital bed for the downstair living room, as Sara would be unable to traverse stairs nor care for her children. Sara had limited outpatient physical, occupational, and speech therapies to address straightforward skills, such as getting in and out of bed, communicating rudimentary needs and wants, and how to walk with a walker. She existed with very low capabilities at home (e.g., "watching television and sitting in a chair") and required 24-hour supervision. As she was totally unable to tend to her children, her 24-year-old sister-in-law, Betty, moved from Oregon to "mother" the children (and newborn son) and run the household.

In this medical and family context, it is instructive to observe the lived experience of a patient of this sort. These patients are required, of course, to navigate a range of medical challenges, physical and intellectual, often when their own intellectual and emotional capacities are restricted by the stroke itself. In addition, there are the issues surrounding rehabilitation and uncertainties about recovery and disability. And finally, and perhaps most importantly, there is the dramatically changed *interpersonal* world that they are forced to face – where their roles as a parent and partner can be changed beyond imagining.

3.1 Case vignette I

Tim was distraught. Betty mustered her dwindling energies and desperately searched for neurorehabilitation for Sara. After a circuitous route, they landed at a holistic treatment program almost one year post stroke. The first step was to delineate Sara's neurological status. Neuropsychological and speech and language testing, in conjunction with clinical observations, revealed that relative to her pre-stroke level of functioning, she demonstrated moderate-to-very severe impairments in visuoconstruction and visuoperceptual skills, and visual recall and executive functions (characterized by deficient complex attention, planning, flexible problem-solving, decision-making, judgment, time management, prioritization, organization, multitasking, "disconnection between knowing and doing," impulsivity, not seeing the "big picture" (Gestalt), and perspective taking). Mild-to-moderate self-relative deficits were observed in her higher level inferential reasoning (written expression and writing fluency), and mild challenges were identified in her oral–motor coordination (phonation) and higher level verbal thought formulation. Retained strengths included her auditory comprehension, verbal expression, reading comprehension, sustained attention, speed of information processing, verbal learning and recall, and math. The occupational therapy evaluation revealed left-sided decreased sensory awareness, impaired visuoperceptual abilities (e.g., visual scanning, visual memory, and visual discrimination), fine and gross motor incoordination, abnormal tone, and visual neglect. The physical therapy evaluation indicated mild difficulties in her lower extremity range of motion and strength, motor timing and coordination, lack of stamina, and high-level balance (without visual input).

All too often, such patients are asked to navigate the world of neurological disability without much in the way of formal psychological support. Sara was in the more fortunate position of having access to psychotherapy, and it was instructive to see how she used this process to gradually adapt to her changed circumstances.

4 The beginning of the psychotherapy process

4.1 Case vignette 2

In the first few psychotherapy sessions with Dr. K., Sara wistfully reminisced about her pre-stroke life:

> My children are my world. Life isn't fair – I took care of my health. I was the CEO of my family, living my dream. I was super independent and now I'm dependent on others. I miss my old life. Everything has been taken away and I'm fighting to get better. I am a supermom, now with a broken wing. I feel anxious and defeated. This has been the year from hell; this stroke sucks.

She aptly referenced the lyrics from the song "Paralyzed" (Tucker, 2013).

Sara's assumptive world was shattered. Her massive right-hemisphere stroke produced fragmentation and a sense of emptiness; she was unable to maintain a clear sense of herself in the face of adversity (Brown, 2010; Wolf, 1988). Compounding this was an absence of psychotherapeutic and other interventions translating to a dearth of crucial selfobject transferences to help restabilize her. Yet, Sara's despondency fluctuated with glimmers of hopefulness, especially once she initiated psychotherapy. Employing attunement with building insight, Dr. K. introduced her to a "road map to recovery," the Patient Experiential Model (PEM) of Recovery (Klonoff, 2010), emphasizing how intensive holistic treatment would create a new "tool kit." Dr. K. emphasized how cognitive remediation exercises, assistance for her mood and adjustment struggles, and relatives' support and education would undoubtedly improve her performance as a mother and wife. Incremental goal setting and the promise of compensation training by the speech and occupational therapists, also directly in the home, provided solace and new prospects. Dr. K. empathically validated Sara's fears and grief, reframing a self-critical perception of succumbing to a "pity party." Following the first few sessions, including beginning to establish rapport with the program psychiatrist, Sara mentioned at the end of the session:

> I feel like a part of the movie, "Mine, Ours, and Yours" (Nathanson et al., 2005). I'm at my one year anniversary – "life day" and my ten year wedding anniversary is next week. There's a case around my head and I'm still healing.

Within the context of a budding idealizing transference relationship, the next several sessions focused on helping Sara regulate her "roller coaster" of emotions. Adages of "trust the process," "patience, trust, and collaboration," and a "wait and see attitude" regarding her long-term prognosis (Klonoff, 2010) were calming. Sara agreed to do some self-ratings and identified profound problems with fatigue (9/10; 1=small problem; 10=large problem), guilt (8/10), and feeling overwhelmed (5/10). The complexities and perplexities associated with improving her awareness and acceptance of her condition were normalized. Cohesiveness was promoted through the fundamentals of proper rest, "brain foods," and energy conservation. Given the preeminence of exercise in her life as self-sustaining, and her dearth of time at home for this endeavor, Dr. K. advocated for more physical therapy on the unit. Her occupational therapist integrated state-of-the-art modalities to treat Sara's upper extremity hemiparesis (e.g., the Empi® and Bioness®). Sara was outwardly appreciative – evidence of a sustaining self–selfobject relationship (Wolfe, 1989). During one session, Sara erupted into laughter recollecting how she had let her four-year-old daughter measure flour for cookies they were baking, culminating in a "baking debacle." She quipped: "who does that?" Through an empathic mirroring transference, Dr. K. was able to validate the humorous side of her often chaotic existence at home.

It is often helpful to see how this growing use of the therapeutic process can itself be helpful for the process of rehabilitation, and indeed for *managing* the process of rehabilitation.

4.2 Case vignette 3

The self psychological approach was amalgamated with sharing knowledge about Sara's neurological status. At her request, two months after beginning holistic rehabilitation, Sara's magnetic resonance imaging (MRI) scans were reviewed by her physiatrist, with her, Tim, Betty, her occupational therapist, and Dr. K. present. Specific limitations, and their localization in the right hemisphere, were sensitively explored. In follow-up psychotherapy sessions, Dr. K. reviewed Middle Cerebral Artery (MCA) distribution strokes, including the homunculus. Also, to give Sara a perspective of retained skills, "what if" scenarios were reviewed, including the greater debilitating effect on parenting if she had suffered a left-hemisphere stroke, producing severe aphasia. Alternatively, she was educated that given the "massive" nature of the stroke, her initial survival was in fact perilous. Through her personal journaling and discussions in psychotherapy, Sara periodically returned to entertaining these other "worst-case scenarios" as these created better perspective taking and a more grateful attitude.

5 Narcissistic rage and catastrophic reactions

How might these neurologically induced changes be linked to the self psychology perspective? Reactions of the self to physical illness constitute secondary disturbances of the self (Kohut & Wolf, 1978). Narcissistic rage emanates from feelings of utter helplessness, loss of integrity, humiliation, vexation, and resentment (Kohut, 1972; Wolf, 1988). The rage and need for revenge are directed toward selfobjects who threaten or damage the self through ridicule, contempt, or defeat (Kohut, 1972; Strozier, 2001; Wolf, 1988). Narcissistic injury causes the self to experience "disintegration anxiety" or fragmentation of the self, characterized by a sense of falling apart, and the loss of self, humanness, and wholeness (Baker & Baker, 1987; Kohut, 2009). Self-esteem is taxed, with no replenishing sustenance (Kohut & Wolf, 1978). A working definition of narcissistic rage after brain injury is "rage engendered by an assault (due to the injury) on the patient's sense of inner being, resulting in a shattering of his or her core essence and self-defining capabilities" (Klonoff, 2010, p. 83).

Catastrophic reactions (CRs) were first described by Goldstein (1952). He described behaviors related to impairment in the abstract attitude when patients fail to perform tasks, where "they appear dazed, become agitated, change color, start to fumble, become unfriendly, evasive, and even aggressive" (Goldstein, 1952, p. 255). A working definition of CRs is the patient's "strong emotional reaction to current difficulties in accomplishing tasks that were easy before the injury. Usually, the failure is sudden and unexpected" (Klonoff, 2014, p. 358). CRs shatter the coherence and continuity of the self (Salas, 2012), and when they are frequent and intense, they can precipitate a depressive state (Klonoff, 2010).

Previous articles have juxtaposed CRs and narcissistic rage through the sharing of underlying experiences of shame and anxiety over injury-based impairments (Klonoff & Lage, 1991; Klonoff, Lage & Chiapello, 1993; Strozier, 2001). However, narcissistic rage is an explosive reaction to the loss of "me-ness" as well as global disintegration of one's sense of self, whereas CRs are short-lived emotional reactions to specific stimuli (Klonoff, 2010; Kohut, 1972). Manifestations of CRs or "meltdowns" include feeling: overwhelmed, frustrated, impatient, angry, furious, sad, depressed, guilty, embarrassed, devastated, helpless, hopeless, snarky, defensive, tearful, anxious, fearful, and panicky, in possible conjunction with avoidance, minimization, blaming of others, withdrawal, shutting down, disavowal, and concealment (Klonoff, 2014; Klonoff et al., 1993). These changes to the nature of the self have the potential to be hugely challenging. What then is the subjective perspective on such dramatic losses, and how might the patient manage these changes with their now-depleted resources?

5.1 Case vignette 4

Sara experienced a profound narcissistic injury, in that she could no longer mother her children. She had endured several miscarriages interspersed with the birth of her five children. Her identity and *raison d'etre* were a devoted mother raising greatly loved and cherished children. Her stroke had stripped and ripped this life passion and mission from her. She bemoaned that it was a "stab in her heart" that she could no longer homeschool.

Sara's stroke-related left hemiparesis, visuoperceptual, memory, and executive function deficiencies, and her consequent inability to care for her children, precipitated an assault on her self-esteem (Klonoff, 2010). Sara's sister-in-law, Betty, was the "lightning rod" for the vengefulness, as she was the constant reminder of Sara as a "pre-stroke consummate mother." Sara was assailed by "disintegration anxiety" and frequent fragmentations, characterized by enfeebled depression and raging scapegoating attacks (Baker & Baker, 1987). She was plagued by feelings of emptiness, depression, worthlessness, and hopelessness (Klonoff, 2010). One day, three months into her psychotherapy she brought in a poem:

Brain Injury

> There is so much loss
> Isn't God the boss?
> Then why did my right brain have to die?
> As I lay in a hospital bed weakened and cry
> My kids at home with no Mamma
> How do I explain this trauma?
> For you, my sweet children I fight
> Every single day and unending night
> My heart carries so much hurt and pain
> I pray for the day that I will again
> Have my life back
> As I run around this track
> Alas, tears stain my cheeks as they fall from my eyes
> Mourning a life that is no more
> I wish I could stop keeping score
> When I return home broken and worn
> I look to gather strength to fight for my life another day

No therapeutic process is without its challenges – though the capacity to recognize the powerful feelings, and to find some sort of control over them, is a clear sign of progress.

5.2 Case vignette 5

Early on in the treatment process, Sara shared that she felt disheartened about her shortcomings and perceived that she was disappointing others. This created a CR cycle of guilt and anger. She engaged in "hindsight is 40/40 thinking" (Klonoff, 2010), blaming herself for things she could not know regarding her medical condition. With increasing awareness came CRs and emotional deterioration; the more she learned, the greater her resentment and hostility. She felt she was a punished "innocent victim." She was livid with God – asking "Why did he let this happen; he doesn't care about me."

Narcissistic rage was projected onto Betty and Tim, with allegations telltale of "killing the messenger" (Klonoff, 2010) when they tried to provide constructive feedback. Comments of feeling "criticized and micromanaged" and "hating the observation, as everyone is waiting for me to make a mistake" were indicative of her distrust of the therapists and family members. Her mood disintegrated into a "doom-and-gloom" depressed outlook and by her own admission, she viewed the world with a "tinted lens."

6 Treatment for narcissistic rage and CRs

6.1 Clinical vignette 6

The injured, enraged self needs to feel understood through the enduring, empathic responsiveness of the psychotherapist (Wolf, 1988). Dr. K. quietly listened while Sara ranted and sobbed about her lousy state of affairs. This was not the time to try to allay her intense emotionality with platitudes. Watching Betty day in and day out expertly mother five children using both working limbs and her cognitive repertory infuriated Sara, who was relegated to simple activities usually with one child at a time and punctuated with frequent rest periods from physical exhaustion. Gradually over time, Sara was guided to realize that her jealousy of Betty was actually externalized self-loathing of her condition and buried in deep grief and loss. Dr. K perceived that the reemergence of a cohesive self was predicated on Sara regaining competencies to be a top-notch mother and wife. Her family's involvement was posited as a crucial component of minimizing "disintegration anxiety," as their "auxiliary frontal lobes" helped Sara reconstitute (Klonoff, 2014; Salas, 2012). Her caregivers, as selfobjects, provided regulatory interventions in the form of external parameters to contain disorganized thinking and behavior, impulsivity, and poor planning (Klonoff, 2014; Salas et al., 2014). Case in point, Betty would often ask "leading" questions and create worksheets to help Sara with stepwise problem-solving for activities of daily living (e.g., meal planning) and parenting duties. At one point, when her mother visited the home, she bought and assigned different colored towels to simplify the bathing routine for the young children.

There are many therapeutic interventions that are designed to be relatively brief. To some elements of the theraputic community, there is an expectation that much can be achieved in treating a psychiatric disorder in perhaps 10 or 15 sessions. In the context of the enormous changes produced by a substantial neurological disorder, this seems far less likely.

6.2 Case vignette 7

Sara was educated about her unique CRs (Klonoff et al., 1993), displayed as feeling down, frustrated, discouraged, defensive ("kill the messenger"), misperception (the "tinted lens"), guilt, and anxiety for the future. Her CRs were compounded with feeling remorseful and dejected due to disappointing others. Interventions were two home visits per week by the occupational and speech therapists for 12 months, simplifying home duties to be manageable, and psychotherapy to teach Tim and Betty to remain empathic when Sara was withdrawn, uncooperative, minimizing, resistant, or hostile (versus lapsing into confrontations or counterattacks) (Klonoff, 2014; Klonoff et al., 1993). Other antidotes for avoiding CR cascades were predicated on "errorless learning" (Glisky, 2004; Wilson, 2009), as the more Sara achieved in the home environment, the less frequent the episodes of emotionally depleting CRs. So as to create more external orderliness and lessen internal disorganization (Salas, 2012), a myriad of checklists and a sophisticated datebook system were developed in collaboration with Sara's occupational and speech therapists and family (e.g., for the morning, after school, evening, lunch preparation, kids' bath time, day trips, and left upper extremity usage).

Collaborative evidentiary techniques (Klonoff, 2010) strengthened her abstract attitude. Detailed error logs were incorporated into cognitive retraining to instruct Sara to self-monitor her rate and types of mistakes, with an eye to generalizing precision into the home. She was given energy conservation pointers (e.g., adaptive equipment for the kitchen to compensate for her left hemiparetic arm and easy-to-prepare versus complex multistep recipes). Notable was that after struggling to make German pancakes from scratch, she opted for prepared batter with creative fruit decorations, so as to decrease multitasking and relish the activity with her children. Pros and cons lists were employed to improve realistic decision-making (Klonoff, 2010); this staved off new CRs. For example, Sara was aided in contemplating the "pluses" and "minuses" of homeschooling versus a charter school experience.

Sara appreciated the psychoeducation process. Handouts on CRs and depression were provided to characterize her emotional repertoire (Klonoff, 2014). Initially, she was astonished at the number of symptoms pertinent to her predicament, as she endorsed 20 types of CRs and 24 signs associated with depression (e.g., low energy, psychomotor agitation, social withdrawal, crying, low self-esteem, self-deprecation, shame, worthlessness, brooding, gloominess, pessimism, sorrow, disillusionment, and despair). Comprehending the physiological and reactive bases to her emotional turbulence and "helpful hints" (Klonoff, 2014) was illuminating to Sara.

Three months into the psychotherapy relationship, Sara was introduced in more detail to specific challenges with executive functions, also through an educational handout that defined typical indicators in "user-friendly language" (Klonoff, 2014). She performed insightful self-ratings, identifying sizeable problems in flexibility (8/10), perseveration (7/10), impulse control (6/10), planning and problem-solving (4/10), judgment (5/10), complex attention and distractibility (6/10), generating strategies (7/10), decision-making (5–7/10), multitasking (5–7/10), abstract reasoning (8/10), and seeing the big picture (6/10).

Throughout neurorehabilitation, Sara continued with regular psychiatric care (with Dr. K. present) so as to delve into catalysts of her CRs and narcissistic rage and sensitively dialogue about her propensity for depressive symptomatology. Coping tools to reestablish a more cohesive self included thought stoppage when she became flooded with bleak assumptions, remembering the reference point of the day after (versus before) the stroke to keep the perspective of improvement and healing, and adjusting expectations to small bite-size steps, with a "things take time" outlook (Klonoff, 2010, 2014).

Clearly, then, a successful therapeutic outcome has much to do with a number of specific, and highly tailored, interventions. But much has also been written on the importance of specific treatment approaches versus the influence of generic therapeutic factors, such as the therapeutic alliance.

7 The therapeutic relationship

Maintenance of the cohesive self and inner self-regulation is challenged during life transitions and traumatic occurrences (Banai et al., 2005). The therapist serves as a selfobject through sustained and empathic understanding and "vicarious introspection" (Baker & Baker, 1987; Kohut, 2009; Wolfe, 1989). This has been described as "interested attentiveness," "understanding acceptance," "reciprocal empathic resonance," or an "echoing-mirroring presence" of someone else who projects a calming, reassuring, or uplifting presence (Wolf, 1988; Wolfe, 1989). The therapeutic relationship scaffolds the "restoration of self" (Schore, 2009) and focuses on restoring a sense of vitality, harmony, and cohesion after either a threat by the disruption of a significant selfobject or some form of narcissistic insult (Baker & Baker, 1987).

The curative process has two steps: the first is predicated on the analyst's grasp of the patient through clinical perceptiveness, attentiveness, and reflective listening in a "relational climate of security" (Kohut, 2009; Lewis & Rosenberg, 1990; Wolfe, 1989). Secondarily, the therapist utilizes "experience-near" interpretations for understanding the nature of the selfobject disruption and narcissistic insults (including the provoked rage), followed by how to restore a feeling of vitality to the threatened self (Baker & Baker, 1987; see Wolfe, 1989, for a review). There is a dynamic process with often rapid oscillations between the understanding and interpreting phases (Kohut, 2009). In the context of substantial empathy and validation of the individual's subjective reality, occasionally the therapist fails in his or her content or timing of an interpretation (Kohut, 2009). This process of disruption and reestablishment of the selfobject bond (or transmuting internalization) enables the patient to better regulate self-esteem (Baker & Baker, 1987; Kohut, 2009).

A key element of all the treatment process is resistance – a theme that is especially interesting in light of neurological impairment, selectively affecting, as it does, only some elements of the mental apparatus.

8 Resistance

Resistance is usually a rich interplay of organicity (e.g., memory and executive function deficits), psychodynamic considerations (e.g., adaptive for psychological survival), mood factors (both physiologically based and reactive), and dispositional traits (Klonoff, 2010; Kohut, 2009). In self psychology, defensiveness protects a vulnerable developing self from trauma (Terman, 2014). The patient needs the analyst for constructive growth through mirroring, idealizing, and alterego transferences (Terman, 2014). These narcissistic transference demands represent the functional rehabilitation of the self and are considered tentative moves toward maturity and the reconstruction of a viable, vigorous self (see Terman, 2014, for a review; Wolfe, 1989). Many of these elements can be observed in Sara's case.

8.1 Case vignette 8

Transference and countertransference reactions had to be navigated throughout the psychotherapy process. Given that Sara's father was a police officer and Tim is a fire fighter, Sara was hypersensitive to what she considered overly conservative and restrictive ultimatums, feeling the pinch from her past of familial selfobjects being hypervigilant about danger. Dr. K. needed to be mindful about a countertransference reaction of overidentification with Sara's "motherhood mission," falling folly to "unwarranted leniency" about injury-related ineptitudes versus maintaining empathic, but "clinical objectivity" to ensure the safest and healthiest therapeutic stepping stones for Sara and her family. This meant thoughtfully "picking battles" and accepting "being unpopular" some of the time (Klonoff, 2010).

Therapy targeted Sara's stress tolerance and regulation of her self-esteem in the context of a pre-stroke cohesive healthy self (Klonoff et al., 1993). Six months into the psychotherapy process, sessions fluctuated between understanding and interpretation. Sara wrestled with acceptance as synonymous with resignation and doing what is being asked of her (by the therapists) versus her internalized desire to do what is necessary. She lamented that she wished she would wake up from a bad dream. Through a "listening stance," this venting fortified the working relationship, as she felt safe and affirmed in the privacy of the office in spewing her built-up exasperations. She once conveyed to Betty, "Dr. K. has a way of making hard thinking not seem like the end of the world."

Mirroring transferences with Dr. K. as well as her occupational and speech therapists were predicated on the praise, admiration, and encouragement she received in her reattainment of skill sets, based on her unending quest for neurological gains and concrete improvements as a wife and mother. Based on the idealizing transferences, she was building trust with her therapy team, perceiving their wisdom and good intentions. Alterego (twinship) transference relationships with her main therapists (whom Sara perceived as competent mothers in their own right) heightened her attentiveness and acceptance of feedback. Sara was developing compensatory psychic structures and reclaiming her sense of self, efficacy, competency, and well-being as a wife and mother (Kohut, 2009).

Through twinship selfobject relationships, the holistic milieu environment was a steady source of emotional nurturance, characterized by commonalities of a tumultuous journey with her peers. Group pychotherapy sessions four times per week, facilitated by Dr. K., represented a "relational climate of security" for mutual sharing (see Klonoff, 2010, for a review). During one "milieu session," (with all patients and staff present), she chose the song, "This is Your Life" (Foreman, 2003) to inspire herself and others to keep trudging. During the "experience near" interpretation phases, outside readings were introduced to counteract her "concrete" and "black and white" assumptions that, based on Facebook posts by her non-injured cohorts, they had the "perfect, unruffled lives." These exemplified "universal suffering," including excerpts from "When Bad Things Happen to Good People" (e.g., the "Mustard Seed" story) (Kushner, 1981) and "Finding Meaning in Life" (Frankl, 1984) as well as artwork and poetry from former rehabilitation patients grappling with their mortality and vulnerabilities. A beneficial mantra became "a new normal" versus "back to normal," typifying the need for a healthy adjustment to her redefined life circumstances.

Therapy is always a complex and challenging process. However, there are specific issues that are faced by those with a brain injury. These are clarified throughout Sara's journey.

8.2 Case vignette 9

Sara plummeted into periods of defensiveness throughout the psychotherapy process, albeit, with a gradual dwindling of the intensity of her emotional torrents. Typically, Sara's resistance embodied refusals and "slippage" (i.e., veering away from the consistent use of tools) and disavowal, especially in the home, and "flight into health" (i.e., I'm "cured" and I don't need the regimen) (Klonoff, 2010). She complained of her therapists and family "babysitting her" and "nitpicking."

Remnants of organic unawareness and executive dysfunction, especially in "seeing the big picture" and self-monitoring, propagated cycles of adherence and rejection. After 14 months, a vital awareness, acceptance, and realism tool devised collaboratively with Sara (with opinions from Tim and Betty) was the "Funk Cycle" (see Figure 6.1). Articulation of this assisted Sara in recognizing a recurring self-defeating pattern that was demoralizing to her and agonizing to Tim and Betty. Underlying themes included cultivating internal versus external loci of control, a disconnection between "knowing and doing," a breakdown in recognizing how actions relate to consequences, a self-centered (versus other-centered perspective), and judgment lapses.

Sara was gently counseled to recognize the deleterious upshots of her resistance, particularly on her family life, the crux of her identity. Cognitive distortions which were contributing to the adversity were discussed,

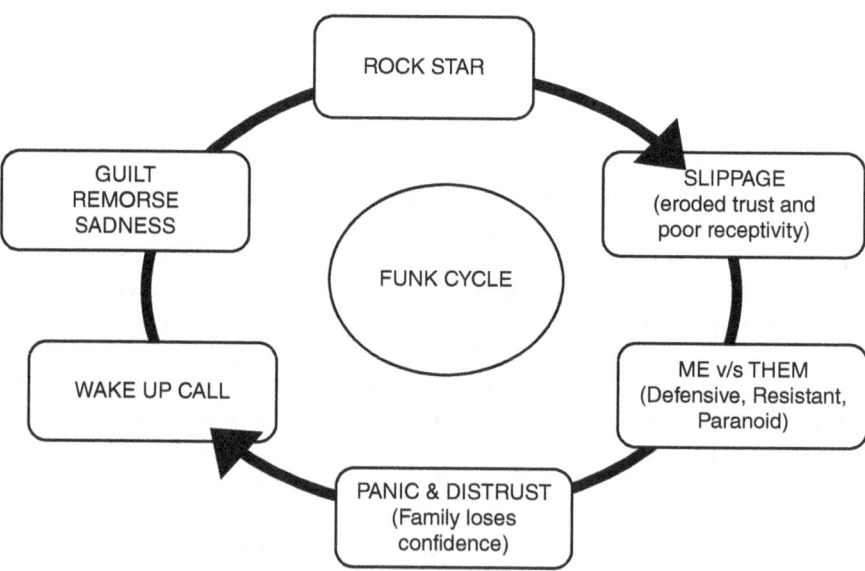

Figure 6.1 Funk Cycle.

including "all or nothing" thinking, overgeneralization, discounting the positives, jumping to conclusions, magnifying or minimizing situations, and blaming (Burns, 1999). Peer feedback in a psychoeducation group of blaming and rebellious behavior indicative of lagging acceptance was a "wake-up call." Sara was guided to recalibrate the compensations as "tools for success" rather than "silly crutches." Handouts entitled "Mean Moms?" and "Mean Therapists?" illustrate that taking a "diligent" versus "lenient" approach ultimately pays off in her (and her children's) self-regulation. Concepts of Sara's resiliency and growing internalization of principles were often revisited compassionately to bolster her spirit.

MEAN MOMS?

We had the meanest mother in the whole world! While other kids ate candy for breakfast, we had to have cereal, eggs, and toast. When others had a Pepsi and a Twinkie for lunch, we had to eat sandwiches. And you can guess, our mother fixed us a dinner that was different from what the other kids had, too. Mother insisted on knowing where we were at all times. You'd think we were convicts in prison. She had to know who our friends were, and what we were doing with them. She insisted that if we said we would be gone for an hour, we would be gone for an hour or less! We were ashamed to admit it, but she had the nerve to break the Child Labor Laws by making us work. We had to wash dishes, make the beds, learn to cook, vacuum the floor, do laundry, and all sorts of cruel jobs. I think she would lie awake at night thinking of more things for us to do. She always insisted on us telling the truth, the whole truth, and nothing but the truth. By the time we were teenagers, she could read our minds. Then life was really tough! Mother wouldn't let our friends just honk the horn when they drove up. They had to come up to the door so she could meet them. While everyone else could date when they were 12 or 13, we had to wait until we were 16. Because of our Mother, we missed out on lots of things other kids experienced. None of us have ever been caught shoplifting, vandalizing other's property, or ever arrested for any crime. It was all her fault. Now that we have left home, we are all God-fearing, educated, honest adults. We are doing our best to be mean parents just like Mom was. I think that is what's wrong with the world today. It just doesn't have enough Mean Moms anymore.

(Unknown Author)

MEAN THERAPISTS?

We had the meanest therapists in the whole world! While some therapists are lenient about attendance and punctuality, CTN therapists expect us to attend therapy every day and be on time. If we are sick, they even expect us to call in and notify them. While some therapists don't care if I use a datebook, CTN therapists are obsessed with my datebook. They expect me to carry it around everywhere AND consult it regularly. They not only want me to take notes constantly, but they expect me to use particular protocols and procedures they have developed. And they won't even let me use sticky notes, or shove lots of loose papers in the front of the book.

CTN therapists also expect us to work and/or go to school! They are always harping at us about "awareness, acceptance, and realism." It's like that's the only thing that matters now. They make such a big deal of our "communication pragmatics," even having us attend a specific therapy group. And then the Speech Therapists AND psychotherapists give us feedback about our behavior, as if that will really matter at the job – after all, my personality is no different now than before the injury, and I did just fine then.

It seems the therapists are always looking over our shoulders....it's like we are under a microscope. The Occupational Therapists even come to our home and watch what we do AND talk to our family members. The Recreational Therapists go on Community Outings with us.... we thought these were just for fun...then we find out we all have specific jobs, responsibilities, and goals AND we get graded on how well we do. Nothing can be a secret here....those therapists are always talking about us in their staff meetings....if we don't accomplish our goals or are not keeping up, they all band together and "get on our case." I thought therapy was going to be a lot easier and more fun than this! It's all their fault that I have to work so hard now... I miss my old life so much.... don't they get that? But then because of our therapists, we realized that we CAN be independent and productive. We can contribute in a meaningful and healthy way to our families. We feel empowered and content about the new direction of our lives. We've even changed how we live and consider ourselves to be better people and citizens. Okay, we didn't realize it while we were in treatment....but now after being back in that "real world" for a while, it all makes a lot more sense. I guess we're pretty appreciative of our Mean Therapists.... It seems they do really care about us after all!

In part because of Sara's right hemisphere deficits, she was encouraged to shift from a "self-absorbed" mindset to joint attention with others (Salas, 2012). She was helped to reframe Tim's and Betty's interactions as "checking in" versus "checking up." Upon contemplation, Sara referenced the "story of Saul" and pledged to practice more mindfulness and consistency, recognizing the "wear and tear" on her tiers of support (Klonoff, 2014) and notably her beloved children. At times, Sara became disenchanted and aggravated by Dr. K., feeling demeaned and constrained. Through the disruption-restoration processes and "transmuting internalization," Dr. K. urged her to relinquish the "me versus them" mentality, listen to her "wise voice," and "be the wife and mom she knows how to be." The children's story, "The Carrot Seed" (Krauss, 1945), was shared to epitomize the role of trust and faith. She took this home to read to her children, feeling heartened by Dr. K.'s "interested attentiveness."

Furthermore, through her deepening relationship with the psychiatrist, Sara introspected about being "irky" and "perturbed." She developed respect and faith in the psychiatrist's advice, as she "spoke the same language" regarding holistic living. After 14 months of therapy, Sara embraced the need for Zoloft and Vistaril "to be her best" (i.e., a cohesive self).

9 The role of self psychology and neuroscience on marital and parenting skills

The complexities of a case such as Sara's should not blind us to the universal themes that are perhaps inevitable in every therapeutic journey. Kohut proposed that individuals have a lifelong need for narcissistic support or sustaining self–selfobject relationships (Wolfe, 1989). In addition to the individual developing endopsychic structures which assume the functions of the external selfobjects, selfobjects evolve over one's life span. They include the parents throughout childhood; parental substitutes (e.g., grandparents, teachers, friends, and neighbors); the peer group during adolescence; and the spouse, friends, and career colleagues during adulthood (Baker & Baker, 1987).

Secure attachment is embedded in empathy, defined as the ability to intrinsically comprehend the feelings, thoughts, and motives of others using cognitive and affective components (Baker & Baker, 1987). Caregivers' empathic responses to children's narcissistic needs generate stability, security, self-cohesion, and internal self-regulation of self-esteem and ambitions (Banai et al., 2005). In a generally responsive environment with "good enough" parenting, and through the developmental process of "transmuting internalization" (i.e., the experience of optimal stressful frustrations in combination with interactive repair), the infant is able to perform drive-regulating, adaptive, and integrating functions that were previously performed by the external object (Baker & Baker, 1987; Kohut, 2009; Schore, 2009). The process involves internalization of self-regulation functions originally fulfilled by parents and the gradual acquisition of the capacity to perform these autonomously (Banai et al., 2005). Then the child's selfobject needs evolve from archaic demands for perfection and constant attention to self-confidence and healthy selfobject needs for intermittent and suitable appreciation and recognition (Baker & Baker, 1987).

Conversely, early trauma and disrupted transmuting internalization becomes a growth-inhibiting environment for the developing self, which generates an "impoverished psychic organization" and a deficit in empathy (Banai et al., 2005; see Schore, 2009, for a review). Repeated failures in meeting the child's legitimate selfobject needs, such as destructive interchanges, impede the development of internal structures to regulate self-esteem (Baker & Baker, 1987). Recurring empathic failures (e.g., excessive criticism, indifference, or hostility) can also be caused by external occurrences, for example, illness in the parent (Baker & Baker, 1987).

Schore (2009) purported that the self–selfobject relationship is embedded in the right hemisphere's mirroring intercommunications between the infant and the mother. This is due to the preeminent role of the right hemisphere (especially the orbital prefrontal areas) in emotional and visual-facial, auditory-prosodic, and tactile-gestural affective processing; face processing; auditory perception; self-awareness; empathy; self-recognition; integration; and self-regulation (see Schore, 2009, for a review; Siegel, 2012). Secure attachment is a developmental relationship whereby there is integration of the two hemispheres, both between the child and caregiver and within the child's brain; right hemisphere-to-right hemisphere communication allows for primary emotional states to be shared using nonverbal signals (Siegel, 2012). Damaged or deficient mothering selfobject functions, manifesting as inaccessibility to the infant or inappropriate or rejecting interactions, can result in early relational trauma in the infant, including his or her attachment security, right brain maturation, and sense of self (Schore, 2009; Siegel, 2012). Therefore, this causes a "developmental arrest" and an inability for the child to self-regulate the intensity and duration of emotional states (Baker & Baker, 1987; Schore, 2009).

Of note, right hemisphere damage also impedes social cognition, including joint attention and intentional attunement in the marital domain (Salas, 2012). Themes include lost familiarity, distance, and alienation in the relationship (Yeates, Edwards, Murray, Creamer & Mahadevan, 2013). Therapy (e.g., emotionally focused couples therapy (ECF)) and self psychology constructs should target attachment crises, ameliorate the neuropsychological difficulties that undermine emotional attunement, and diminish emotional withdrawal in the uninjured partner so as to reduce fragmentation and rebuild structural cohesion and vigor of both selves (Wolf, 1988; Yeates et al., 2013). Emotion recognition ability and the capacity for mentalizing improve interconnectedness (Yeates et al., 2013). External scaffolding is a valuable strategy to rekindle connections (Salas, 2012).

The difficulties encountered by patients such as Sara are especially complex when they map onto the interpersonal world, where the challenges of social cognition are so stark. Not only do these impede Sara's ability to be a good partner and mother, but we should also recall how central these elements are to her sense of self – especially her role as a mother.

9.1 Case vignette 10

Based on the interplay of self psychology and neuroscience constructs, the psychological development and well-being of Sara's five children were clearly precarious. A monumental undertaking was teaching Sara to regain the attunement critical for effective parenting. Sara had wonderful parenting talents pre-stroke, which she needed to rekindle during this phase of her treatment. Together with Dr. K. and the treating occupational and speech therapists, a painstaking journey was taken to incrementally rebuild Sara's skill set using external scaffolding. Hundreds of hours spanning almost two years were spent developing as many practical compensations as possible, while at the same time helping Sara rediscover her "mother radar" which was so refined pre-stroke. Using principles from self psychology and incorporating her cognitive challenges, she was aided in developing a "new job description." The overarching goal was to move the role of Betty from the "front line" to the "side line." "Jobs" were predicated on her strengths and the saliency of relating properly to her children based on active listening, healthy limit setting, and "together time" with individual and subgroups of her children, rather than overextending herself with extra obligations (e.g., homeschooling, driving with the children). Paramount was fostering attachment relationships through physical care (e.g., holding, carrying, and snuggling) and adaptive equipment and techniques (e.g., diapering, community ventures, etc.) (Rogers & Kirshbaum, 2011) as well as motherly intuition about her children's internal states (Schore, 2009).

Specific criteria to increase duties and unsupervised time (with some and all of the children) were laid out on a weekly/monthly basis. Safety was always the supreme factor, and Sara was prepped to take a Cardiopulmonary resuscitation (CPR) and first aid class. At least weekly "milieu meetings" (Klonoff, 2010) were held with Sara, Tim, and Betty to review the "operational" and parenting components of family life. Minutes from these meetings were brought to psychotherapy sessions for discussion. The form also included "mood ratings" of each party and "psychotherapy topics" to allow for investigation into the underlying emotions of each party. This format provided the necessary structure Sara required secondary to her executive function, visuospatial, and incidental memory difficulties, while developing metacognitive, global parenting, and relational skills.

Related to the impact of Sara's right-hemisphere stroke on her cognitive, perceptual, and emotional status, her biggest challenge was consistently using her tools, without "drift." The deleterious consequences of this were twofold: she was much less efficacious in performing her wifely and parenting endeavors. And importantly, she was inadvertently setting a poor example for her children, as "willy nilly" follow through created "wiggle room" for her children's behavior and expectations. Theoretical and real-life materials were used through the incorporation of user-friendly dialogue (e.g., "domino effect," "trickle down," and "ripple effect") to clarify this tendency. Sara actually witnessed a lack of ownership incident in her eldest child, reinforcing the saliency of being an optimal role model. Multiple collaborative methods were utilized to inculcate constancy, including checklist ratings by Sara, Tim, Betty, and the speech and occupational therapists with strict contingencies for increasing unsupervised time with her children. Indices included similar weekly self-assessment executive function ratings for parenting proficiencies relative to those of therapists and family members, and harmonious communication at home. Dr. K. proposed a metaphor of Sara as the foundation of a sturdy (versus collapsible) building, fortifying six floors (one for her husband and each child). The visual imagery of preventing any "cracks in the foundation" was inspiring to Sara in "cementing" the use of her protocols.

Given the wealth of tools, but Sara's residual deficits, a priority of treatment was "good enough parenting" (Bettelheim, 1987). To avoid a "growth-inhibiting environment," Sara and Tim needed to hire a part-time (25 hours per week) "personal assistant" (selfobject) with a prior background as a mother and teacher. She aided with mechanical aspects of home life (e.g., driving, errands) and served as a resource to Sara for complex parenting skills and strict adherence to her checklists and home systems. After 18 months of neurorehabilitation, Dr. K. and the speech and occupational therapists all joined in the instruction of this individual. In addition, Dr. K. and the speech therapist conducted in-service education at the children's school so that kindhearted parents (selfobjects) would continue part-time homeschooling on Sara's behalf. Accepting these parental substitutes was and is an ongoing emotional struggle, as it catalyzes periodic CRs and "lingering sadness" (Patrick-Ott & Ladd, 2010) about her residual limitations. A therapeutic perspective-taking exercise was proposed for both Sara and Dr. K., where Sara was invited to write a letter to herself reflecting her anguish (see below). Her gradual acceptance and adjustment to outside involvements are driven by her will, empathic attunement, and recognition of the need to do what is best for her children's cohesive self-structures.

Dear Sara

How are you? Last time we talked, you seemed very discouraged and in a lot of despair. How can I help you? Don't give up. You have come so far. There are six incredible people counting on you. March was a rough month, I know, (and) that you want to give up. I cannot stress enough; keep putting one foot in front of the other. Don't look back, but forward. Work hard, not easy. This is the hardest, saddest road you have ever traveled, and it is so lonely.

I am here for you. I am painting a picture of your kids for your binder. Keep running because victory will taste so sweet. I know you are sad, but I care about you so much. I know your smiles hide so much pain. I love you dear friend.

Love, Me.

To facilitate healthy narcissistic development in her children, Sara and Tim were encouraged to restart professional reading pertinent to their evolving age-related phases and needs. The weekly visits by both her occupational and speech therapists (as sustaining selfobjects) were instrumental in reorienting Sara's "mom smarts" based on the modeling of nurturing and attentive behavior and retraining Sara's right hemisphere in mirroring intercommunications. Dr. K. also performed a home visit and met periodically with the children. Positive indicators of loving interactions were reinforced, including Sara's capability to lead home craft projects, clear directions and redirection, flexibility, "teachable moments," and lovely patience. This was all evident in the context of some left-sided neglect (e.g., spilling paint during a project) and some decreased multitasking.

Sara's perspective-taking abilities were enhanced using "feeling journals" created by her older children. Written scenarios included what upset the child, perceived consequences, and what the youngster wanted his or her mother (and father) to fathom. Sara has become a "teamwork master" by involving her children in age-appropriate helpfulness, for example, chipping in on meal setup and cleanup, and following their own checklists to keep their rooms tidy. Figure 6.2 depicts a "home functioning" checklist developed collaboratively with Sara, Tim, Betty, and her therapists. Her "mother aptitude" and self-appraisal were honed by comparing self-ratings with those of her speech therapist. Post-treatment, Sara became adept at creating her own new checklists, indicating sound employment of executive functions (including metacognition and updating mental models), excellent "buy-in," and a mature psychological organization.

Throughout Sara's psychotherapy, she and Tim were seen conjointly weekly and then twice per month. Fortunately, and in some ways surprisingly, the fundamental elements of a reconstituted marriage were evident mostly throughout the therapy. This appeared related to the solidity of the marriage pre-stroke with secure attachment (mature selfobject relations), strong pre- and post-stroke intercommunication and conflict resolution skills, their religious faith and core beliefs about everlasting marital vows, and their mutual pledge to address any marital challenges "head-on." Despite the severity of her right-hemisphere stroke, behaviorally, she evidenced a number of key attributes necessary for connectedness, including relatively intact attention, memory, and language skills; emotion-recognition/responsivity; affective attunement; and the capacity for mentalizing (Yeates, 2013). Tim's emotional distress was heightened, not by relationship challenges per se, but by the overwhelming amount of parenting duties that were unexpectedly thrust upon him. The more that Sara resumed the mother role, the better his outlook and demeanor.

Tim was reticent about engaging in marital therapy, as he was private and tended to downplay emotions, in keeping with his chosen profession. However, Tim, like Sara, responded positively to Dr. K.'s "echoing-mirroring

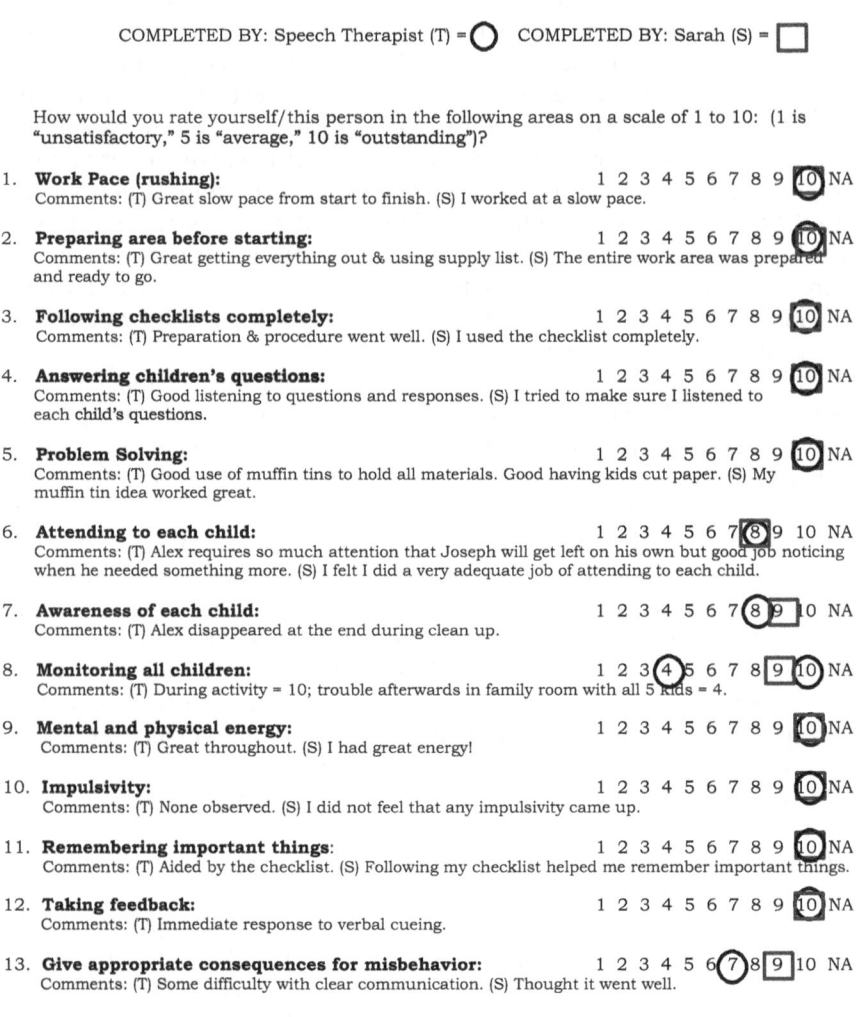

COMPLETED BY: Speech Therapist (T) = ◯   COMPLETED BY: Sarah (S) = ☐

How would you rate yourself/this person in the following areas on a scale of 1 to 10: (1 is "unsatisfactory," 5 is "average," 10 is "outstanding")?

1. **Work Pace (rushing):**   1 2 3 4 5 6 7 8 9 ⑩ NA
   Comments: (T) Great slow pace from start to finish. (S) I worked at a slow pace.

2. **Preparing area before starting:**   1 2 3 4 5 6 7 8 9 ⑩ NA
   Comments: (T) Great getting everything out & using supply list. (S) The entire work area was prepared and ready to go.

3. **Following checklists completely:**   1 2 3 4 5 6 7 8 9 ⑩ NA
   Comments: (T) Preparation & procedure went well. (S) I used the checklist completely.

4. **Answering children's questions:**   1 2 3 4 5 6 7 8 9 ⑩ NA
   Comments: (T) Good listening to questions and responses. (S) I tried to make sure I listened to each child's questions.

5. **Problem Solving:**   1 2 3 4 5 6 7 8 9 ⑩ NA
   Comments: (T) Good use of muffin tins to hold all materials. Good having kids cut paper. (S) My muffin tin idea worked great.

6. **Attending to each child:**   1 2 3 4 5 6 7 ⑧ 9 10 NA
   Comments: (T) Alex requires so much attention that Joseph will get left on his own but good job noticing when he needed something more. (S) I felt I did a very adequate job of attending to each child.

7. **Awareness of each child:**   1 2 3 4 5 6 7 ⑧ ⑨ 10 NA
   Comments: (T) Alex disappeared at the end during clean up.

8. **Monitoring all children:**   1 2 3 ④ 5 6 7 8 ⑨ ⑩ NA
   Comments: (T) During activity = 10; trouble afterwards in family room with all 5 kids = 4.

9. **Mental and physical energy:**   1 2 3 4 5 6 7 8 9 ⑩ NA
   Comments: (T) Great throughout. (S) I had great energy!

10. **Impulsivity:**   1 2 3 4 5 6 7 8 9 ⑩ NA
    Comments: (T) None observed. (S) I did not feel that any impulsivity came up.

11. **Remembering important things**:   1 2 3 4 5 6 7 8 9 ⑩ NA
    Comments: (T) Aided by the checklist. (S) Following my checklist helped me remember important things.

12. **Taking feedback:**   1 2 3 4 5 6 7 8 9 ⑩ NA
    Comments: (T) Immediate response to verbal cueing.

13. **Give appropriate consequences for misbehavior:**   1 2 3 4 5 6 ⑦ 8 ⑨ 10 NA
    Comments: (T) Some difficulty with clear communication. (S) Thought it went well.

(T) Really good job with all three kids doing the same activity. Next, each child will do a different activity. Sara, continue to do planning and preparing at home, not in the clinic.

Figure 6.2 Collaborative home functioning checklist.

presence" (Wolfe, 1989). Psychotherapy sessions focused on selected detrimental elements of executive functions, including cognitive rigidity, synthesis of information related to social consequences (for the family), and de-escalation techniques for affect dysregulation due to occasional misattribution of Tim's intensions (Yeates, 2013). Gradually, the marital relationship was recalibrated from a "hierarchy" to a "partnership" (Klonoff, 2010) or the reemergence of mature selfobject relations which were self-sustaining and kindling of balanced harmony (Wolf, 1988). Sessions enabled the elucidation and clarification of each member's perspectives and affective states within a safe haven. Tim and Sara were given social cuing devices to enhance open communication; Sara responded well to prompts to contemplate the "big picture," while Tim benefited from reminders for more frequent verbalizations about Sara's progress (versus deficits). Through external scaffolding exercises (Salas, 2012), Sara and Tim deepened their ties and intimacy, for example, by restarting weekly "date nights." Frequent marital "milieu meetings" enabled a healthy "communication platform" or shared space for functional communication (Klonoff, 2010; Yeates et al., 2013). Eventually all of the key constructs were integrated into "Nugget notes" and a list of "C words" (e.g., CRs, CRs by proxy (Klonoff, 2014), concrete thinking, corner cutting, collaboration, communication, consistency, confidence, and courage) for Sara's (and her family's) easy reference.

10 Late phase of therapy

Sixteen months after starting psychotherapy and 2.5 years post-stroke, Sara and her whole family went to a church camp where they all participated in sports activities (e.g., swimming, diving, and hiking). An overarching theme was the "season of survival," and she found the experience "rejuvenating" and "healing." She poignantly recounted to Dr. K. sharing her story of her stroke and recovery process, ending with "my brain injury is part of my life, but does not define me." After two years of psychotherapy, Sara was discharged from holistic treatment. She had made profound improvements in her functional skills, awareness, acceptance, and realism. And most prominently she also improved in her capacity to be an exceptional mother and wife. She now has a healthier, more harmonious sense of self and a sense of "wholeness" (Klonoff & Lage, 1991). Through her courageous and persevering efforts (with backing from her "tiers of support"), there was a consolidation of Sara's cohesive self-structure, including identity, meaning, and actualization of her potential (Banai et al., 2005; Klonoff, 2014). Sara and Tim have maintained periodic follow-up psychotherapy visits with Dr. K. to reinforce her progress and address issues and concerns as they arise; there is a fortified, mutually respected and appreciative working relationship.

Taken together, this chapter blends concepts from the neurosciences and self psychology for a worthy process of psychotherapy after brain injury. We have followed the psychically turbulent foray of a vibrant mother and wife, endowed with a solid structural self, able to sustain its coherence, continuity, and self-esteem. Regardless of this good starting position, her severe right-hemisphere stroke catapults her into a state of fragmentation and narcissistic rage. We then follow a journey as she integrates a range of psychic and neurologically based compensatory structures. Through mirroring, idealizing, and alterego transference relationships with her psychotherapist, and occupational and speech therapists, she comes to be far more embedded in a reality of healthy and sustaining selfobject relations, within an empathic treatment milieu and her home life. Ultimately, we see that she was able to reconstruct a sense of self-cohesion, wholeness, and identity as a nurturing and loving, albeit neurologically altered, wife and mother. It is an impassioned journey, and also one which offers insights into the way that a healthy mind can be radically changed by stroke, with additional insights into the neuropsychological basis of psychotherapy.

References

Árnadóttir, G. (2011). Impact of neurobehavioral deficits on activities of daily living. In: G. Gillen (Ed.), *Stroke rehabilitation: A function-based approach (3rd ed.)* (pp. 456–500). St. Louis: Elsevier Mosby.

Baker, H. S., & Baker, M. N. (1987). Heinz Kohut's self psychology: An overview. *The American Journal of Psychiatry*, 144(1), 1–9.

Banai, E., Mikulincer, M., & Shaver, P. R. (2005). "Selfobject" needs in Kohut's self psychology: Links with attachment, self-cohesion, affect regulation, and adjustment. *Psychoanalytic Psychology*, 22(2), 224–260.

Ben-Yishay, Y., & Diller, L. (2011). *Handbook of holistic neuropsychological rehabilitation: Outpatient rehabilitation of traumatic brain injury*. New York: Oxford University Press.

Bettelheim, B. (1987). *A good enough parent: A book on child-rearing*. New York: Alfred A. Knopf.

Brown, J. (2010). Psychotherapy integration: Systems theory and self-psychology. *Journal of Marital and Family Therapy*, 36(4), 472–485.

Burns, D. D. (1999). *Feeling good handbook*. New York: Penguin.

Byars, J. A., & Heilman, K. M. (2015). Right hemispheric neurobehavioral syndromes. In: J. Stein, R. L. Harvey, C. J. Winstein, & R. D. Zorowitz (Eds.), *Stroke recovery and rehabilitation (2nd ed.)* (pp. 225–240). New York: Demos Medical Publishing.

Capruso, D. X., Hamsher, K., & Benton, A. L. (2006). Clinical evaluation of visual perception and constructional ability. In: P. J. Snyder, P. D. Nussbaum, & D. L. Robins (Eds.), *Clinical neuropsychology (2nd ed.)* (pp. 547–571). Washington, DC: American Psychological Association.

Festa, J. R., Lazar, R. M., & Marshall, R. S. (2008). Ischemic stroke and aphasic disorders. In: J. E. Morgan & J. H. Ricker (Eds.), *Textbook of clinical neuropsychology* (pp. 363–383). New York: Taylor & Francis Group.

Foreman, J. (2003). *This is your life* [Recorded by Switchfoot]. On: *The beautiful letdown* [CD]. US: Columbia/Sony BMG.

Frankl, V. E. (1984). *Man's search for meaning (3rd ed.)*. New York: Simon & Schuster.

Gillen, G. (Ed.). (2011). *Stroke rehabilitation: A function-based approach (3rd ed.)*. St. Louis: Elsevier Mosby.

Glisky, E. L. (2004). Disorders of memory. In: J. Ponsford (Ed.), *Cognitive and behavioral rehabilitation: From neurobiology to clinical practice* (pp. 100–128). New York: Guilford Press.

Goldstein, K. (1952). The effect of brain damage on the personality. *Psychiatry*, 15(3), 245–260.

Gottesman, R. F., & Hillis, A. E. (2010). Predictors and assessment of cognitive dysfunction resulting from ischaemic stroke. *The Lancet Neurology*, 9(9), 895–905.

Klonoff, P. S. (2010). *Psychotherapy after brain injury: Principles and techniques.* New York: Guilford Press.

Klonoff, P. S. (2014). *Psychotherapy for families after brain injury.* New York: Springer Science & Business Media.

Klonoff, P. S., & Lage, G. A. (1991). Narcissistic injury after traumatic brain injury. *Journal of Head Trauma Rehabilitation*, 6(4): 11–21.

Klonoff, P. S., Lage, G. A., & Chiapello, D. A. (1993). Varieties of the catastrophic reaction to brain injury: A self psychology perspective. *The Bulletin of the Menninger Clinic*, 57(2), 227–241.

Kohut, H. (1972). Thoughts on narcissism and narcissistic rage. *Psychoanalytic Study of the Child*, 27, 360–400.

Kohut, H. (1977). *The restoration of the self.* New York: International Universities Press.

Kohut, H. (2009). *How does analysis cure?* Chicago: University of Chicago Press.

Kohut, H., & Wolf, E. S. (1978). The disorders of the self and their treatment: An outline. *The International Journal of Psychoanalysis*, 59, 413–425.

Krauss, R. (1945). *The carrot seed.* New York: HarperCollins Publishers.

Kushner, H. (1981). *When bad things happen to good people.* New York: Avon Books.

Langer, K. G., Laatsch, L., & Lewis, L. (Eds.). (1999). *Psychotherapeutic interventions for adults with brain injury or stroke: A clinician's treatment resource.* Madison: Psychosocial Press.

Levine, B., Schweizer, T. A., O'Connor, C., Turner, G., Gillingham, S., Stuss, D. T., Manly, T., & Robertson, I. H. (2011). Rehabilitation of executive functioning in patients with frontal lobe brain damage with goal management training. *Frontiers in Human Neuroscience*, 5(9), doi: 10.3389/fnhum.2011.00009.

Lewis, L., & Rosenberg, S. J. (1990). Psychoanalytic psychotherapy with brain-injured adult psychiatric patients. *The Journal of Nervous and Mental Disease*, 178(2), 69–77.

Matano, A., Iosa, M., Guariglia, C., Pizzamiglio, L., & Paolucci, S. (2015). Does outcome of neuropsychological treatment in patients with unilateral spatial neglect after stroke affect functional outcome? *European Journal of Physical and Rehabilitation Medicine*, 51(6), 737–743.

Nathanson, M., Shuman, I., Simonds, R., Suckle, R., Trench, T., & Zubick, K., (Producers), & Gosnell, R. (Director). (2005). *Yours, mine, & ours* [Motion picture]. United States: MGM.

Newby, G., Coetzer, R., Daisley, A., & Weatherhead, S. (Eds.). (2013). *Practical neuropsychological rehabilitation in acquired brain injury: A guide for working clinicians* (1st ed.). London: Routledge.

Oliveira, C. R., Pagliarin, K. C., Calvette, L. de F., Gindri, G., Argimon, I. I., & Fonseca, R. P. (2015). Depressive signs and cognitive performance in patients with a right hemisphere stroke. *Codas*, 27(5), 452–457.

Ownsworth, T., & Shum, D. (2008). Relationship between executive functions and productivity outcomes following stroke. *Disability and Rehabilitation*, 30(7), 531–540.

Patrick-Ott, A., & Ladd, L. D. (2010). The blending of Boss's concept of ambiguous loss and Olshansky's concept of chronic sorrow: A case study of a family with a child who has significant disabilities. *Journal of Creativity in Mental Health*, 5(1), 73–86.

Ponsford, J. (Ed.). (2004). *Cognitive and behavioral rehabilitation: From neurobiology to clinical practice.* New York: Guilford Press.

Prigatano, G., P., Fordyce, D. J., Zeiner, H. K., Roueche, J. R., Pepping, M., & Wood, B. C. (1986). *Neuropsychological rehabilitation after brain injury.* Baltimore, MD: Johns Hopkins University Press.

Purdy, M. H. (2014). Executive functions: Theory, assessment, and treatment. In: M. L. Kimbarow (Ed.), *Cognitive communication disorders* (pp.77–128). San Diego, CA: Plural Publishing.

Rogers, J., & Kirshbaum, M. (2011). Parenting after stroke. In: G. Gillen (Ed.), *Stroke rehabilitation: A function-based approach (3rd ed.)* (pp. 583–597). St. Louis: Elsevier Mosby.

Ruff, R. M., & Chester, S. K. (2014). *Effective psychotherapy for individuals with brain injury.* New York: Guilford Press.

Salas, C. E. (2012). Surviving catastrophic reaction after brain injury: The use of self-regulation and self-other regulation. *Neuropsychoanalysis,* 14(1), 77–92.

Salas, C. E., Radovic, D., Yuen, K. S. L., Yeates, G. N., Castro, O., & Turnbull, O. H. (2014). "Opening an emotional dimension in me": Changes in emotional reactivity and emotion regulation in a case of executive impairment after left fronto-parietal damage. *Bulletin of the Menninger Clinic,* 78(4), 301–334.

Schore, A. N. (2009). Relational trauma and the developing right brain: An interface of psychoanalytic self psychology and neuroscience. *Annals of the New York Academy of Sciences,* 1159, 189–203.

Siegel, D. J. (2012). *The developing mind (2nd ed.).* New York: Guilford Press.

Stöttinger, E., Filipowicz, A., Marandi, E., Quehl, N., Danckert, J., & Anderson, B. (2014). Statistical and perceptual updating: Correlated impairments in right brain injury. *Experimental Brain Research,* 232(6), 1971–1987.

Strozier, C. B. (2001). *Heinz Kohut: The making of a psychoanalyst.* New York: Farrar, Straus, and Giroux.

Ten Brink, A. F., Matthijs Biesbroek, J., Kuijf, H. J., Van der Stigchel, S., Oort, Q., Visser-Meily, J. M., & Nijboer, T. C. (2016). The right hemisphere is dominant in organization of visual search-A study in stroke patients. *Behavioural Brain Research,* 304, 71–79.

Terman, D. M. (2014). Self psychology as a shift away from the paranoid strain in classical analytic theory. *Journal of the American Psychoanalytic Association,* 62(6), 1005–1024.

Tucker, J. (2013). *Paralyzed* [Recorded by Rock Kills Kid]. On: *Are you nervous* [CD]. US: Reprise Records/Warner Music Group.

Wilson, B. A. (2009). *Memory rehabilitation: Integrating theory and practice.* New York: Guilford Press.

Wilson, B. A., Gracey, F., Evans, J. J., & Bateman, A. (2009). *Neuropsychological rehabilitation: Theory, models, therapy and outcome.* New York: Cambridge University Press.

Wolf, E. S. (1988). *Treating the self: Elements of clinical self psychology.* New York: Guilford Press.

Wolfe, B. (1989). Heinz Kohut's self psychology: A conceptual analysis. *Psychotherapy,* 26(4), 545–554.

Yeates, G. (2013). Towards the neuropsychological foundations of couples therapy following acquired brain injury (ABI): A review of empirical evidence and relevant concepts. *Neuro-Disability & Psychotherapy,* 1(1), 108–150.

Yeates, G., Edwards, A., Murray, C., Creamer, N. Z., & Mahadevan, M. (2013). The use of emotionally-focused couples therapy (EFT) for survivors of acquired brain injury with social cognition and executive functioning impairments, and their partners: A case series analysis. *Neuro-Disability & Psychotherapy,* 1(2), 151–197.

Chapter 7

When the RIGHT hemisphere goes WRONG

Reality and phantasy following right hemisphere lesion

Kobi Tiberg

I Introduction

Winnicott (1960) wrote that "there is no such thing as an infant...without maternal care there would be no infant". This sentence echoes in my mind whenever I treat patients with vast lesions in the territory of the right middle cerebral artery (RMCA) that also extend to prefrontal areas. These 'right hemisphere patients' usually suffer from left-sided hemiplegia, left hemi-spatial neglect (reduced awareness of stimuli on the left side of space) and disorders of visuospatial perception and cognition. Interestingly, some of these patients seem not to be able to acknowledge their disabilities and/or the consequences of these disabilities. In other words, they are unaware of them, a phenomenon commonly known as anosognosia.

Research has shown that at some deeper level, below the observable unawareness, some of these patients do have knowledge about their disabilities and sad consequences (Ramachandran & Blakeslee, 1998; Kaplan-Solms & Solms, 2000; Nardone, Ward, Fotopoulou & Turnbull, 2008). This knowledge appears to remain implicit and inaccessible most of the time, but can be temporarily brought to conscious awareness using diverse means, such as caloric vestibular stimulation (Ramachandran & Blakeslee, 1998) or psychoanalytic interpretation (Kaplan-Solms & Solms, 2000). Usually, patients lack the capacity to attend to this knowledge or to 'allow' it to enter conscious awareness from where it seems to be 'rejected', 'organically repressed' or 'dissociated', due to the right hemisphere lesion.

In a model that integrates neurocognitive and emotional factors, Fotopoulou (2010) suggested that anosognosia for hemiplegia may reveal the exaggeration of 'self-serving' emotional mechanisms. According to this model, after a stroke to the right hemisphere, denial coping strategies can be exaggerated, due to a dysfunction of basic neurocognitive mechanisms required for body awareness. These neurocognitive mechanisms, which allow individuals to appreciate the situation in realistic terms, also control and inhibit emotional influences on body awareness. When impaired, a body perception that is distorted by an uninhibited emotional need to perceive the body as normally functioning can prevail. Anosognosia, then, could be conceptualized as a neurological equivalent of a psychodynamic defense. Ramachandran and Blakeslee (1998), in a similar way, suggest that these patients' defense mechanisms are 'amplified tenfold'.

It is important to note here that anosognosia is not a unitary phenomenon. There are different kinds of deficits comprising anosognosia for hemiplegia, and although superficially the same, they can be distinguished amongst patients (Marcel, Tegnér & Nimmo-Smith, 2004). And yet, at least in some anosognosic patients, motivation and emotion seem to play a key role (Turnbull, Fotopoulou & Solms, 2014). In this group of patients, it doesn't take much more than a few minutes of conversation to notice that this 'unawareness' involves defending, sometimes desperately, against a very unwelcome truth that crawls underneath.

There is a growing literature on the fluctuating nature of anosognosic patients' unawareness and the way in which psychological variables can change the presentation of these patients (Turnbull & Lovett, 2012). In some of them, what is 'organically repressed' at one point in time, because it threatens the pre-injury self concept, can surprisingly be gathered into a new updated body-ego schema at another; what is 'neglected' and forcefully denied in one situation can be painfully admitted and even mourned in another. This evasive allocation and withdrawing of attention from different aspects of knowledge about the disability, 'getting in and out of awareness', seem to represent different 'bargains' or points of balance between the patient's aversive reality 'asking' to be realized and his defensively compromised perception 'wishing' to hide it. Environmental factors may have a crucial influence on setting these balance points.

Kaplan-Solms and Solms (2000) suggest that, following right perisylvian damage, being unaware or 'organically denying' the paralyzed left side (anosognosia) is only one of the many ways in which patients can deal with the painful reality of hemiplegia. Other forms described in their book are 'not minding' the paralyzed side (anosodiaphoria), disowning it and perceiving it as 'not-me' (asomatognosia) or even becoming negatively obsessed with it, thus hating, harming and wishing to get rid of it (misoplegia).

The connection between these emotional aspects and the visuospatial deficits exhibited by patients with right perisylvian damage has been conceptualized by Kaplan-Solms and Solms as a narcissistic regression. According to the authors, a key element of this syndrome involves an alteration of *space itself*, which is treated "narcissistically". In other words, space is treated "as if it were arranged as the patient wished it to be, rather than how it actually is" (p. 184). In various ways, the loss of function can then be avoided and the grief for the loss spared. The authors offer several descriptions of how this 'narcissistic regression' can occur. In the case of Mr. C, for example, "it was as if he had withdrawn into a cocoon of self-sufficiency, and yet he was simultaneously very needy and demanding" (p. 163). In spite of Mr. C's need to be looked after and cared for "he consciously abhorred dependence and vulnerability of any kind and wanted to be treated as if he were the chairman of a public company" (p. 163). According to the authors, Mr. C "tended to ignore, minimize, and rationalize the paralysis" (p. 161), and he treated the left side of his body "as if it were merely another piece of external reality that was refusing to do his bidding" (p. 163). In the case of Mr. D, whose right hemisphere lesion was not just parietotemporal but also involved frontal areas, "the fact of the paretic hand represented a narcissistic injury that was intolerable to him" (p. 192). Mr D's way of dealing with it was "to expel the hand...into the hated external reality...There, it was attacked ruthlessly and relentlessly, sometimes by actual physical violence" (p. 192). "At one point, Mr. D actually stated that the hand felt as if it did not belong to him" (p. 191).

An important observation of Kaplan-Solms and Solms (2000) was that when the injury involves ventromedial prefrontal areas, it is not just the body and space arrangement that is altered, but reality itself can be heavily influenced by the patient's wishes and phantasy world. In what seems to be a breakdown of ego processes, the patient's reality becomes dramatically distorted by confabulations (false memories), often of 'wish-fulfilling' nature (Turnbull, Berry & Evans, 2004; Fotopoulou, 2008; Tiberg, 2014).

From a Freudian point of view (1911), some confabulations can be considered as anchored in 'primary process' or dreamlike thinking. Primary process is characteristic of the unconscious system, and the governing purpose obeyed by it is the 'pleasure principle', which strives towards gaining pleasure and releasing tension. This tendency towards immediate gratification is often implemented by taking the most direct route to discharge, and the paradigmatic example of this process is hallucination. In contrast, secondary process is characteristic of the preconscious–conscious system and is governed by the 'reality principle'. Here, the direct route is not sought in order to obtain gratification, but instead detours are taken and thinking is used to postpone gratification in order to comply with the conditions imposed by the outside world. According to Kaplan Solms and Solms (2000), a key function of the ventromedial frontal cortex is inhibiting the primary process. In consequence, individuals with lesions to this area seem to function according to the principles that Freud described as the characteristics of the system unconscious, one of them being the primary process (Freud, 1915). The authors refer to the state of prefrontal patients with ventromedial lesions as "psychosis-like", and often we see that their symptoms overlap with delusional symptoms of 'psychiatric' nature.

The ego disequilibrium theory (Feinberg, 2010) also proposes, as an explanation to the behavioral and psychological changes observed in patients with right prefrontal damage, a form of regression to developmentally earlier, or more primitive, stages of mental functioning. Feinberg (2011) proposes that such regression causes a recrudescence of primitive defense mechanisms, so denial, projection, splitting, fantasy and paranoia become frequently used by patients. Importantly, Salas and Turnbull (2010) elaborate on this model by noting that such recrudescence does not imply that mature defenses are completely abolished, but that immature defenses are rather exacerbated.

Neurologically, what can be observed after vast right hemisphere lesion is a left 'verbal' hemisphere that is disconnected from information about the body, space, time and reality-monitored episodic self. In consequence, the patient's coordinates of reality are dramatically severed, and the remaining talking left brain is fed by pleasure principle laws that put almost no limit to what is possible. The gaps are sometimes huge: the patient may be able to engage in insightful, intellectual conversation, based on this intact semantic knowledge and language abilities; however, when conversation ends, he is helplessly left in his wheelchair, his left side of the body dysfunctional and neglected, along with that whole side of space. Due to his physical disability and flawed visuospatial perception, he cannot navigate himself anywhere. However, in his unmonitored, fantasized reality, he may sail away in time and space, creating much better circumstances for his body and for himself. At the price of losing grip on shared reality, mourning of his grave losses is spared.

Similar to Winnicott's infant, who is totally dependent on his environment and doesn't exist without maternal care, our anosognosic patient cannot survive without his significant other or caregiver. However, the patient's relationship with his significant other is often much less harmonious and natural than that of a mother and her infant. Due to the lesion, the patient may become egocentric and demanding. Following impairment to mental functions such as mentalizing and empathy (Salas, 2012), he may also have difficulties considering other people's perspectives and needs. Furthermore, he may equate internal and external reality, thus, treating what is inside his head as equivalent to what is out there in the physical world (see the concept of 'psychic equivalence' by Fonagy and Luyten, 2012). Finally, often he may not be able to acknowledge upsetting, actual aspects of reality, which are dramatically distorted by his lesion in the service of his wishes and needs.

To his misfortune, the carer or significant other often becomes the representative of a hated reality, who (inevitably) exposes the fraud of fantasy and confabulation. As such, he is the one who gets most of the fire – or the narcissistic rage - for 'ruining the party'. This fire is kindled by the (organically dictated) regressive defenses of the patient, who can situate the significant other at the wrong end of a splitting mechanism. The spouse, who until the minute of the stroke could be a beloved lifelong partner, may suddenly find herself an object of ruthless unrealistic accusations, and even of paranoid ideation (e.g., Yeates et al., 2008; Salas, 2012). As a consequence, the couple dynamics often become the most problematic issue and the main subject of psychotherapy, in which the therapist needs to bridge between two realities, very different from one another.

The main goal of this chapter is to describe different interventions aimed at managing this type of clinical problem, using the case of a patient with a large right hemisphere lesion as an example. I will first present the patient and his wife, as well as the couple dynamics that emerged after the stroke. Following that, I will describe moments of the psychotherapy process, which I believe illustrate different types of therapeutic interventions. Finally, I theoretically elaborate on the clinical material presented, this, using Freudian and Winnicottian ideas.

2 Dan and Sarah

Dan was 67 years old at the time of admission to the neurorehabilitation ward. He was a tall man with a large physique, thick blond hair and a big beard. Dan was married to Sarah, and they had two grown-up daughters. Twelve days before admission Dan suffered an ischemic stroke in the territory of the right middle cerebral artery (MCA), with a large area of infarction that affected the parietal, temporal and frontal (including prefrontal) lobes.

Dan was referred to me for psychotherapy a month after admission, due to the impact that anosognosia was having on his behavior and his relationship with his wife. The psychological intervention, almost from its beginning, was couple-oriented. Sessions were usually held once a week over a period of four years, initially at the hospital and then at the outpatient clinic.

A consequence of Dan's stroke was a dense left hemiplegia, which left him wheelchair bound and physically dependent on others – mainly his wife, Sarah. The stroke also caused several cognitive deficits, which can be summarized by in the classical 'right hemisphere syndrome': hemi-spatial neglect, anosognosia and constructional apraxia. To demonstrate the severity of his visuospatial problems, while riding his car with his wife once, he asked her why she was driving from the back seat of the car.

Dan was very eloquent, thus suggesting a preservation of language skills. He was an intellectual, with a great wealth of knowledge in many areas, which also seemed to be preserved after the stroke. Neuropsychologically, the huge gap between his 'left' verbal and 'right' visuospatial abilities was evident in his performance on the Wechsler Adult Intelligence Scale (WAIS-3). While Verbal Comprehension Index was in the high average range (79th percentile), Perceptual Organization Index was in the extremely low range (0.1 percentile).

Dan had a good, witty sense of humor, which according to his wife improved after the stroke. However, his behavior following the stroke was similar, in many aspects, to that of the right hemisphere patients, described by Kaplan-Solms and Solms (2000), who hated their paralyzed limb, and in whom the boundaries of the perceived body seemed to have retreated to disowning that hated, paralyzed limb:

DAN: This hand is not mine. Two criteria should exist to prove that it's mine. First it should obey my orders and second it should be connected to my body. Maybe it is connected to my body but it doesn't obey my orders. It's a corpse. A doll hand…I have no use in it. No control of its muscles… I don't know what happened to my original hand. One of my complaints to the institution in which I work is that they didn't tell me under what circumstances my hand was detached… Did they run a DNA test to see that it's really mine? Was there a car accident? I want details about how I was detached from my dear hand… They tell me the hand is mine and it is nonsense. My wife uses this excuse whenever she's not willing to put the hand somewhere else in the house, when I ask her to temporarily store it somewhere…

So the paralyzed hand could not be accepted as part of Dan's body. This implied, sadly, that he could not mourn the loss of his functional arm and integrate it to his new body schema. Dan experienced his paralyzed hand as 'alien-to-the-body' and believed that his old functional hand was kept securely in an unknown place.

Most of the time Dan was unaware of his hemiplegia and cognitive deficits. However, when confronted with his physical disability, he denied it adamantly or blamed his wife as the cause of his limitations. For example, there was a barrier at the side of Dan's bed that prevented him from falling at night. When asked to explain his difficulty to get out of bed by himself, Dan said:

> The removal of the barrier that prevents me from getting out of bed in the morning is the whole problem, and Sarah wouldn't take it away. 'Let's chain him' she says…all I want is for her to take it off in the morning so I can get out of bed…

However, Sarah wasn't blamed only for Dan's physical limitations, but also for more cosmic, tragic facts of nature. In one session, Dan said that he wanted to bring his mother to his grandson's birthday. Sarah was surprised: "but your mother died 22 years ago". "You kill everyone!" Dan protested, "and anyway, so what? She still has a right to meet her great-grandson". As the reader can see here, Dan's logic had all the characteristic elements of the "system unconscious": exemption from mutual contradiction, timelessness and replacement of external by psychical reality (Freud, 1915).

3 Where am I?

Another field of dispute was Dan's numerous geographical confabulations. Dan could wake up one day in Paris, the next day in London and on yet another day in Tokyo, while staying at home, in Tel Aviv, all along.

DAN: I know I'm in the south of England but Sarah doesn't agree with me. Yesterday I was sure I'd been in Paris.
SARAH: Yesterday we were in Bangkok, the day before we had been in Paris.
DAN: Shhhh… they might hear that and give us the bill…

As I mentioned earlier, Sarah claimed that Dan's sense of humor improved after the stroke. This fact is not surprising if we think of Freud's writings about the joke's relation to the unconscious (1905) or Lacan's writings on the joke as "a signifier which would reveal an unconscious truth which the person concerned was trying to conceal" (Quinodoz, 2013). In Dan's case, it seemed that due to the brain lesion, huge parts of reality became unconscious. Humor, which is quite an advanced defense mechanism, seemed to serve as a very efficient and unthreatening bridge that continuously sent 'memos', in the guise of jokes, to the conscious mind. We will develop further this point later in the case.

As for the geographical confabulations, how did Dan decide where he was? Here is a clue to the answer. One day Dan and Sarah went to a cinema in Tel Aviv, the city where they lived, to see a film that took place in New York. When they got out of the cinema, Dan suggested that since they were already in New York, they should go visit Anna, a friend of theirs who lived there. On another occasion, while in the car, the couple heard on the radio that the prime minister had visited Paris. Immediately after hearing that, they were in Paris. So according to Dan's 'primary process' logic, it was enough to be exposed to a signifier of a place, through auditory or visual channels, in order to be immediately transmitted to the actual signified place.

DAN: I expect every morning that Sarah would say that we're in New York or Paris and I'm very frustrated when she doesn't say what I feel.
SARAH: Is it important for you to know where you **really** are?
DAN: **You** think we are in Tel Aviv.
SARAH: It's a fact! I showed you the address sign: Bialik St.
DAN: It's true. This I really couldn't explain. The only explanation was that heaven is also doing what Sarah wants. Or that Bialik Street is chasing us wherever we go!

In the end, Dan arrived at a conclusion that was inevitable from his point of view, by projecting his confusion into his wife:

DAN: For Sarah every place we are at is Bialik Street and I say it's not possible that every place on earth is Bialik Street. I think Sarah has lost hold on reality. I ask myself, do I give her the help she needs, psychological help that would get her out of this condition? She's a logical woman who's dealing a lot with mathematics, an academic field with clear rules. And, it's as if she's not with us, something has happened to her…

4 Who am I?

Equally interesting to Dan's confabulations about place were confabulations about who he was. These confabulations appeared to have a function in compensating for his 'narcissistic injuries' via wish fulfillment. Let's consider the following example. During his compulsory military service, Dan dropped out of the officer's training course after a mistake he had made. This was experienced by him as a great loss and a narcissistic injury that never healed. In one of our sessions, Dan, who believed he was still working at his company, declared:

DAN: I was offered by the CEO of my company the position of special adviser to the chief of general staff, with the rank of brigadier general. The CEO will do anything to keep me in the company, and he knows how important this is to me so he said: 'I will arrange it for you'.

SARAH: Everything they offered you is nonsense.

DAN: The people who offered it are too important to think it is nonsense. This week the defense minister will correct the injustice that was made to me by the Israeli defense force 30 years ago. I asked my new secretary to find out what my new salary would be and she said, '300,000 dollars a minute'. I said, 'What? Taxi drivers work by the minute, not brigadier generals'. But today I got reinforcement for that. A direct commander had told me the same thing. In the ceremony I will be given the rank by the chief of general staff on the one side and by Sarah on the other.

THERAPIST: It's important for you that Sarah is there to give you the rank

DAN: Only so she will have to eat her hat afterwards...

During therapy Dan was offered numerous dream jobs all over the world and accepted them without hesitation. He was angry and frustrated with Sarah, for she did not support him and kept contradicting his stories, 'out of envy' – as he saw it. When I tried to understand Dan's motive in accepting all these hard work jobs after retiring, he explained: "Someone wrote it was the money, but it's so untrue. It's the right acknowledgement of my abilities! For years I felt hurt for not finishing the officers' training course, for being expelled a month before it ended. Now I will have proof from the chief in command that I finished with honors. The army is making amends after all these years. My company is saying, 'Here's the globe. Choose wherever you'd like to work and go there for a salary of 2 million dollars a month for an unlimited period'. They correct what they should have a long time ago. 'What is so bad in retiring?' Sarah asked, somewhat desperately, and added, "Your motto has always been, 'How good it is to do nothing and then to rest!'" "When you don't work you don't exist!" Dan declared:

You are worthy of contempt! I enjoy my retirement but I'm afraid of isolation... that my whole functioning will be between me and the toilet. A man is defined by his profession. The first question that you are asked is 'what are you doing for a living?' I want to be able to say, 'I work at my previous job and expand it'.

However, it was not just military or work-related issues that were the topic of Dan's confabulations:

DAN: Three months ago I was sent an email, saying: 'Dan, be careful! The hunting season has started. Girls are looking for grooms and your name was mentioned in many forums as a good catch, so be careful!' Why should I be careful? I should lie on my back and say, come, you girls, just don't tear me to pieces....

Dan usually held on to his cool version of reality quite strongly and rigidly. For much of the time, he could not accept alternatives to his view. However, as in many cases of anosognosia following right hemisphere lesions, there were moments in which he could accurately acknowledge different aspects of his limitations or some of their consequences. Here is an example of a grandiose confabulation that also contained a touching reference to Dan's actual condition.

DAN: I was appointed as the commander of the military colleges. I thought what I should say in the opening speech and I have it more or less pre-pared now. I'd like to tell them that my life experience in the last one and a half years has taught me that the transition from being healthy to being sick is very quick, and that they should take care of their health.... There is almost complete dependence on other people. Today I can't make myself coffee. Driving a car is a whole story but **I do it in spite of Sarah's protest**. Dependency is much bigger than it used to be. You need a very close relationship with the person who gives you service, so you better start building the relationship.

As mentioned earlier, the evasive allocation and withdrawing of attention from different aspects of knowledge about the disability, this 'getting in and out of awareness' in anosognosia, seem to represent different bargains, or different points of balance, between the patient's aversive reality 'asking' to be realized and his defensively compromised perception 'wishing' to hide it. In the last confabulation described, when Dan acknowledges his dependency on Sarah, it seems that he can live with the fact that he can't make himself coffee. Driving, on the other hand, seems to be a more sensitive issue. He does acknowledge that it is 'a whole story' today to drive. But this seems to be the limit of what can be accepted by his organically narcissistically regressed ego, at that spe-cific point in time: "I do it (driving) in spite of Sarah's protest", Dan asserts.
    It is interesting to note here that in the anosognosia study by Marcel and colleagues (2004), it was found that overestimation of the ability to drive a

car was significantly more common in men than in women, consistent with cars being socially more important for men than for women.

5 Psychotherapy: what worked and what didn't

How do we deal in therapy with such a fantastically regressed and fluid reality? In this section, I will present examples of 'types' of interventions that were employed throughout the years of therapy. I hope something can be learned from this couple therapy. For reasons of clarity, I will start with interventions that targeted Dan's problems, and then I will describe my work with Sarah.

First, what didn't work? Situations in which I was tempted to 'educate' Dan and inform him about the 'real world' were often rejected and interpreted by him as me teaming up with Sarah and giving her a 'weapon against him'. This led to the risk of losing him as a partner in therapy. In relation to this observation, it is interesting to point to ideas by Ogden who warns against interventions that tend to erode analytic space by stating 'facts' instead of inquiring into the patient's mode of constructing his personal symbolic meanings. Nevertheless, it is important to clarify that some 'explanations' and 'neuropsychoanalytic education' were better received when Dan himself invited them. For example, after watching the film *A Beautiful Mind*, which tells the story of a renowned mathematician, John Nash, Dan curiously asked whether he, Dan, was also schizophrenic. The movie then worked as a 'third object' that enabled the analytic couple to open a discussion about not only differences but also similarities between delusions and confabulations, for example, the common experience of 'losing reality'.

Another path that sometimes proved to be effective was offering careful interventions that were made in an attempt to connect Dan's confabulatory perceptions with the motivation behind them. In these cases, following validation of the underlying motivation, the fluid balance between what could be accepted by Dan and what had to be rejected sometimes seemed, unexpectedly, to change in favor of the former. For example, in one session, Dan protested about the fact that he was asked to explain why he had wanted to stand up when he was trying to do that by himself, unaware of his disability: "I won't spend the rest of my life in this chair!" he said, "But why do I have to explain every little thing?" "Maybe", I suggested, "you just **want** to be able to stand and walk and sometimes we want something **so much**, that it's hard to see that it's not possible". Dan sighed and said, "It's a pity you can't turn the wheel backwards. The consequences of this stroke are too hard!" "So hard that it's sometimes hard to realize them", I said and now I sighed. "I cannot see any progress", Dan continued, "I reached a stage so painful that it's unbearable. There is no indication of where I am in the rehabilitation effort. The most difficult question is: "How long it will last? When will I get up?"

Another way of dealing with fantastic confabulations was asking Dan to freely associate in order to figure out its meaning, just like in working with dreams – another creation of the unconscious. In one of our sessions, Dan told me about an enema he had had a few days before at the neurorehabilitation ward. This is how he described his memory of it:

> One day a monkey jumped on my back, pushed me to bed, and before I could say anything, a long pipe was pushed up my buttocks, it was turned on and... yes, it was indeed an enema! Then I went out and found the newspaper on the floor. The headline said: "the citizens of Israel were surprised this morning by what the government had sent them. Everyone got an enema to their home" I was offended as a citizen. They've gone crazy! There's no limit to what they do!

When I asked Dan to associate with different elements of this fantastic, dreamlike confabulation, he said: "An enema is a very massive invasion of privacy; an intrusion to processes that I'm responsible for. The result is relieving, but, essentially this is a violation of freedom, of the control you exert on your body". Through this subjective definition of enema, Dan's experience became clearer. It was as if his associations decoded the dreamlike, imaginary memory, and turned it from a symbolic riddle into a very comprehensible human experience. It could be suggested then, that the invasion of privacy and the violation of freedom and control of the body were depicted in the confabulation by the animalistic attack of the enema-enforcing monkey that was sent by the governmental (nursing staff) 'Other'. Another possibility is that **I** was experienced, in the transference, as that intrusive monkey. The fact that **everyone** got an enema to his or her home might have represented Dan's wish not to be alone in his idiosyncratic experience and to share it with others.

Trying to understand the symbolic meaning of fantastic confabulations through free association and interpretation proved to be a fruitful enterprise on some occasions. With time, in moments of higher insight, Dan himself was spontaneously pointing to the symbolic meaning of a confabulation or even the latent wishes behind them.

All in all Dan's mood was positive. For much of the time he passively enjoyed the good fortune that his wish fulfilling confabulations offered. The confabulations were sent to him through various channels, such as written messages on walls and on the floor. When he seemed to be sitting in his wheelchair, doing nothing, he was often busy receiving these messages. When his confabulations dictated actions that he insisted he and Sarah should do, such as going to a party to which they were invited at the Chief of General Staff's house or going to a ceremony in which Dan should have received his new rank, solutions had to come from within his world (e.g., 'cancelation phone calls' that had been 'received' from the military). However, it is important to note that some of Dan's confabulations were also paranoid and required to be concretely managed. For example, when he confabulated that terrible things had been done to one of his daughters, a phone call from the daughter, asserting that she was ok, helped him calm down.

6 Sarah

An aspect of Dan's confabulatory experience that constantly disturbed him was Sarah's difficulty to share his fantastic world. In one session, he reported a dream he had in which he was eating special bread. He described how much he had wanted to be able to pass the bread from the dream to reality so he could bring it to Sarah. Dan's wish that Sarah would be fed by the same 'bread', that his senses and memory were fed by, was one of the focuses of the work with Sarah.

At the beginning of therapy, and for quite a long time, Sarah was very distressed and often broke into tears. It was very hard, if not impossible, for her to accept Dan's condition and frequent confabulations. It seemed that if she had let Dan 'be' in Paris or New York or Tokyo, she would have been left alone in Tel Aviv, and this was unbearable for her. She used to argue with Dan, trying to persuade him how unreasonable his perceptions were, urging him to 'correct' his thoughts and behavior. This often irritated Dan and made him fight back and hold onto his confabulations. Dan experienced Sarah as enviously trying to control him and as devaluating his marvelous achievements. Accepting Sarah's opinion was experienced as a humiliating surrender. It is important to note here that it seemed that this pattern of interaction did not start with the stroke; however, it was painfully intensified afterward.

When Dan was still hospitalized, Sarah found it most difficult to accept his passivity and lack of initiation and cooperation in the different rehabilitation therapies. Sarah was a doer, who believed that 'not doing something is a crime'. So it was hard for her to accept that, due to the unawareness of deficits caused by his stroke, Dan did not fight to get better. When Dan and Sarah went home, she used to read him books in order to keep him active. She often protested about the fact that he preferred wasting his time reading unreal messages on walls to watching TV.

In one session, when Dan was more in touch with his disability, he described Sarah's attitude: "Sarah wants a 'deus ex machina' solution, an 'old Dan pill' that I would take and become who I used to be once again"..."She thinks", he said, "that I need retuning". "That's why we are here", Sarah commented. "We're here also to retune your expectations and hopes", Dan corrected. Helping Sarah retuning her expectations and hopes was with no doubt a main goal of the psychotherapeutic process. This was accomplished mainly by helping her to get in touch with her terrible loss so she could mourn it. Negative feelings that were related to this loss seemed to lie underneath the many defenses that made it so difficult for her to accept Dan's condition.

Another direction of the treatment with Sarah was to provide 'neuropsychoanalytic education'. For example, explaining how Dan's behavior – dealing with feelings of loss and worthlessness by using regressive defense mechanisms – was directly related to his right hemisphere lesion. At times, there was no need to say much about this issue as Dan's motives were transparently revealed through his words. For example, when Sarah stated in one session that years ago Dan received a letter from the Israeli Defense Force saying they didn't need his services anymore, Dan protested and said that Sarah had no interest in adhering to these claims but stabbing him with a knife and twisting it. "So you managed to prove there's another system that doesn't need me. Does this mean that the next system that will no longer need me is the family?" Through this painful question, Dan's grandiose confabulations seemed to have a compensatory rationale that shielded him from feeling useless and rejected; these confabulations seemed to help him maintain his self-esteem and dignity. Such an understanding helped me see how important it was not to disarm Dan of these defense mechanisms by contradicting him or proving him wrong, and I tried to explain that to Sarah.

Sarah was endlessly devoted to Dan. She had left a career as a scientist and dedicated all her time to care for him. Dan was aware of such sacrifice and told her at different occasions that he was full of admiration for her devotion, that she was the whole world to him and that he would be lost without her. However, Sarah's role as a wife and carer 24/7 generated a lot of tension and frequent arguments. Sarah, who had said that "accepting all these things is like giving up, admitting there's no chance it would get better", forcefully fought against Dan's confabulations, while Dan often experienced Sarah's corrections and help as attempts to control him, diminish him and limit his freedom. "Let go Sarah, let me live my life", Dan yelled in one session, "because if you won't do that out of free will, I have already proven to you there are 6 women who want to be Mrs. M number 2!". When, following an argument, Sarah once asked Dan to hug her so she could help him get up from his wheelchair, Dan said it was easier for him to strangle her than to hug her.

Although (and maybe because) there seemed to be no space between them, it was very difficult for Sarah and Dan to accept help, to let a stranger into their life. In therapy we worked through the difficulties and fears that were involved until finally they hired Maria. Besides the physical help that Maria offered, she proved to be an important 'third' that enabled some physical and psychological space between Dan and Sarah. Gradually, tutors who studied with Dan subjects he was interested in, such as philosophy, offered additional activities. These also replaced Sarah, who could back off a little from the position of Dan's 'therapist', a position that often made her frustrated and angry and was experienced by Dan as demanding and controlling. While quenching Dan's intellectual interest, these lessons also relieved Sarah and helped her to see that Dan was 'doing something meaningful'. In time, Dan and Sarah also found ways to explore activities together more peacefully.

Dan's separate activities appeared to have given Sarah more time and space for herself. Nevertheless, she still struggled adjusting to a routine where she was able to decide what to do and enjoy it. In one session, Dan saw a bag on the floor and asked Sarah if she was going on a trip. "No", Sarah replied, "would you like me to?" "Yes", Dan answered, "And what will you do?", she asked, "I will miss you!" Dan responded, maybe implying his need for more opportunities to miss Sarah.

Dan supported Sarah's going out on her own and having more activities. He said he was worried that if she occupied herself only with him, she would get bored. "I'm afraid about what would happen to Sarah on the day I close my eyes. It will be very difficult for her to recover", Dan predicted.

Sarah had usually rejected suggestions to go out on her own. She explained that she belonged to a generation that needed to dedicate its time to family and work and not to oneself. When I tried to understand more, much guilt came onto the surface. Sarah said that leaving Dan at home alone was a **betrayal**. Here I looked for a voice that would come from the same realm but would counter Sarah's 'super ego command' and give some legitimacy to her own, separate needs. So following her self-accusation of betraying Dan, I suggested that staying with Dan at home all day might be betraying herself.

In yet another session, Sarah maintained that she couldn't leave Dan at home sitting in his chair, "He needs stimuli all the time", she claimed. This, I felt, was a good moment to demonstrate the separateness of Dan's desires from hers. I turned to Dan and asked him how **he** had felt while sitting in his chair at home. Dan's very different needs strikingly appeared as he answered that he had felt perfectly fine sitting in the chair half asleep... "I just couldn't understand", he continued, "how Sarah couldn't see that we are in London with the dripping rain and thought we are in Bialik St...She takes me back there all the time..." Dan's experience of his life, as it was, seemed to be not so bad for much of the time and I tried to reflect that to Sarah.

Sarah's urge to constantly take Dan back to Tel Aviv was meaningfully processed in one of the next sessions. In that session, when the issue of Sarah's corrections of Dan came up, she suddenly said that accepting Dan's condition was for her like separating from him. Through this insightful comment, the needs behind Sarah's Sisyphean fight against Dan's confabulations became clearer, and the grave meaning of accepting them could finally be empathically processed. Different aspects of 'separateness' vs. 'separation' were discussed in that session along with Dan's satisfaction with just 'being', in contrast to Sarah's great need for 'doing'.

In one of the next sessions, Sarah excitedly reported that she had heard a radio interview with the son of a famous Israeli couple. The famous couple had broken up at that time, after many years of living together. The son had talked in the interview about his parents' separation and had claimed that "sometimes you have to separate in order to go on with your life". Upon hearing that, Sarah said, she had realized that "life is too short to waste it on crying at night whether I was hurt or not". She had told that to Dan and started to look for a volunteer job with children for a few hours a week. This activity was followed by a trip abroad with her grandson and more and more things that she did 'separately'.

And yet, Sarah's great difficulty in accepting Dan's condition was sometimes still expressed in her denial of it. In one session, she said about herself and Dan that "both of us have a lot of energy and Dan is a healthy man", to which Dan commented: "of course, a symbol of health!" When, in another, later session, Sarah maintained that "Dan has no mental disability", and that he can realize reality, I felt very frustrated. After all the work that has been done, hearing Sarah say that made me somewhat lose my empathic, understanding position: "Pretending Dan has no mental disability has a great price you pay every day", I said to Sarah. "I don't feel there is progress", Sarah protested after a short silence. "I know how difficult this is for you", I said, "but I think that for progress to occur something has to change in your attitude because Dan just can't". When Sarah asked what she should do when Dan says all these unrealistic things, I suggested, in an acceptance-and-commitment, 'buddhistic' spirit, that maybe she should try to just 'let them be', and we discussed things that can be changed and things that cannot.

I wasn't sure about these last interventions, but in the next session, something different happened. Dan opened: "I was sent a letter this week saying that I was going to be appointed as commander of the Air Force and the navy". At this point I expected Sarah to stop Dan and explain why it couldn't be so, as she had usually done, but instead there was silence. I was surprised. Dan continued: "I'm not familiar with these things. I told two people I know in the navy and in the Air Force that I'm going to recommend them as commanders to the commander in chief of the Israel defense forces". Now I was even more surprised and also excited. It was the first time ever Dan had refused a job he was offered. "Beautiful!" I couldn't hide my enthusiasm, "Maybe you understood that these jobs were not suitable for you and so you referred them to more suitable people and. . ." Dan interjected: "And the commander in chief said, 'Well done!' . . .finally a man with the balls and the courage to execute these appointments!"

Sarah then said that life was calmer the last week, "I internalized some of what you had told me". I suggested that there might have been a connection between Sarah's attitude of not correcting Dan, Dan's reaction of rejecting the grandiose jobs and the calmer week. Dan then added that he also realized that being a pilot is not his real desire (after starting flight training a week earlier).

I wish I could say here that at this point of treatment Dan's confabulations had stopped, but this would be a confabulation. However, in the following sessions, Dan's position vis-à-vis his confabulations seemed to change a bit. For example, when Sarah referred to a negative, distressing confabulation that Dan had had about his parents and asked him whether he could see that it wasn't reasonable, Dan answered: "I wish I could". As another example, Dan protested that Sarah didn't let him rest. "She has a comment about everything. What's most annoying", he added, "is that she is right in her comments!" Finally, in a few cases, Dan said that his confabulations sounded unreasonable and that maybe he was 'fucked up in the head' because of the cerebro-vascular accident (CVA). All these examples appeared to indicate some weakening of Dan's 'psychic equivalence' (Fonagy & Luyten, 2012).

In therapy, there were fewer and fewer 'crises' to take care of. We gradually reduced the frequency of sessions, until we had only sporadic follow-up sessions and finally we decided to end therapy. The last-year follow-up sessions were usually warm, playful and full of humor. Although Dan did not have full insight into many of his confabulations, they seemed to be more contained and 'well handled' by Sarah. Dan seemed to be more curious about his lesion and its consequences, and more open to explanations about them. When, in one of the last sessions, Dan said that he did not get so many job offers as before, and that a few countries did not offer him to be their king, I suggested that they might have finally heard about his retirement and they let him enjoy it. Dan and Sarah definitely knew how to enjoy retirement. They have gone out together a lot to the theater, to concerts and to many lectures. They told me once that at the end of a play, they used to clap hands together – Dan's right, healthy hand to one of Sarah's hands. This, I thought, could offer a terrific answer to the ancient Zen quan, mentioned in Ramachandran and Blakeslee's chapter about anosognosia (1998): "What is the sound of one hand clapping?" Well, it is loud and clear, when another's – a significant other's – hand meets it in attunement.

7 A few thoughts about playing, reality and phantasy

"Why can't I be your right hemisphere?" Sarah asked Dan at one time. "Because you sit to my left", Dan replied. What was right and what was left – in both senses of both words – was highly debatable in this therapy. The 'rightness' of Dan's memories and perceptions and the nature of what his left-brain tissue could achieve were the target of bitter arguments between Dan and Sarah, as described. This couple's dynamics can be viewed as a meeting between two ways of dealing with unwanted reality, as described by Freud (1924a, 1924b), neurotic and psychotic.

According to Freud (1924a, 1924b), both in neurosis and in psychosis, there are attempts to replace a disagreeable reality by one which is more in keeping with the subject's wishes. However, neurosis does not disavow the reality; it only ignores it. Psychosis, on the other hand, disavows it and tries to replace it. In neurosis, a piece of reality is avoided by a sort of flight, whereas in psychosis, reality is remodeled. This 'remodeling' through delusion, Freud suggests, "is found applied like a patch over the place where originally a rent had appeared in the ego's relation to the external world" (1924a, p. 151). In our case, it seemed that Dan's organic narcissistic 'patches' were exactly the pieces of reality Sarah was neurotically trying to avoid. One way of 'flying away' from the reality of a confabulator husband was by constantly arguing with him about the veracity of his confabulations. Dan's 'backfire' at Sarah, on the other hand, can be viewed as an externalization of his inner struggle against the rejected piece of reality, the truth about his abilities. This truth, Freud suggests, constantly forces itself upon the mind in psychosis just as the repressed does in neurosis. In this case, both Dan and Sarah acted as psychic mirrors which painfully reflected and exaggerated exactly those parts of reality that the other was desperately trying to hide or hide from.

The world of phantasy, Freud suggests, plays a pivotal role in both neurosis and psychosis. It is the storehouse from where the materials for building the new reality are derived in psychosis, and it is also the place from where the neurosis draws the material for its new wishful constructions. In this spirit, we can say that in our case, there was a clash between the two areas of phantasy – Dan's and Sarah's.

The concept of 'phantasy area' takes us back to the Winnicottian world and the Winnicottian baby. As I suggested earlier, there is something about neurologically regressed patients like Dan, who sustain a vast right hemisphere lesion, which can be viewed as a 'smart version' of that Winnicottian, totally dependent baby, who does not exist without maternal care (1960). Interestingly, Dan once said that while being intensely taken care of by Sarah, he had thought to himself, "So this is how kings that everybody obeys their orders live". More concretely, he had been crowned as a king in many countries through confabulation. This royal theme may remind us of Freud's 'his majesty the baby' and also of Winnicott's no-less-majestic baby's needs, in the early dyad dynamics.

One of the most essential ideas in the Winnicottian interactional world is that of play (Winnicott, 1971). Play, according to Winnicott, is always on the border between the subjective and that which is objectively perceived. It is neither a matter of inner psychic reality nor a matter of external reality. It takes place in the potential space between the baby and the mother, which is contrasted with the inner world and the external one. Into the play area the child gathers objects or phenomena from external reality and uses them in the service of inner or personal reality. Put differently, the child manipulates external phenomena in the service of the dream and invests chosen external phenomena with dream meaning and feeling. In this process, there is an interplay of personal psychic reality and the experience of **control** of actual objects. The mother here has an adaptive function. She needs to fit in with the baby's play activities.

We, of course, do not expect a grown-up man's wife, after more than 40 years of marriage, to start treating her husband as a baby or small child. However, I find Winnicott's model quite useful in understanding the nature of the needs and reactions of right hemisphere and right prefrontal patients. These patients can sometimes get out of their minds when their needs are not being met or their 'reality' is being challenged. The danger, back to Winnicott's baby, is that the potential space may become filled with what is injected into it from someone other than the baby. It seems, Winnicott (1971) suggests, that whatever is in this space that comes from someone else is persecutory material, and the baby has no means of rejecting it; exploitation of the potential space leads to a pathological condition in which the individual is cluttered up with persecutory elements of which he has no means of ridding himself. This can explain why Dan could accept Sarah's reports about 'phone calls' that were 'received' from the army and cancelled his planned meetings, but could not accept her contradicting the very veracity of these meetings. It was crucial for him that Sarah also played (along) within his potential space. It seemed that within this space, there was much more capacity for acceptance and containment on his side. This can also explain my counter-transferential 'motherly' need to sometimes protect Dan from Sarah's reality-based 'impingements'. Interestingly, at a moment of more insight, Dan once said: "maybe the stroke **plays** with me".

When Dan said he had accepted all the jobs he had been offered because he was afraid that "my whole functioning will be between me and the toilet", he might have feared that his potential space would be shut down, and his existence would be limited only to concrete physical needs. His consequent saying that "when you don't work you don't exist" can be accordingly paraphrased: "When you don't play you don't exist". And Dan was an expert in playing. Sometimes, when an argument was starting to build between him and Sarah about his perceptions, endangering their mutual play zone, he used to say something that returned the conversation back to play-track. This was often done through the use of humor, sometimes spiced with a slight tease towards Sarah. For example, when Sarah complained once that whenever she got out of bed to drink water, Dan looked for her on his right side (because of the left-sided neglect); while she has always slept to his left, Dan answered that she should be happy that at this age, after so many years, she was still looked for.

Sarah also knew a few things about the magic of humor and playing. When, for example, she corrected Dan once about his **real** military rank, he said to her: "Stop talking nonsense. In the madhouse where I will be hospitalized you will also be hospitalized in the bed next to me!" Sarah turned to Dan surprisingly and asked: "Even there we won't be separated?"

"The same nurse will take care of both of us!" Dan answered from within the same playground, and playing could be resumed. Such corrections of 'play failures' convinced me that Winnicott had a point in saying that play belongs to health; that only in playing is communication possible and the person is free to be creative; and above all, that playing is itself a therapy.

We can probably say now that much of the work that was done with Dan and Sarah was ultimately aimed at helping them not step too much on each other's phantasy area or potential space and rehabilitate their capacity for playing together, which in the end becomes self-therapy. Actually, this therapy started as individual psychotherapy with Dan. However, very soon Dan asked that Sarah would join the sessions, "because she also needs therapy". Sarah wasn't enthusiastic about either having separate sessions or going to individual psychotherapy herself. And so, I saw them together. In retrospect, there were probably issues – like Sarah's loss and her difficulty in accepting it – that could be worked through more in depth and efficiently in individual sessions. And yet, seeing them together enabled 'online' work in the mutual play area and its breakings, which was priceless.

Dan and Sarah's talent for playing was evident also in the broader sense of the term: that is in their usage of cultural phenomena. According to Winnicott (1971), play expands into creative living and into the whole cultural life of man. Cultural experience, which is also located in the potential space between the individual and the environment (originally the object), is actually a derivative of play. As mentioned earlier, in spite of Dan's disabilities, Dan and Sarah continued to be very enthusiastic culture consumers. They went together to numerous lectures about a great diversity of subjects: from history and philosophy to art and geography and many more. They went to the theater, to music concerts and even on urban trips! All this enabled enjoyable time together in potential, 'conflict-free' areas. It seemed they were able to enjoy things together very much, as long as they were not questioning each other's realities.

From a personal point of view, Dan and Sarah's incredible wealth of cultural knowledge, passion for it and talent to play with it, entwined with their sense of humor and wits, made our sessions enormously enriching, playful and sometimes 'fun' – alongside all the great challenges, pains and hardships they contained. Counter-transferentially, throughout this therapy I often found myself tossed between identifying with Dan – not understanding how Sarah did not let him be wherever he had wanted – and Sarah – feeling angry about Dan's 'reluctance' to see reality and about his being offensive towards her. This sometimes aroused strong feelings of frustration and anger in me. However, Dan and Sarah's ability to resume play through shared enthusiasm about a cultural experience (a book, a play, a concert), or through a humorous diversion, kept me optimistic even through very difficult sessions.

I cited many interactions between Dan and Sarah in this chapter because I very much wanted this unique therapy to come to life through it. However, allow me one last example that I think captures beautifully this ability to resume play, which was so essential to the therapeutic power of this couple. In one session, when, following a dispute about their location, Sarah finally let Dan be where he had wanted, Dan turned to her and said: "You know, I have always said that wherever you are, that's home for me, so I shouldn't argue with you about it".

Except for play, this last dialogue, as well as the whole therapy, brings to mind Loewald's (1974) beautiful definition of reality testing as "far more than an intellectual or cognitive function. It may be understood more comprehensively as the experiential testing of fantasy – its potential and suitability for actualization – and the testing of actuality – its potential for encompassing it in, and penetrating it with, one's fantasy life. We deal", Loewald concludes, "with the task of a reciprocal transposition" (1974).

8 Final words

In this chapter, I tried to suggest different ways of working with right hemisphere confabulating and anosognosic patients, through my experience of psychotherapy with such a patient and his wife. Several interventions appeared to facilitate the therapeutic process, such as (a) working through 'the denied'; (b) using material brought up by the patient as a 'third' or a 'bridging' object (e.g., a film); (c) connecting the confabulation with the underlying motivation so the patient can temporarily grasp how motivation alters perception of reality; (d) deciphering the meaning of confabulations through free association, as when working with dreams or other unconscious material; (e) helping the patient's significant other mourn his or her losses; (f) educating partners on how the patient behavior is heavily influenced by the type of brain injury; and (g) helping partner understand patient's new behavior, in order to create a social environment that doesn't constantly challenge the patient's misperceptions, thus enabling positive and rewarding interactions. I believe that further publications of clinical case studies and research that integrate neuropsychological and psychoanalytic understanding of right hemisphere (RH) and prefrontal cortex (PFC) patients will help provide these difficult neurological patients and their families with more effective and accurate interventions that would enable a better quality of life for all involved.

References

Feinberg, T. E. (2010). Neuropathologies of the self: A general theory. *Neuropsychoanalysis*, *12*(2), 133–158.

Feinberg, T. E. (2011). Neuropathologies of the self: clinical and anatomical features. *Consciousness and cognition*, *20*(1), 75–81.

Fonagy, P., & Luyten, P. (2012). The multidimensional construct of mentalization and its relevance to understanding borderline personality disorder. In

A. Fotopoulou, D. Pfaff & M.A. Conway (Eds.), *From the Couch to the Lab: Trends in Neuropsychoanalysis*. Oxford: Oxford University Press, doi: 10.1093/med/9780199600526.003.0023

Fotopoulou, A. (2008). False selves in neuropsychological rehabilitation: The challenge of confabulation. *Neuropsychological Rehabilitation, 18*, 541–565.

Fotopoulou, A. (2010). The affective neuropsychology of confabulation and delusion. *Cognitive Neuropsychiatry, 15*(1–3), 38–63.

Freud, S. (1905). Jokes and their relation to the unconscious. In J. Strachey (Ed.), *The standard edition of the complete psychological works of Sigmund Freud* (Vol. 8, pp. 9–238). London: Hogarth Press.

Freud, S. (1911). Formulations on the two principles of mental functioning. In J. Strachey (Ed.), *The standard edition of the complete psychological works of Sigmund Freud* (Vol. 12, pp. 215–226). London: Hogarth Press.

Freud, S. (1915). The unconscious. In J. Strachey (Ed.), *The standard edition of the complete psychological works of Sigmund Freud* (Vol. 14, pp. 161–215). London: Hogarth Press.

Freud, S. (1924a). Neurosis and psychosis. In J. Strachey (Ed.), *The standard edition of the complete psychological works of Sigmund Freud* (Vol. 19, p. 149). London: Hogarth Press.

Freud, S. (1924b). The loss of reality in neurosis and psychosis. In J. Strachey (Ed.), The standard edition of the complete psychological works of Sigmund Freud (Vol. 19, pp. 181–188). London: Hogarth Press.

Kaplan-Solms, K., & Solms, M. (2000). *Clinical studies in neuro-psychoanalysis*. London: Karnac Books.

Loewald, H. W. (1974). Psychoanalysis as an art and the fantasy character of the psychoanalytic situation. *Papers on Psychoanalysis*. New Haven, CT: Yale University Press, 1980, pp. 352–371.

Marcel, A. J., Tegnér, R., & Nimmo-Smith, I. (2004). Anosognosia for plegia: Specificity, extension, partiality and disunity of bodily unawareness. *Cortex, 40*(1), 19–40.

Nardone, I. B., Ward, R., Fotopoulou, A., & Turnbull, O. H. (2008). Attention and emotion in anosognosia: evidence of implicit awareness and repression?. *Neurocase, 13*(5–6), 438–445.

Quinodoz, J. M. (2013). *Reading Freud: A chronological exploration of Freud's writings*. Hove: Routledge.

Ramachandran, V. S., & Blakeslee, S. (1998). *Phantoms in the brain: Probing the mysteries of the human mind*. London: Fourth Estate.

Salas, C. E. (2012). Surviving catastrophic reaction after brain injury: The use of self-regulation and self-other regulation. *Neuropsychoanalysis, 14*(1), 77–92.

Salas, C. E., & Turnbull, O. H. (2010). In self-defense: Disruptions in the sense of self, lateralization, and primitive defenses. *Neuropsychoanalysis, 12*(2), 172–182.

Tiberg, K. (2014). Confabulating in the transference. *Neuropsychoanalysis, 16*(1), 57–67.

Turnbull, O. H., Berry, H., & Evans, C. E. (2004). A positive emotional bias in confabulatory false beliefs about place. *Brain and Cognition, 55*(3), 490–494.

Turnbull, O. H., Fotopoulou, A., & Solms, M. (2014). Anosognosia as motivated unawareness: The 'defence' hypothesis revisited. *Cortex, 61*, 18–29.

Turnbull, O. H., & Lovett, V. E. (2012). Emotion and delusion: Seeking common ground between neuroscience and the psychotherapies. In A. Fotopoulou, D. Pfaff & M. Conway (Eds.) *From the couch to the lab: Trends in psychodynamic neuroscience.* Oxford: Oxford University Press.

Winnicott, D. W. (1960). The theory of the parent-infant relationship. *The International Journal of Psycho-Analysis, 41,* 585.

Winnicott, D. W. (1971). *Playing and reality.* London: Psychology Press.

Yeates, G., Hamill, M., Sutton, L., Psaila, K., Gracey, F., Mohamed, S., & O'Dell, J. (2008). Dysexecutive problems and interpersonal relating following frontal brain injury: Reformulation and compensation in cognitive analytic therapy (CAT). *Neuropsychoanalysis, 10*(1), 43–58.

Chapter 8

Neuropathological inertia and re-mobilisation of cathexes

Brief psychodynamic therapy after basal ganglia lesions

Aonghus Ryan and Giles Yeates

I Introduction

I.I Overview

Neuropsychoanalytic theory holds that emotions are an inextricable part of conscious experience (Solms, 2013) that have evolved as a feedback system to help the organism understand how it is doing with respect to evolutionary imperatives, i.e., to survive and propagate our genes (Solms & Zellner, 2012). Through experiencing the external world, we learn to associate different objects (people, things, events) with different emotions. Libidinisation (or cathexis) is the fusing of emotion with cognition and is a central aspect of learning in that recalling objects *along with* the associated emotional traces orientates us to the importance and relevance of previously experienced objects in our environment. This also frees up mental resources for new learning by increasing predictability and reducing surprise (Solms, 2013). Underlying these emotions is a fundamental binary; things feel good or they feel bad, which is Freud's pleasure principle (Strachey, 1961).

However, there is another important principle that is fundamental to the organism getting these pleasurable and unpleasurable emotional experiences and learning about the world – the impetus to explore. The pleasure principle in itself is insufficient to prompt "goalless seeking" (Solms & Zellner, 2012). An organism must be able to (or somehow be rewarded to) go out into the world in the first place so it can experience external reality, feel its way through the problems it encounters, experience pleasure and unpleasure and learn about the world. In this chapter, we consider a useful theory for conceptualising the impetus to explore Panksepp's SEEKING system. We hope to use an unusual case, a case not best served by traditional cognitive neuropsychology explanations, of psychotherapy in the context of neuropathological apathy and inertia secondary to basal ganglia damage to explore the relationships between cathexis/libidinisation and the SEEKING system.

1.2 Dopamine, self-stimulated exploration and the SEEKING system

Many researchers in the role of dopamine have shown that it is a pivotal neurotransmitter in encouraging exploration in terms of subjective experiences of expectation, reward, wanting, liking, incentive salience, and appetitive motivation (Berridge, 2009; Berridge & Robinson, 1998; Panksepp, 1998). Berridge (2009) reviewed the literature and delineated the differing neurobiology of 'wanting' and 'liking', and Solms and Zellner (2012) suggested that expectancy and anticipation are associated with dopaminergic mesolimbic centres, whereas pleasure itself is more associated with opioid transmission.

Perhaps the clearest exemplification of the role of dopamine on the impetus to explore is Panksepp's SEEKING system. Drawing on his extensive research in affective neuroscience, Panksepp proposed emotional systems to conceptualise the basic emotions in mammals. Panksepp's emotional systems are SEEKING, RAGE, FEAR, sexual LUST, maternal CARE, separation-distress PANIC/GRIEF and joyful PLAY (Panksepp, 1998). For clarity, capitalisations are used for these terms to differentiate between emotions and emotional systems (Panksepp, 2010). SEEKING is an ethological term that "implies a psychological dimension as opposed to a mere behavioral process... a neuro-emotional system" (Panksepp, 1998, p. 145). The SEEKING system is the appetitive motivational system that:

> makes animals intensely interested in exploring their world and leads them to become excited when they are about to get what they desire... In other words, when fully aroused, it helps fill the mind with interest and motivates organisms to move their bodies effortlessly in search of the things they need, crave, and desire. In humans, this may be one of the main brain systems that generate and sustain curiosity, even for intellectual pursuits.
>
> (Panksepp, 1998, p. 52)

Panksepp also stated that SEEKING is a major source of life "energy", sometimes called "libido" (Panksepp, 2010). Indeed, the SEEKING system has been described as correlating closely with Freud's libidinal drive:

> both [SEEKING system and libido, *author's insertion*] energizes the behaviour that makes you want to go out into the world and get what you need, and energizes a learning system to associate particular things, people and situations to particular pleasures and need gratifications. This system, which underlies objectless desire, "a goad without a goal", as Panksepp calls it.
>
> (Solms & Zellner, 2012, p. 140)

The interconnectedness of SEEKING to different elements of Panksepp's emotional systems is of particular interest. SEEKING is considered to represent a separate form of objectless desire from attachment PANIC/GRIEF and "subserves affectionate attachment" (Solms & Zellner, 2012). There is also evidence that prolonged activation of the PANIC/GRIEF system is associated with the "dysphoria of depression which may be due largely to abnormally low activity of the reward-SEEKING system" (Panksepp, 2010, p. 539; Panksepp & Watt, 2011). Each aspect of Panksepp's emotional system has associated neurocircuitry. For the SEEKING system, critical circuits are concentrated in the extended lateral hypothalamic corridor, specifically the fronto-striatal-thalamic dopaminergic circuits.

1.3 Abnormal function in dopaminergic systems

The dopaminergic neurotransmitter system is the most important for the normal functioning of the SEEKING system (Panksepp, 1998), and damage to these critical areas frequently results in the opposite of energised behaviour. Bilateral globus pallidus damage is associated with changes in motivation, initiation and emotion (Miller et al., 2006; Vijayaraghavan, Vaidya, Humphreys, Beglinger & Paradiso, 2008) and apathy (Murakami et al., 2013; Rochat et al., 2013). Following acquired and/or progressive damage in the globus pallidus, profound changes in the initiation and flow of mental processes are observed, an absence of what we might call the person's 'mental spark'. This has been described by Niv and Rivlin-Etzion (2007) as "paralysis of the will" and by Sacks (1973) as adynamia. Sacks contrasted patients' ability to respond to stimuli from the external world with a core limitation in self-stimulation, internal initiation and maintenance of goal-directed and reflective activity. Sacks also emphasised the existential nature of the patient's pause in the absence of a potent environmental cue to trigger further action:

> The essence of this passivity lies in peculiar difficulties of self-stimulation and initiation, not in capacity to respond to stimulation... The problem, then, is to provide continual stimulus of the appropriate kind. And if we can achieve this we can recall... from inactivity into normal activity, and from the abyss of unbeing into being. *'Quis non agit non existit'...* *when is not active he does not exist – when we recall him into activity ...* *we recall him to life.*
>
> (Sacks, 1973, pp. 345–346)

Such changes in motivation and initiation are in many ways similar to depressive symptoms. Indeed, apathy has been posited as dissociable from depression in Parkinson's disease (PD; Kirsch-Darrow, Fernandez, Marsiske, Okun & Bowers, 2006), a disease associated with the loss of the dopaminergic neurons in the basal ganglia (e.g. Blum et al., 2001). By contrast, an oversupply of dopamine in the treatment of PD with dopamine agonists is frequently associated with impulse control disorders (ICDs), increased reward-seeking behaviour and problematic behaviours including pathological gambling, compulsive shopping, binge eating and hypersexuality (Wolters, van der Werf & van den Heuvel, 2008). Sinha, Manohar and Husain (2013) place impulsivity and apathy at opposite ends of a dopamine-dependent spectrum of motivated decision-making in patients with PD.

The neurological changes associated with carbon monoxide (CO) poisoning occur because the affinity of haemoglobin is 210 times higher for CO than for oxygen (O_2). CO displaces O_2 in haemoglobin, leading to hypoxic injury. Carbon monoxide poisoning is associated with changes in cerebral cortex, cerebral white matter and basal ganglia, and especially in the globus pallidus (Prockop & Chichkova, 2007). CO poisoning is also associated with parkinsonian syndrome and mild or moderate intellectual impairment (Prockop, 2005).

1.4. Thresholds to self-stimulation

A related concept to abnormal function in dopaminergic systems and the SEEKING system is the "elevated threshold for self-stimulation and reward" (Panksepp, 2010, p. 538). Apathy traits in the normal population have been described as a "decreased willingness to exert effort when rewards are small, or below threshold" (Bonnelle, Veromann, Heyes, Sterzo, Manohar & Husain, 2015). Animal research suggests that rats with basal ganglia lesions are less likely to direct higher levels of effort towards achieving larger rewards, compared to controls, opting instead for easier though much smaller rewards (Salamone &Correa, 2012).

In terms of treatments, speech and language therapists and physiotherapists have been employing and researching techniques focussing on high-intensity training of movement and vocalisation amplitude (i.e. bigger and louder) in PD (Ebersbach et al., 2010; Ramig et al., 2001) to overcome thresholds to activity, with promising results in terms of reported symptom severity. The dependence of such patients on external stimuli to trigger successive phases and continuation of complex mental activity in the context of psychotherapy also means that the neuropsychoanalytical therapist may act as the patient's 'auxiliary ego' (Kaplan-Solms & Solms, 2000), to invite the patient across the threshold into activity and to support, compensate and enliven patients' psychological work during sessions.

1.5 Aggression, RAGE and the SEEKING system

As regards the relationship to the range of basic emotion systems, two neurobiologically distinct categories of aggression are typically identified: SEEKING/assertive/predatory 'quiet biting attack' and defensive/offensive RAGE 'affective attack' (Panksepp, 1998; Weinshenker & Siegel, 2002; see Table 8.1). Panksepp and Zellner (2004) observed that self-stimulated

Table 8.1 Categorisation of two types of aggression

Category of aggression	Types included	
SEEKING/assertive/predatory	Controlled	Proactive
	Instrumental	Predatory
Defensive/offensive RAGE; affective attack	Irritable	Defensive
	Impulsive	Explosive
	Reactive	Territorial
	Hostile	Maternal

Adapted from Panksepp and Zellner (2004).

exploratory behaviours, similar to those associated with the SEEKING system, can be seen in both predatory exploration in more predatory species (hunting) and assertive aggression in non-predatory species (foraging), based on the shared neurobiological substrate:

> We believe it is significant that in all species studied, predatory aggression is elicited by stimulating the lateral hypothalamus from sites where self-stimulation reward is typically evoked, and it is now well known that this brain system is confluent with the mesolimbic dopamine circuit which runs from the ventral tegmental area through the lateral hypothalamus to the nucleus accumbens and other forebrain zones. This overall circuit has been called the "reward system," the self-stimulation system, or the term that we prefer, the SEEKING system...
>
> (Panksepp & Zellner, 2004, p. 43)

In humans, Panksepp and Zellner (2004) also identified a possible subgroup within these categories: those who can channel RAGE into controlled behaviour, best described as the sociopathic or the psychopathic. This may be relevant with the current case study:

> Perhaps certain people (especially those with a sociopathic or alexithymic streak) are able to shift into a predatory aggressive or SEEKING mode in response to irritations and frustrations, while more emotionally arousable people may tend to cope with them by remaining in the affective mode.
>
> (Panksepp & Zellner, 2004, pp. 51–52)

1.6 Freudian drive theory

Drive is traditionally described as the demand for work on the body, arising from the relationship between mind and body. Drives usually conceived of as without intrinsic representational content, but can be conceptualised as creating 'pressure', which is experienced as unpleasure, while drive

Table 8.2 Components of Freudian drive theory

Component	Definition	Neurobiological correlates
Source	Giving rise to drive: demands on body for work	Hypothalamic need detection mechanisms
Aim	The experience of satisfaction when the drive demand is met	Activation of the mesolimbic dopamine system
Object	The object or representation which, through learning, is associated with the aim	Cortical encoding and representational processes interacting with sub-cortical areas

From Solms and Zellner (2012).

satisfaction experienced as pleasure (Freud's pleasure principle; Solms & Zellner, 2012). One way to conceptualise Freudian drive theory is to break it down into distinct elements, as described by Solms and Zellner (2012): source, aim and object. The source gives rise to the drive demand (unpleasure); the aim is the experience of satisfaction when the drive demand is met (pleasure), and the object is that object which has been associated with the aim through learning. Table 8.2 summarises the definition of source, aim and object with the neurobiological correlates. With regard to the current case study, we might reasonably expect that due to dopaminergic deficiency the specific drive element to be affected is the aim.

1.7 Key questions to be addressed by the current case:

– What light does this case shed on the role of dopaminergic SEEKING in everyday psychic experience?
– Does the concept of thresholds to self-stimulation assist our understanding of patients with damaged dopamine systems?
– Does RAGE activate the SEEKING system in some individuals with damaged dopaminergic systems?
– Does the current case shed light on Freudian drive theory, in terms of the role of dopaminergic substrates in the source, aim and object of the drive system?

2 Case details

2.1 Nature of injury

The patient, PA, was a 48-year-old male survivor of carbon monoxide poisoning, following a suicide attempt in 2007. A magnetic resonance imaging (MRI) scan revealed damage to the globus pallidus bilaterally, the neural circuitry understood to be crucial to dopaminergic pathways and the SEEKING system. The principal unusualness of the case is that, despite damage to the neuroanatomical regions subserving the SEEKING system, many other functions were relatively well preserved, enabling the patient to engage in psychotherapy. However, as we shall see, his ability to make use of psychotherapy was quite limited in the early years after his injury.

2.2 Relevant background

The neuropsychological consequences of PA's injury stood alongside significant pre-injury psychological complexity. He witnessed his biological father die suddenly from an aneurysm when he was six years old. His stepfather, who moved in to the family home within weeks of his father's death, demeaned and physically abused him throughout the rest of his childhood. He did not recall ever-receiving warmth, affection or protection from his mother, but spoke of positivity and warmth from his two older sisters. To survive, he learned to cut himself off from unbearable feelings. Indeed, making himself impervious to rejection or hurt appeared to be the organising principle of his interactional style. He reported employing sociopathic interpersonal patterns, particularly using superficial charm to 'play the game', to keep himself aloof and others at a safe distance in social interactions. He eschewed many interpersonal and societal norms: romantic relationships typically lasted a matter of months, and he spent time in prison for fraud.

At the time of his injury, he was self-employed, buying and refitting old computers with more up-to-date software, and selling them on at a good profit. The emotional distress he experienced following rejection from a woman with whom he had had a tempestuous and antagonistic on and off relationship, a woman who was also carrying his unborn child, culminated in an impulsive suicide attempt. Suddenly plunged into the emotions he had been keeping at bay for years, perhaps into the pit of unresolved grief for his father, he was unable to calm or soothe himself. Despite never contemplating suicide before, to escape this emotional distress he attempted to gas himself in the garage. He was discovered some time later by the cleaner.

2.3 Post-injury presentation

The patient presented with primarily a lack of initiation and flat affect: amiable but detached from all others around him. Inertia pervaded his personal, social and vocational worlds, and his thoughts, planning, reasoning and memories did not get started or developed without external cues. When cues were present – the right questions from others, a key pad to prompt the entry of a code – the right response could be triggered. It was as if the internal 'mental spark' to get thoughts and actions started was missing. His over-learned routines were the most powerful influences – he was on 'auto-pilot'

Table 8.3 Neuropsychological data at baseline (2008)

Domain	Task	Scaled scores and percentiles
Initiation	D-KEFS Letter Fluency	10
	D-KEFS Category Fluency	5
	D-KEFS Design Fluency	4
	Hayling Sentence Completion 1	5
Inhibition	Hayling Sentence Completion 2 Speed	4
	Hayling Sentence Completion 2 Accuracy	2
Working memory	WMS-III Letter-Number Sequencing	3
Attentional switching	Test of Everyday Attention (TEA) Visual Elevator Accuracy	<1
Spatial anticipation	Brixton test	2

in these routines and struggled to shift into 'manual' to try something new or adapt to a situation. An illustrative example of these automatised routines was the volume of shower gel used by the patient. While showering, seeing the bottle prompted the action to squirt some out to wash with. It appeared he would get somehow lost in this routine and, without the presence of mind to monitor how he was doing, would finish the entire bottle of gel, meaning he got through several bottles a week.

Selected neuropsychological assessment results are outlined in Table 8.3. One year post-injury he demonstrated a marked dysexecutive pattern, with poor initiation, inhibition, deficits in auditory-verbal working memory, cognitive flexibility and pattern recognition and prediction. The changes in his cognitive abilities post-injury also modified his relationships with other minds. In particular, his globally slowed speed of processing meant he could no longer 'play the game' of keeping others at an emotionally safe distance by dissembling as effectively in social situations. He reverted to a more primitive defence of avoiding social situations almost entirely. In addition, he reported that feelings of shame at having tried to take his own life had led to a withdrawal from practically his entire former social circle. He rarely left his apartment and had very little mental of physical exercise. He was morbidly obese at the beginning of the therapeutic work.

3 Intervention

3.1 Rehabilitation history

PA was initially referred for community neuro-rehabilitation in January 2009, and he received occupational therapy, and group, individual and family psychotherapy over the course of three years. However, his use of occupational and vocational therapy was limited. He did not employ compensatory strategies to assist with initiation of functional tasks. In addition, he did not engage very much in individual or group psychotherapeutic interventions. Even the significant stimulus of others (clinicians and fellow survivors) appeared insufficient to trigger the development of new coping repertoires, adjustment positions and updated, realistic goals. He eventually disengaged from the service, once he was settled into supported independent accommodation.

A one-year hiatus in service involvement was brought to an end as his family reported a sudden resumption of mental activity, six years post-injury. The historic vulnerability of a family member, revealed through a disclosure of past abusive actions perpetrated by the patient's stepfather, triggered significant levels of anger and rage in the patient (affects not present in the five years previously). This was soon followed by new, unprecedented levels of exploratory mental activity and overt behaviour on the part of the patient, extending to both emotional and functional domains of life. These included both creative ways to verbally attack and publically shame his stepfather, and neutral creative activity such as developing e-commerce activity following a long pause of productivity. He had been somehow 'goaded' into action. Given both the patient's emotional concerns and his new mental vitality, new possibilities within psychotherapy seemed likely.

Nine months of fortnightly therapy was re-offered and accepted by the patient (17 sessions in total). The therapeutic intervention was based on the Brief Dynamic Interpersonal Therapy (DIT; Lemma, Target & Fonagy, 2011) model, which incorporates (among other influences) Kleinian object relations theory and mentalisation-based approaches. DIT encourages therapeutic warmth and a collaborative approach to formulation and interpretations.

3.2 Psychometric assessment

Session-by-session paper-and-pen psychometrics were administered. The Hospital Anxiety and Depression Scale (HADS; Zigmond & Snaith, 1983) is a well-validated psychometric questionnaire yielding two subscales: anxiety (HADS-A) and depression (HADS-D). The range on each subscale is 0–21, and a score of 8+ is considered a reliable cut-off for possible anxiety disorder or depression for each subscale (Bjelland, Dahl, Haug & Neckelmann, 2002). The Patient Health Questionnaire (PHQ-9; Kroenke Spitzer &Williams, 2001) is based on each of the nine criteria of depression in the Diagnostic and Statistical Manual of Mental Disorders IV – Text Revised (DSM IV-TR; APA, 2000; DSM-IV). The range is 0–27. The Generalised Anxiety Disorder (GAD)-7 is a brief seven-item clinical measure of GAD (Spitzer, Kroenke, Williams & Löwe, 2006), and the range is 0–21. Social, agoraphobic and specific phobic avoidance was assessed using the three-item Improving Access to Psychological Therapies (IAPT) phobia scale, based on the Fear Questionnaire (Marks & Mathews, 1979). Ratings are on a 0–8 scale (e.g. 0 = would not avoid it; 4 = definitely avoid it; 8 = always avoid it). A score of 4 or greater suggests possible clinical disorder (IAPT National Programme Team, 2011).

3.3 Initial sessions

While the prompt for the work to begin was evidence of increased self-motivated activity, a change from inertia to activity, numbness to rage towards his parental figures, the initial sessions were nonetheless characterised by a disengagement from emotions, from the therapist, and to some extent from external reality. The patient was experienced by the therapist as friendly, yet detached, with something of an adolescent air of emotional naivety and frequent mental shrugs. Things were 'fine'. Early sessions were often lethargic, with many long silences, which were challenging to interpret. Were these pregnant pauses or inert nothingnesses? Were they neuropathological or psychopathological in origin, or both?

The therapist (AR), who was in training at the time, experienced anxiety about his own vulnerabilities that he was failing the patient – perhaps he was missing some crucial element in the therapeutic approach. At times, the therapist ended up with the patient in the inert fog; at other times, he felt drawn to a parental, fatherly role with the patient. Later, it became clearer that the hypothesised neuropsychological deficit and historic tendencies to repress feelings and to keep people at a distance formed a 'double lock' for the patient, over-determining and maintaining a guarded, yet often empty, internal state. The therapist was working against the grain of both the historic psychological resistance to feeling and the neuropathological inertia due to the brain injury. He needed to activate the patient with questions, to act as an auxiliary ego to help overcome the threshold to activity.

At this stage in the work, the therapist focussed on establishing an alliance with the patient, which included hearing the patient's narrative of key events, such as the death of his father, the circumstances leading up to his suicide attempt and the birth of his son (whom he had only once met). However, in recounting these deeply significant moments, the absence of palpable emotions was striking. There were some somatic indications of anxiety: fidgeting with the end of his shirt and unusual movements of the eyes, which were possibly anxiety-reducing motor discharges, but otherwise the patient appeared largely detached from his emotions. The patient articulated his resistance to feeling: "If I think about those things [past events], I'll go mad". This was taken up by the therapist, and permission was sought and received from the patient to return to emotional moments, to stay with difficult topics to see if emotions would surface.

The major exception to this detached presentation was the patient's conflicted contemptuous rage towards his living parental figures, and this topic tended to energise the patient, and in turn the conversation. In the early sessions, the rage towards both living parental figures was undifferentiated; the intentions and mind of his mother had been absorbed into the denigrated stepfather. The parental objects of mother and stepfather were fused, and he talked about 'them'. "I f***ing hate them"; "They're so f***ing tight[1]".

The end of the initial phase culminated in a map of the patient's emotions, defences and ways of relating to self and to others, called the Interpersonal Affective Focus (IPAF; Lemma, Target & Fonagy, 2011, see Figure 8.1), which was shared and agreed with him. His defences included social avoidance, numbing out his emotions and withholding self and emotions from others, which he achieved using his social skills and by manipulating others. The effects of his brain injury reinforced his avoidance, his withholding of self from others and his numbing of emotions. However, he was also more emotionally vulnerable in social situations, as he was less able to use his social skills and quick wit to manipulate others. His experience of psychological and physical abuse by his stepfather (unprotected by his mother) meant the patient often related to himself as a failure (feeling powerless) and mentalised others as likely to be contemptuous of him. In terms of emotions, which as we shall see were uncovered and explored in the middle sessions, the patient moved from activated rage towards accessing his own vulnerabilities and needs, and his fear of not having these needs met.

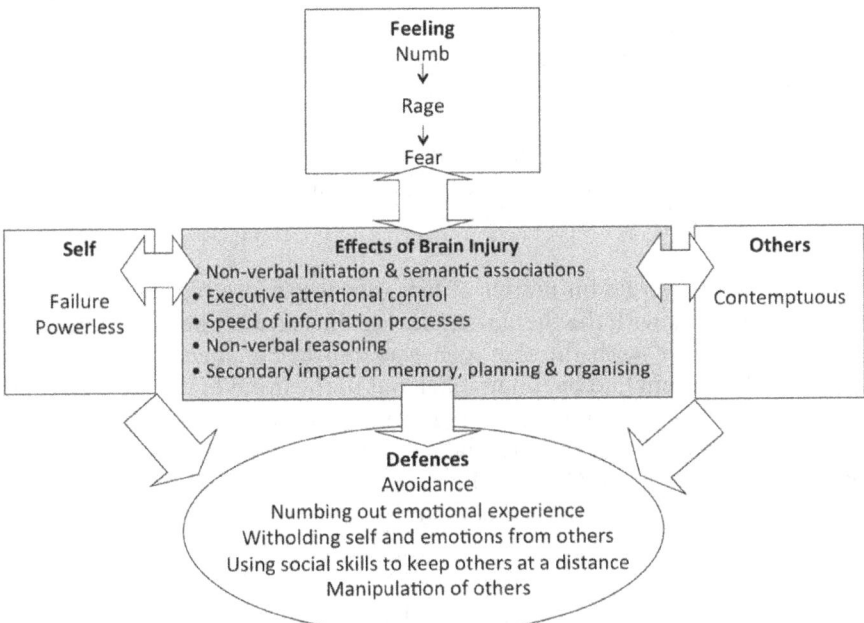

Figure 8.1 PA's case formulation using an IPAF approach.

3.4 Middle sessions

The middle sessions of the work used the IPAF to orientate the patient towards his processes. There was an initial focus on validating the patient's defences and making sense of them in the contexts in which they emerged. With the patient's permission, the therapist focussed on deepening emotions in the room, by circling back around to topics when it appeared the patient numbed out his feelings. This opened the door to exploring other emotions. Here, the patient gave voice to his regrets:

P: I wish I hadn't treated A [former girlfriend who was kind to him] like s**t, I wish I had never got with B [mother of his child], I wish I'd never tried to kill myself. There's a lot of regret in my life.

T: What's it like now to think about those things, to say those words?

P: It's horrible really, it's not very nice.

T: What goes on for you when you think of those horrible things?

P: I feel sad.

T: And what's that like? [PAUSE 15 secs]

P: I don't know really, I can't explain that, sorry.

The therapist noticed with the patient that he seems to have "numbed out" from feeling and sought permission to return to the emotions of regret and sadness.

T: What does sad feel like?

P: I feel deflated, don't feel like doing anything, don't feel like going out sometimes, feel like being on my own - does that make sense?

T: Yes... why don't you want to go out?

P: I don't want others to see that I am sad or to share my feelings with other people... because if people see I'm sad they will be concerned about me... and I'll have to explain myself to them.

The statements were a bit matter of fact, but this was a big step for the patient. He checked with the therapist, seeking reassurance he has made sense. This 'checking in' with the therapist was another change from the initial sessions: the patient had begun to reach out to the mind of the therapist. The patient showed some signs of having anxiety spikes here and was looking sideways in a peculiar way, potentially an anxiety-related somatic discharge or fleeting dissociation. Clearly, the patient has put himself in a vulnerable position by opening up to the therapist.

T: Why are you sad?

P: Basically, because six years ago I nearly lost everything, nearly my life, as well. I don't want to relive it really, not with others... it's a raw nerve, it feels quite fresh in my mind. It brings it all back.

T: What else comes up for you... if it brings it all back?

P: Hatred, lust, love... fear.

T: Tell me more about those things, hatred, lust, love and fear.

These words surprised the therapist, particularly the speed at which they emerged. The therapist had a mental image of a glacier that had suddenly and unexpectedly shifted. Was it going to collapse? Nonetheless, it was still hard to be confident about the level of emotional resonance the patient experienced with his words. It still felt superficial, detached. He continued exploring these themes, largely unprompted now for a few minutes. There appeared to be an internal spark that was energising his inner exploration.

P: I hate myself for what I tried to do. I hate myself for how I treated A [PAUSE 40 secs]... I hate myself for the way I was, the way I treated people... It was mainly lust but a little bit of love for A [PAUSE 35 secs]... I feel sad for what I have lost... the shame of it.

T: You mentioned fear...

P: Yeah, fear of getting hurt.

T: What sort of hurt?

P: Being alone.

T: Is that your biggest fear?

P: Yeah.

The therapist also worked with the patient to defuse and separate the parental objects by enhancing and encouraging the mentalisation of his mother's intentions and perspectives behind her concrete behaviour. He was then, in the middle sessions, able to explore differential feelings towards each living parental object. His mother's absence, complicit passivity and withholding were as painful to the patient as the active abuse of the stepfather. The embodied, sexual, nurturing/barren themes were evident in his words: "Cold c**t; cold f**k" in reference to his mother. Here he talks about yesterday's visit from his mother:

P: My mother came around yesterday. She brought two f***ing doughnuts.[2] Tight f***ng bitch. I dropped her home, there's nothing left to her, she's dead. I feel nothing, actually, I felt nothing towards for her. I feel empty, complete emptiness, towards her, boredom really.

T: I hear you saying you feel nothing, yet I sense that there is at least some anger about her, too...?

P: She is so in-f***ing-credibly mean... 20% (of me) absolutely hates her, 30% feels sorry for her and the other 50% has total contempt for her. I said to her, he [step-father] has totally f***ed you, hasn't he? You're dead aren't you, you've died. She said, no I haven't, no I haven't.

T: Have you ever had a conversation like that before, where you have let your mother know how you feel?
P: No, never.

He then moves on to his projected rage:

P: She (mother) was so tight and mean to my sister. I probably would have tried to kill her [laughs]... bitch". "He's killed my mum basically, it's sad...

He appears to be disengaged from this feeling so the therapist is quick to agree with him to see if it will help him to connect with the feeling:

T: That *is* sad. That's your mum.
P: Mmmm

He then gives voice to his murderous rage towards his stepfather:

P: If I could flick a switch right now [leaning over to flick the switch of a socket on the wall on and off again], and I thought I'd get away with it, I'd do it. The trouble is, it's too risky. I have the rest of my life to think about.

3.5 Concluding sessions

The main themes from the concluding sessions were to consolidate learning, to encourage self-acceptance and forgiveness and to communicate counter-transferential feelings. To consolidate learning, the IPAF was frequently used in order to help the patient understand what defences he had dropped and how this had allowed the therapist into his inner world. This is then reflected upon in the countertransference:

T: Not letting people in, telling white lies, in this relationship you have dropped that, you've opened up, that has felt like a connecting experience, and that's been really lovely.
P: Yeah, you're right.

The patient's scores on the standardised questionnaire suggested a slight shift in his symptoms of depression/apathy, and this comes across in his energy levels and his self-description:

T: How are you?
P: I'm fine, happy, content. Yeah, fine actually, at the moment. I feel like something so bad has happened in my life. I've had enough of feeling down and depressed and low. I feel brighter every morning, a bit more enthusiastic about things.

The patient expressed transferential feelings of attraction and love towards the therapist:

P: If you were a girl, I'd ask you out on a date. Nah… only kidding.

During the penultimate session, where the therapist is exploring how the patient feels about ending, we see evidence that the feeling of connectedness with the therapist has evoked object love in the patient:

T: I'll miss seeing you, I have hopes for you and anxieties about how you'll go and how it will reflect on our work. It's been a real privilege to have been let in. How do you feel coming to the end of our work together?
P: A bit sad, I'll miss you, you've been a great person to talk to, someone who doesn't judge me, to listen to me. I love you for that, thanks very much.

4 Results

4.1 Neuropsychological assessment

The results of repeat neuropsychological assessment, carried out six months after the ten months of psychotherapy had ended, suggested largely unchanged cognitive abilities, with two exceptions: Category Fluency (Delis-Kaplan Executive Function System [D-KEFS]; Delis, Kaplan & Kramer, 2001), which assesses initiation and working memory for verbal information, and Letter-Number Sequencing (Wechsler Memory Scale [WMS-III]; Wechsler, 1997), which assesses the ability to hold information in mind and perform mental manipulations, working memory. The scaled score differences (4 and 5, respectively) were both greater than the standard error of measurement for the sub-tests (3.58, 95% confidence interval – Delis, Kaplan & Kramer, 2001; 3.01, 95% confidence interval, UK sample norms – Wechsler, 1997, respectively), meaning the scores probably reflect an actual change (Table 8.4).

4.2 Psychometric assessment

There was modest improvement in the patient's mood, as suggested by the reduced scores on the HADS-D subscale: 13 at the outset of therapy to 8 by the last session. He continued to indicate through the questionnaire that he did not "look forward with enjoyment to things" as much as he used to, which appeared to echo the core deficit in SEEKING. He consistently reported laughing much less than he used to, sometimes feeling slowed down, but often having good levels of enjoyment (pleasure). His scores on the HADS-A subscale suggested minimal symptoms of anxiety. His scores on

Table 8.4 Neuropsychological data at baseline (2008) and follow-up (2014)

Domain	Task	Scaled scores and percentiles (September 2008)	Scaled scores and percentiles (December 2014)	Verbal description	Behavioural correlates
Initiation	D-KEFS Letter Fluency	10	11	No change	Conversant in therapy
	D-KEFS Category Fluency	5	9	Significant improvement	Improved fluency between ideas in therapy
	D-KEFS Design Fluency	4	4	No change	N/A
	Hayling Sentence Completion 1	5	5	No change	Poor initiation in speech
Inhibition	Hayling Sentence Completion 2 Speed	4	6	No change	Frequent automatic phrases, e.g. "Things are fine"
	Hayling Sentence Completion 2 Accuracy	2	1		
Working memory	WMS-III Letter-Number Sequencing	3	8	Significant improvement	Improved ability to work with ideas in therapy (less inertia or shutting down)
Attentional switching	TEA Visual Elevator Accuracy	<1	3	No change	N/A
Spatial anticipation	Brixton test	2	3	No change	Stereotyped, compulsive behaviours (shower gel)

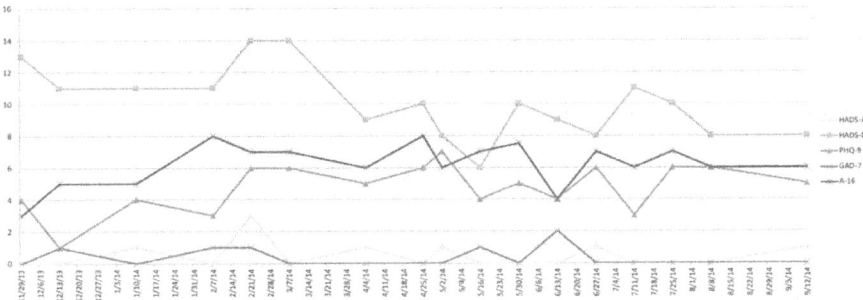

Figure 8.2 Psychometric data before, during and after therapy. HADS-A, Hospital Anxiety and Depression Scale Anxiety subscale; HADS-D, Hospital Anxiety and Depression Scale Depression subscale; PHQ-9, Patient Health Questionnaire-9; GAD-7, Generalised Anxiety Disorder-7; A-16, social phobia item.

the PHQ-9 were 4 at baseline and 5 by the last session. The PHQ-9 incorporates one question about "Having little interest of pleasure in things", which encompasses both interest (wanting/dopaminergic SEEKING) and pleasure (liking/opioid reward); PA endorsed this item in every session. PA's scores on the GAD-7 were very low throughout therapy. However, social anxiety, as measured by the single item A-16, began on 3 and ended on 6 (Figure 8.2).

4.3 Other markers of change

Observationally, PA demonstrated more self-motivated internally focused exploration in the presence of the therapist. This self-exploration was in the context of significant character resistance to experiencing his emotions. Another observable change was the reduced latency in the patient's responses to the therapist's questions. In terms of countertransference, the therapist found himself far less often in that inert fog from earlier sessions. The energising of PA's mental world also allowed him to begin to work through some of past pain towards object love towards the therapist. In terms of subjective experience, PA's words that "I feel brighter in the morning" matched improved scores on mood questionnaires. His family also reported new vocational activity while PA was in therapy; he attended a job interview and continued to engage in ecommerce.

5 Discussion

5.1 Overview

In this unusual case, we present evidence of a reactivated RAGE system reinvigorating the SEEKING system in a patient with neurological damage to brain area understood to be most important to the normal function of the SEEKING system. The reinvigoration of the SEEKING system energised the patient's mind and body, which presented an opportunity for him to mobilise his mental faculties and operations towards the therapist, to experience closeness with the therapist, enabling the exploration of historic difficulties within the enriched relational intersubjective field of the therapeutic situation. The patient's process began with inertia giving way to an external goad at the emergent, exposed historical vulnerability, which allowed projection of the patient's similar disowned feelings of rage, and then continued to the re-introjection (internalisation of the goad) and working through of rage to access anxieties, vulnerability and yearning to connect with others. In summary, we posit there was a process from neuropathological inertia "on pause" → projected rage "I can't believe what he has done" → owned rage "I f***ing hate them" → working through → reaching out to the mind of the therapist → accessing own vulnerabilities "I am anxious, lonely, ashamed, have needs".

The revitalisation was evidenced by the patient's reported subjective experiences of change, his words, psychometric measurements, observations in session and the views of his family. As he became more aware of his needs and vulnerabilities, so his anxiety about meeting others (social anxiety) increased. There were also limits to this revitalisation. He remained emotionally detached, perhaps due to the historic resistance to feeling, or the neuropathological limitations in the SEEKING system, or both – a double lock against experiencing emotions. The interpersonal gains in therapy and attempts to connect with others in his life outside of therapy, to leave his flat, were also modest.

Another change was seen in auditory–verbal working memory and initiation, which may have been due to natural spontaneous recovery or test–retest effects. These improvements do appear to overlap with the reduced latency in PA's verbal responses and may to some degree be a reflection of practice in sessions exploring his inner world, putting words on his thoughts and crossing the threshold into engaging with another mind through conversation. What is more striking is the continued presence of the core cognitive impairment, particularly in initiation. The fact that RAGE appears to have enabled some activation of the SEEKING system in the context of this static picture is, we think, the most remarkable feature of this case.

5.2 Implications

5.2.1 Does RAGE activate the SEEKING system in some individuals with damaged dopaminergic systems?

In contrast to previously reported findings that over-activation of the PANIC/GRIEF system can lead to a *suppression* of SEEKING (Panksepp, 2010; Panksepp & Watt, 2011), we present evidence of an initially quite narrowly focused activation of RAGE prompting a *reinvigoration* of SEEK-ING. The activation of the RAGE system towards a hated object mobilised the energy and movement associated with this system to cross the threshold of a neuropathologically and historical psycho-developmentally maintained global mental inertia. This new mental momentum and outward direction was then channelled through the relational experience of the therapeutic situation, the safety and then the potency of the mind of the therapist guiding the mentalising activity of the newly mobilised patient's mind.

We suggest that this case supports Panksepp and Zellner's (2004) prediction that people with sociopathic tendencies may be able to shift into a predatory aggressive or SEEKING mode in response to RAGE. Here, a patient with sociopathic characteristics channelled RAGE into predatory SEEKING – the back door to SEEKING through RAGE-fuelled predatory exploration. While the SEEKING behaviour went beyond the hated object, into explorations in vocation, there were also limits to this energisation in that it remained necessary for an auxiliary ego (therapist) to draw him over the threshold into exploration of emotional and self-reflective topics.

5.2.2 What light does this case shed on the role of dopaminergic SEEKING in everyday psychic experience?

We believe this case draws our attention to the role of the dopamine SEEK-ING system in energising other systems, the mental spark to light up other aspects of the mental apparatus and to connect to other minds, with all the possibilities that follow. In this case, mental activity was characterised by mentalisation of other and self to access vulnerable, disowned parts of the patient's own mind and elaborate the nuances of others' actions and intentions. This new path progressively led to enriching and rewarding intersubjective experiences (the warmth and love for the therapist) and the disentangling of the mother from the stepfather and softening to her vulnerabilities. We believe this to be a striking illumination of the activating possibilities of this association in the context of neurological damage. We hypothesise that RAGE, with its energising effects, constructively worked on (i.e. with a therapist) can help revitalise suppressed SEEKING systems – anger as an empowering, energising force. This case also supports the idea that SEEKING represents a separate form of objectless desire from attachment PANIC/GRIEF, and that SEEKING "subserves affectionate attachment" (Solms & Zellner, 2012).

5.2.3 Does the concept of thresholds to self-stimulation assist our understanding of patients with damaged dopamine systems?

We propose that another important element in understanding this case is the concept of thresholds to self-stimulation. The goading of the patient into action through external events, and the internalisation of this goad, energised the patient such that he got over some threshold and became available to the therapist, enabling connection and exploration. The therapist acted as a prompter, the auxiliary ego, but also served to amplify the emotions in the room by returning the patient to moments were some degree of emotion was present. When the patient could cross the threshold into activity, the other elements of Panksepp's emotional systems, which closely correspond to Freud's drives, were intact: RAGE activated the SEEKING system, the energy of the SEEKING system allowed, through engagement with the mind of the therapist, an awakening of the PANIC/GRIEF system.

We hypothesise that the dubious *reward* of mental exploration of his emotions ("it is pretty horrible to think about that stuff") and the high level of effort required to overcome historic repression of feeling, in addition to neuropathological inertia, created a pathological and neuropathological double lock to the exploration of feeling for the patient. From this perspective, it is less surprising that for several years post-injury he did not engage meaningfully in difficult, effortful rehabilitation, despite his many losses and underlying longing for connection. The presence of the therapist was a vital element in overcoming thresholds to activity in patients without acquired brain injuries or neurological conditions.

5.2.4 Does the current case shed light on Freudian drive theory, in terms of the role of dopaminergic substrates in the source, aim and object of the drive system?

As predicted, the current case demonstrates the major deficits in libidinal drive/SEEKING due to neuropathological deficits in the dopaminergic system at the level of aim. This was overcome to a degree by activation of RAGE system through predatory self-stimulated exploration (Table 8.5).

Connecting with the therapist and spending time reflecting on his feelings was important, because the patient started to feel his way through his problems, to experience emotions which aim to give feedback on how he is doing from an evolutionary perspective. RAGE reinvigorated his SEEKING system and gave him the impetus to explore his world, to encounter and emotionally experience and libidinise objects within it, with attendant experiences of unpleasure (e.g. old grief) and pleasure (connecting with the therapist's mind; love). He started to become re-orientated to his basic need for connection with others, and increasingly, he reached out to the mind of the therapist. We think this is an elucidating example of the important role the SEEKING system plays in helping us to get out and get the experiences we need to learn and develop. We hope, too, that this experience can help to

Table 8.5 Components of Freudian drive theory neural correlates and patient's presentation

Component	Definition	Neurobiological correlates	Current case
Source	Giving rise to drive: demands on body for work	Hypothalamic need detection mechanisms	Intact in PA. No problem with the hypothalamus, or other biological, hormonal disturbance affecting the ability of the body to place demands on the brain for work
Aim	The experience of satisfaction when the drive demand is met	Activation of the mesolimbic dopamine system	Major deficits in libidinal drive/ SEEKING at the level of aim. Overcome to a degree by activation of RAGE system through predatory actions
Object	The object or representation which, through learning, is associated with the aim	Cortical encoding and representational processes interacting with sub-cortical areas	Functioning well, though with stereotyped, compulsive behaviours (shower gel). However, highly limited self-stimulated exploration

re-orientate PA to his losses and his desires to fulfil his healthy needs and longings.

5.3 Limitations and suggestions for future explorations

There are limitations to the generalisability of the findings due to the single case design. In addition, there were no ways to control for sources of error, such as the influence of spontaneous recovery or other factors individual to PA. The two psychometric assessments that happened to contain items related to SEEKING were hindered by their reliance on the patient's subjective experience and understanding of the question. The PHQ-9 item also conflated wanting/interest and liking/pleasure in the same question, neurobiologically distinct systems. However, we suggest that there is a clear rationale for larger cohort studies with patients having hypoxic injuries to assess for similar energising of emotional systems through external stimulation (e.g. therapist), pharmacological stimulation (dopamine agonists) or encouraging patients over the threshold by increasing the salience of rewards – bigger and larger. We also suggest there is a case for developing a SEEKING assessment tool, incorporating a subjective questionnaire with observational and behavioural elements, for use with clinical populations. Such an assessment tool should assess for apathy, low motivation, mental and physical exploration, creativity and separate wanting from liking, and include elements of impulse control difficulties to consider possible effects of dopamine agonist use.

5.4 Conclusions

We believe this case highlights the potency and relevance of the SEEKING system in invigorating many areas of the mental apparatus. This case also supports the hypothesis that other emotional systems, RAGE, can influence and activate some SEEKING behaviour. In some respects, we are left with the Sacks problem: how to provide continual stimulation to recall the patient to life. However, we believe that a better understanding of the role of the SEEKING system through accurate assessment can help us to appraise the effectiveness of pharmacological and diverse therapeutic interventions on the SEEKING system.

Notes

1 "Tight" is an informal British English phrase meaning "unwilling to spend or give much money; mean".
2 During a video presentation of the case, a psychotherapist in the audience remarked that two doughnuts struck her as a potent image of two hollow breasts, underscoring the lack of maternal nurturance the patient had experienced.

References

American Psychiatric Association. (2000). *Diagnostic and statistical manual of mental disorders - Text Revised (4th ed.)*. Washington, DC: American Psychiatric Association.

Berridge, K. C. (2009). Wanting and liking: Observations from the neuroscience and psychology laboratory. *Inquiry*, *52*(4), 378–398. https://doi.org/10.1080/00201740903087359

Berridge, K. C., & Robinson, T. E. (1998). What is the role of dopamine in reward: Hedonic impact, reward learning, or incentive salience?. *Brain Research Reviews*, *28*(3), 309–369.

Bjelland, I., Dahl, A. A., Haug, T. T., & Neckelmann, D. (2002). The validity of the hospital anxiety and depression scale: An updated literature review. *Journal of Psychosomatic Research*, *52*(2), 69–77.

Blum, D., Torch, S., Lambeng, N., Nissou, M., Benabid, A. L., Sadoul, R., & Verna, J. (2001). Molecular pathways involved in the neurotoxicity of 6-OHDA, dopamine and MPTP: Contribution to the apoptotic theory in Parkinson's disease. *Progress in Neurobiology 65*(2), 135–172. PII: S0301-0082(01)00003-X

Bonnelle, V., Veromann, K. R., Heyes, S. B., Sterzo, E. L., Manohar, S., & Husain, M. (2015). Characterization of reward and effort mechanisms in apathy. *Journal of Physiology-Paris, 109*(1–3), 16–26.

Delis, D. C., Kaplan, E., & Kramer, J. H. (2001). *Delis-Kaplan executive function system: Technical manual.* San Antonio, TX: Psychological Corporation.

Ebersbach, G., Ebersbach, A., Edler, D., Kaufhold, O., Kusch, M., Kupsch, A., & Wissel, J. (2010). Comparing exercise in Parkinson's disease—the Berlin BIG Study. *Movement Disorders, 25*(12), 1902–1908.

IAPT National Programme Team (2011) *The IAPT Data Handbook 2.* London: Department of Health.

Kaplan-Solms, K., & Solms, M. (2000). *Clinical studies in neuro psychoanalysis.* London: Karnac Books.

Kirsch-Darrow, L., Fernandez, H. F., Marsiske, M., Okun, M. S., & Bowers, D. (2006). Dissociating apathy and depression in Parkinson disease. *Neurology, 67*(1), 33–38.

Kroenke K., Spitzer R., & Williams J. (2001). The PHQ-9: Validity of a brief depression severity measure. *Journal of General Internal Medicine, 16*, 606–613.

Lemma, A., Target, M., & Fonagy, P. (2011). *Brief dynamic interpersonal therapy: A clinician's guide.* New York: Oxford University Press.

Marks, I. M., & Mathews, A. M. (1979). Brief standard self-rating for phobic patients. *Behaviour Research and Therapy, 17*, 263–267.

Miller, J. M., Vorel, S. R., Tranguch, A. J., Kenny, E. T., Mazzoni, P., van Gorp, W. G., & Kleber, H. D. (2006). Anhedonia after a selective bilateral lesion of the globus pallidus. *American Journal of Psychiatry, 163*(5), 786–788.

Murakami, T., Hama, S., Yamashita, H., Onoda, K., Kobayashi, M., Kanazawa, J., & Kurisu, K. (2013). Neuroanatomic pathways associated with poststroke affective and apathetic depression. *The American Journal of Geriatric Psychiatry, 21*(9), 840–847.

Niv, Y., & Rivlin-Etzion, M. (2007). Parkinson's disease: Fighting the will? *Journal of Neuroscience, 27*(44), 11777–11779.

Panksepp, J. (1998). *Affective neuroscience: The foundations of human and animal emotions.* New York: Oxford University Press.

Panksepp, J. (2010). Affective neuroscience of the emotional BrainMind: Evolutionary perspectives and implications for understanding depression. *Dialogues in Clinical Neuroscience, 12*(4), 533–545.

Panksepp, J., & Watt, D. (2011). Why does depression hurt? Ancestral primary-process separation-distress (PANIC/GRIEF) and diminished brain reward (SEEKING) processes in the genesis of depressive affect. *Psychiatry: Interpersonal & Biological Processes, 74*(1), 5–13. http://dx.doi.org/10.1521/psyc.2011.74.1.5

Panksepp, J., & Zellner, M. R. (2004). Towards a neurobiologically based unified theory of aggression. *Revue Internationale de Psychologie Sociale, 17*, 37–62.

Prockop, L. D. (2005). Carbon monoxide brain toxicity: Clinical, magnetic resonance imaging, magnetic resonance spectroscopy, and neuropsychological effects in 9 people. *Journal of Neuroimaging, 15*(2), 144–149.

Prockop, L. D., & Chichkova, R. I. (2007). Carbon monoxide intoxication: an updated review. *Journal of the Neurological Sciences, 262*(1), 122–130.

Ramig, L. O., Sapir, S., Countryman, S., et al. (2001) Intensive voice treatment (LSVT) for patients with Parkinson's disease: A 2 year follow up. *Journal of Neurology, Neurosurgery, and Psychiatry, 71,* 493–498.

Rochat, L., Van der Linden, M., Renaud, O., Epiney, J. B., Michel, P., Sztajzel, R., ... & Annoni, J. M. (2013). Poor reward sensitivity and apathy after stroke Implication of basal ganglia. *Neurology, 81*(19), 1674–1680.

Sacks, O. (1973). *Awakenings* (Rev. Ed.). London: Picador.

Salamone, J. D., & Correa, M. (2012). The mysterious motivational functions of mesolimbic dopamine. *Neuron, 76*(3), 470–485.

Sinha, N., Manohar, S., & Husain, M. (2013). Impulsivity and apathy in Parkinson's disease. *Journal of Neuropsychology, 7*(2), 255–283. https://doi.org/10.1111/jnp.12013.

Solms, M. (2013). The conscious Id. *Neuropsychoanalysis, 15*(1), 5–19. http://dx.doi.org/10.1080/15294145.2013.10773711

Solms, M., & Zellner, M. (2012) Freudian affect theory today. In Fotopoulou, A., Pfaff, D., & Conway, M. A. (Eds). *From the couch to the lab: Trends in psychodynamic neuroscience* (pp. 49–63). New York: Oxford University Press.

Spitzer, R. L., Kroenke, K., Williams, J. B. W., & Löwe B (2006). A brief measure for assessing generalized anxiety disorder: The GAD-7. *Archives of Internal Medicine, 166*(10), 1092–1097. https://doi.org/10.1001/archinte.166.10.1092

Strachey, J. (1961). *Beyond the pleasure principle. Sigmund Freud: Translated and newly edited by James Strachey.* London: Hogarth Press and the Institute of Psycho-Analysis.

Vijayaraghavan, L., Vaidya, J. G., Humphreys, C. T., Beglinger, L. J., & Paradiso, S. (2008). Emotional and motivational changes after bilateral lesions of the globus pallidus. *Neuropsychology, 22*(3), 412.

Wechsler, D. (1997). *Wechsler memory scale (WMS-III).* San Antonio, TX: Psychological Corporation.

Weinshenker, N. J., & Siegel, A. (2002). Bimodal classification of aggression: Affective defense and predatory attack. *Aggression and Violent Behavior, 7*(3), 237–250.

Wolters, E. C., van der Werf, Y. D., & van den Heuvel, O. A. (2008). Parkinson's disease-related disorders in the impulsive-compulsive spectrum. *Journal of Neurology, 255*(5), 48–56.

Zigmond A. S., & Snaith, R. P. (1983). The hospital anxiety and depression scale. *Acta Psychiatrica Scandinavica, 67,* 361–370.

Chapter 9

Forgetting, repeating, and working through

Unconscious learning and emotional regulation in a case of profound amnesia

Paul Moore

1 Introduction

This chapter focuses on the problem of amnesia and its contribution to the existing literature on the neuropsychological and psychoanalytical basis of memory systems, and its potential relevance for psychoanalytic theory and praxis. Observations from a *long-term* psychoanalytic process (72 sessions) of an individual with profound amnesia after an anoxic episode are presented in this chapter. Clinical phenomena from the treatment are presented and examined in the context of neuropsychological and psychoanalytic frameworks of understanding.

Interpersonal functioning is a key feature of psychoanalytic work, arguably even more so with individuals who have experienced a brain injury. Content repetition, both conscious and unconscious, was identified across the duration of the therapeutic process as being a cardinal mechanism to the therapeutic work. The forms and functions of these different types of repetitions are examined in this chapter through the focused observation of the phenomena in the context of psychoanalytic psychotherapy with a patient who suffered from profound anterograde amnesia. The relationship of psychoanalytic concepts such as transference and countertransference to these repetitions is examined as functions of the developing therapeutic alliance and transference relationship between the person with amnesia and the therapist. Finally, the implications for psychoanalytic praxis and the area of psychotherapy with brain-injured patients are considered in relation to the material presented.[1]

2 Psychoanalysis and amnesia

The clinical phenomena of profound amnesia, after acquired brain damage, have offered valuable insight into the neurological basis, and the neuropsychological mechanisms, of memory and learning (Milner, Corkin & Teuber, 1968; Schacter, 1992; Squire & Zola, 1997). The most important finding of this line of research has been the increased scientific understanding of the existence of independent memory systems. Individuals who present with profound amnesia – after hippocampal and medial temporal lobe damage – are significantly impaired on explicit recall of new episodic events. However, they simultaneously appear to preserve the ability to retain and utilize data from other sources, such as procedural and non-declarative memories, particularly when this information is of an emotionally salient nature. Persons with profound amnesia are not only able to experience emotions (Damasio, Damasio & Tranel, 2012; Feinstein, Duff & Tranel, 2010), but more importantly, they can learn about the emotional value of experiences and form decisions as a result (Claparede, 1911; Tranel & Damasio, 1990, 1993; Turnbull & Evans, 2006). This preserved capacity is critical to the ability to develop and sustain interpersonal relationships.

No discussion of remembering or forgetting in relation to profound amnesia is complete without reference to the cognitive psychology concept of episodic memory introduced by Endel Tulving (1972) in his seminal paper "Episodic and Semantic Memory". In this groundbreaking publication, Tulving introduced the concept of episodic memory as a specialized memory system involving individual's personal experience of past events. This specialized memory system can overlap somewhat with another concept he termed "semantic memory" – a knowledge of facts. What distinguishes episodic memory from semantic memory, according to Tulving, is the former's unique phenomenology. Episodic memory includes the phenomenon he called "mental time travel", which in other words means that when an event is remembered it is reexperienced; it is as if the person can travel back inside their mind to access the original event from the perspective of having been there. The term "episodic" approximates to our common everyday use of the word "remembering". Tulving devised the labels "noetic" and "autonoetic" to distinguish between the conscious states associated with semantic and episodic memory, respectively (Tulving, 1985). The adaptive function of an episodic memory system has been suggested as being able to generate self-related knowledge between a person and their environment (Mahr & Csibra, 2018), allowing the person to learn from experiences and to strategize looking forward, with the aid of these remembered experiences, and through the use of mental time travel in a temporally forward-and-backward direction.

The neural substrate of episodic memory is suggested to be localized in the medial temporal lobes – specifically the hippocampus and surrounding medial temporal cortices (Cheng, Werning & Suddendorf, 2016). It is reasonable to expect that any damage to this area would impact the process of autonoesis as outlined by Tulving. What happens then to a brain-injured person who has experienced damage to this area? Do they still have the capacity to time travel mentally?

The existence of separate memory systems has clear importance to the theory and practice of psychoanalytic therapy. Such findings in the domain of cognitive neuroscience and neuropsychology align with recent psychoanalytic research and theory regarding the role of conscious and un/ nonconscious processes associated with psychic change (Boston Change Process Study Group, 2008; Charles, 2005; Clyman, 1991; Fosshage, 2005). With this in mind, psychoanalytic therapy with profoundly amnesic individuals can aid in the understanding of these memory systems and their relevance for psychoanalytic theory and practice.

3 Case introduction and presentation

At the time of treatment, J.L. was single and 38 years old. Before the brain injury occurred, and previous to commencing psychoanalytic psychotherapy, J.L. lived on his own, at what was at one time the family home. He had obtained a master's degree and was employed as an engineering professional. Three years before psychoanalytic treatment began, as a result of poor diabetes management, J.L. experienced an anoxic brain injury and suffered three cardiac arrests in quick succession. As is typical of the neuropsychological consequences of such damage, J.L then presented with a significant impairment in laying down new episodic memories (anterograde amnesia), while retaining, to a large degree, the capacity to recall events before the brain injury (retrograde amnesia).

In his intake report, taken at the rehabilitation service, it indicated that prior to the accident, there were premorbid systemic issues relating to his background. J.L. had three brothers (two older and one younger) and two younger sisters. His life had been turbulent and unsteady, with the family moving quite frequently because of work – often emigrating. There was one very long-distance move, during which the family settled for almost ten years. On admission to the rehabilitation services, J.L. reported using and abusing alcohol from the age of 13. However, during treatment, he reported the starting date as being even earlier (ten years).

J.L. was 20 years old when his parents had an acrimonious separation, and he recalls having to help his mother and siblings to leave the country quickly, eventually relocating back home, where they got by through the generosity of friends and family. J.L. met with this adversity well, working during the day as an office clerk and returning to education by night to obtain his master's degree. He also trained for, and eventually worked in, engineering design. However, within a few years of returning (when J.L. was in his early twenties), both parents passed away. He lost his father first, followed three years later by his mother. Soon after J.L. lapsed into a severe alcohol and cannabis addiction, which also led to a deterioration in work performance and subsequent loss of a series of work positions. At the same time, J.L. began to neglect his personal well-being, his living arrangements, and more importantly his diabetes, which had been first diagnosed at 16. This resulted in a series of heart attacks, and eventually the anoxic brain injury.

Since the injury, J.L. has lived in a residential unit for neurological patients. Prior to this, he had spent a year in a rehabilitation hospital, which he appears to have preferred much over his current accommodation. At the hospital, his days were structured and interesting. At the residential unit, he became the youngest service user and did not have much in common with the other patients. He has an older brother who lives nearby and who visits J.L. once a week. However, J.L. had little contact with the rest of his family who live abroad. At the residential unit, his routine was highly repetitive, with much of his day consisting of listening to music, doing jigsaws, and making models. There are further activities organized by the residential unit and the rehabilitation services which he attended twice a week. Because of his diabetes, he was monitored closely by the staff at the unit. This lack of freedom was a great source of frustration, and J.L. repeatedly expressed a strong desire to live independently or to be moved to assisted housing.

4 Neuropsychological assessment

The assessment of general cognitive functioning suggests that J.L. presented with an *average* level of intelligence before the accident (Wechsler Test of Adult Reading (WTAR); Wechsler, 2001), while his post-morbid general intellectual ability appeared at the *low average* level, with a full-scale score of 87 [Wechsler Adult Intelligence Scale (WAIS)-III; Wechsler, 1998a]. No differences were found between verbal (verbal IQ = 88) and performance scales (performance IQ = 87). A more detailed analysis of the indexes offered by the WAIS-III suggests that J.L.'s performance was in the normal range for Verbal Comprehension, Perceptual Organization, and Working Memory, with only Processing Speed significantly below the normal range.

The assessment of memory abilities confirms the clinical presentation of profound anterograde amnesia for both verbal and visual information. Results from the *Logical Memory Task* (Wechsler Memory Scale (WMS)-III; Wechsler, 1998b) show a marked difficulty in recalling verbal information immediately after it was presented, and also after delay. It is important to note that recall did not improve with cues.

His capacity to recognize information previously presented to him was also severely impaired. Results from the *Rey Auditory Verbal Learning Test* (RAVLT; Rey, 1964) offer a similar picture. Consistent with the typical presentation of profound amnesic patients, J.L.'s ability to retain information on *immediate* presentation (on the order of seconds – audio–verbal short-term memory) was largely preserved. However, delayed recall – the capacity to remember previously presented information after minutes – and recognition – the ability to judge whether certain information has been previously presented or not – were severely impaired. In relation to visual memory, a marked difficulty in retaining new information was observed. The copy and recall of visual information in both the *Visual Reproduction task* (WMS-III) and the *Rey-Osterrieth Complex Figure task* (ROCF; Osterrieth & Rey, 1944) offered similar results, showing severe deficits on immediate and delayed recall, as well as recognition. In relation to executive functions, J.L. presented an *average* performance on tasks that assessed working memory (Spatial and Digit Span, WMS III), abstraction, and categorization (*Twenty Questions Task*, Delis-Kaplan Executive Function System (D-KEFS); Delis, Kaplan & Kramer, 2001).

In sum, the results gathered from the neuropsychological assessment are consistent with a classic profile of anterograde amnesia, which is mainly characterized by the inability to register new information (*encoding*). Consistent with other amnesic patients described in the literature (Baddeley, Eysenck & Anderson, 2014; Sacks, 1995; Scoville & Milner, 1957; Wilson & Wearing, 1995), J.L. had relatively preserved executive abilities and working memory.

5 Psychoanalytic observations

5.1 Clinical presentation

The first time I met J.L. he was dressed in old jeans, training shoes, and a football jersey. He wore his hair long and it came to just above the shoulder. Around his neck hung a collection of odds and ends – nail clippers, keys, pens, a miniature torch, a bottle opener, and a mobile phone. The latter J.L. used as a memory aid. Also suspended around his neck were his glasses, attached to what looked like an old piece of chord. A patchy day-old growth of beard revealed the haphazard nature of the previous days shaving. Nicotine-stained fingers betrayed a heavy smoking habit. Intriguingly, the nail of his little finger on the right hand had been allowed to remain longer than its neighbors. This idiosyncrasy endured for the remainder of the therapy, a curiously continuous feature despite J.L.'s amnesia.

At this initial encounter J.L. presented as polite and friendly, and spoke both confidently and clearly, with a foreign accent. He appeared to be lucid and oriented for both time and space. When entering the consulting room, he examined it with what seemed to be an intelligent air. However, after exchanging introductions, the amnesia presented itself almost immediately, and J.L. repeated information to me which he had already mentioned five minutes earlier. The following (transcribed audio-taped) excerpt shows the impact of J.L.'s memory impairment on the continuity of the session, as well as the preservation of higher order executive functions, such as reflexive insight:

P [PAUL MOORE]: Maybe I'll take some notes while we're talking… maybe just start by just telling me about yourself.

J [J.L.]: I was born in XXX… went to (University) at night time. I worked full time and studied part-time. I did that for six years… got my degree in XXXX and worked in the profession and after that it was a bit of mystery for me.

P: What do you remember?

J: How do you mean?

P: What happened to you?

J: What happened me? I don't know.

P: What do you remember of your early life?

J: Oh yeah I remember being brought up I remember everything up to about two years ago...three years ago [*Suddenly the alarm goes off somewhere in the room and we both cannot find the source for a while, and analyst and patient share laughter*]

P: So you don't remember anything after 3 years ago?

J: No

P: So what happened?

J: I have no idea.

P: And would you like to tell me about your life before 3 years ago?

J: I used to be a structural engineer.... [i.e. *J.L had already forgotten that he mentioned his work as a structural engineer..*

J: I can't read... I can't get the information to stay in my head. And I don't know why I could read and read and read and read and I would have to go back and start again... just have to keep repeating it over and over and it just won't stay in my head[*He seemed to be aware of his memory problems, but it did puzzle him why this was so*].

P: And what about listening to audio tapes, watching TV?

J: I can watch TV, but ask me about half an hour of watching and I haven't got a clue about what I've been watching so [*J.L. did not appear to be unduly upset about this*]

P: You can't hold the information?

J: Yeah.

P: It gets dropped.

J: Mmm mmm it goes in one ear and out the other

P: What is that like for you?

J: It doesn't bother me at all... if there is a film on I will watch it and I will really enjoy it but don't ask me about the film a half an hour after I was watching it. I wouldn't even know if I was watching it or not.

J.L.'s presentation during the following sessions extends the clinical picture, regarding the extent of his amnesia, even further. When I collected J.L. from the reception area, he appeared not to remember my name, nor the location of the consulting room where we had met previously the week before, nor the layout of the building. During the initial sessions, he did not formulate questions as to why he was meeting with me, nor about who I was. Neither were there ever any overt references to our previous session, this suggests some level of temporal discontinuity in J.L.'s subjective experience. Nevertheless, he could bring back topics we had discussed during the initial meeting, most notably sports, which seemed to have somehow been "preserved" in memory. Interestingly, even though the topic was similar, the emphasis put by J.L. was different on each occasion. The repetition of certain topics across sessions was to become a significant feature of the therapeutic process:

J: Did you watch any sport over the weekend? [*This was a topic discussed during the previous session*]

P: I didn't...Did you?

J: No, not really. I did watch Rory McIlroy though.

P: Do you like golf?

J: Yes, I used to play it...but I was never really any good at it. That's going back a couple of years now.

P: Did you enjoy it?

J: Oh yeah.

P: How are things in Bellevue [the residential unit, not the actual name]?

J: Same old same old... ticking along... [2 minutes silence] ... Did you watch any of the golf just on there now?

P: No I didn't see any of it.

J: Rory McIlroy did very well. I don't know what happened to Tiger Woods. He's gone off the radar completely.

Repetitive phenomena, such as the above, were to become strikingly prominent and common features in the treatment with J.L., as repetition is in all psychoanalytic treatments; however, it was much more amplified and intensive in this instance. Repetition is a phenomenon that is commonly observed in psychoanalytic therapies, where learnt interpersonal and intrapersonal patterns of behavior are brought by patients into the sessions as part of the transference–countertransference dynamics of the patient–therapist relationship. Classic psychoanalytic theories (Bion, 1962, 1963; Freud, 1914; Klein, 1946) suggest that a main goal of treatment is to help remembering and elaborating of the underlying conflicts (working through) instead of simply repeating the past. The capacity to remember events from the past is often severely impaired in people with profound amnesia (Milner, Corkin & Teuber, 1968; Schacter, 1992; Squire & Zola, 1997). In addition, because of the memory impairment, patients with amnesia tend to repeat contents (Moore, Salas, Dockree & Turnbull, 2017), thus systematically disrupting the remembering–elaborating process. Such repetitions are often understood, and dismissed, in the neuropsychological literature as deficits of cognitive functioning (Hassabis, Kumaran, Vann & Maguire., 2007; Klein, Loftus & Kihlstrom, 2002). While the clinical phenomenon of repetition is well documented in aphasiology research (Hengst, Duff & Dettmer, 2010), a search of the neuropsychological literature, in relation to this phenomenon in amnesic patients, amazingly returns no research literature. But what if these repetitions are meaningful attempts by the person's psyche to navigate and make sense of the world? Might these repetitions represent adaptive efforts to come to terms with a profoundly changed relationship with the environment? Or a profoundly changed self trying to come to terms with a profoundly changed environment? In what ways can a deeper understanding of the nature and function of content repetitions in profoundly amnesic patients assist in the therapeutic treatment of this population? In contrast to neuropsychology, psychoanalysis has a rich, detailed, and abundant literature on the phenomena of repetition in psychotherapeutic treatment (Fonagy & Target, 2004; Freud, 1914; Genovese, 1990; Joseph, 1960). Interestingly, neuropsychoanalytic literature provides a rich source of material that may provide the foundations for bridging this gap and the basis for integrating neurobiological research with clinical neuropsychological therapeutic practice (for a comprehensive review of this research, see Zellner, 2014).

I would like to put forward the argument that a psychoanalytic approach, which places value on repetitions, can use these repetitive phenomena as clinical data, and therefore therapeutically in the treatment of individuals with profound amnesia. J.L.'s case highlights the impact of profound amnesia in a long-term psychoanalytic process, particularly in relation to the nature and function of the phenomena of content repetition and its role in the transferential–countertransferential dynamics. More importantly, long-term psychoanalytic work, as illustrated through J.L.'s experience of psychoanalytic psychotherapy, demonstrates the utility of psychoanalytic concepts and techniques in accessing heretofore uncharted therapeutic domains in profoundly amnesic patients.

Freud (1914) proposed that the main goal of psychoanalytic psychotherapy is to help the remembering and elaborating (working through) of underlying conflicts– as opposed to simply acting out and repeating the past. However, the capacity to remember recent past events is severely impaired in people with profound amnesia (Aggleton & Brown, 1999; Sacks, 1995; Scoville & Milner, 1957; Squire & Zola, 1998; Wilson & Wearing, 1995). Due to the memory impairment, session content is frequently repeated; this repetition disrupts remembering and interferes with the elaborating process. This is consistent with Luria's (1973) neuropsychological description of how people with medial temporal lobe lesions are affected in the area of memory. Luria discovered that stored information is dislodged by the introduction of new information into the system.

J.L. met with me once weekly in the offices of the Brain Injury Support Agency. The sessions were face-to-face and lasted 50 minutes for a period of two years. Sessions were audio recorded and then transcribed. Upon reviewing the transcripts, three clearly delineated and differentiated forms of repetition were identifiable in the sessions – regulatory repetition, epistemological repetition, and implicit repetition – each with its own specific phenomenology and functionality. In the following sections, these three distinct forms of repetition will be examined in further detail through the exploration of clinical vignettes, demonstrating the unique phenomenology and function of each class of repetition.

5.1.1 Regulatory repetition

This is the fixed and rigid repetition of information with no variation in terms of structure or content. This form of repetition was often observed after the abrupt disruption of the session's temporal continuity, when J.L. dropped subjects of conversation, because of his memory impairment. However, this type of repetition was also observed in moments of high emotional arousal. It is proposed that in such instances repetition may, at times, have a defensive character, which helped J.L. to retreat to safe ground when faced with overwhelmingly difficult emotion. Irrespective of the causal factors, the net result was that J.L. was left in a psychic void between narrative memory and temporality. The way in which such breaks in continuity were managed by J.L. was to fill the ensuing voids in thinking by following up quickly with questions. These questions typically related to sport or cinema. This seem to be a kind of mental stop-gap, defending him from the impending threat of anxiety associated with losing a train of thought so suddenly. The repeated use of these questions provided a retreat to emotionally safe and reliable ground. On occasions where the content or the dialog between J.L. and me became meaningful, often when an emotionally difficult or sensitive episode was touched upon, there was a defensive maneuver of shutting down employed. This also had the effect of leaving J.L. marooned in an uncertain subjective mental space (and state), and the lifeline of the question was deployed to me, in an effort to reach a "known" state of mind.

This type of regulatory repetition occurred across the duration of the therapy. For example, in the third session of the treatment following a two-minute pause from JL, he asked "Did you watch any of the football?" Later on, towards the end of the session, following a two and half minute pause JL asked me "So, have you been to the cinema lately?". In the subsequent week's session after a one-and-a-half-minute pause JL asked "So, what's on at the cinemas now?". After a one and half minute pause, twenty-four sessions in to the treatment, the following question was asked "So, did you watch any sport over the weekend?", and again following a particularly charged discussion concerning the frustration J.L. experienced while living in the residential unit, and a subsequent two minute silence J.L. enquired "So here, come on, did you watch any football?". Finally, in the penultimate and ultimate sessions the repetition was again used on both occasions, in response to silences of two minutes or more, "so, have you been to the cinema lately?", and "What's on in the cinema now?", respectively. Even in the final stages of the final session this mechanism was present, when following another silence J.L. asked me "Have you been watching the athletics?".

It is of interest to ask the question, why this content – cinema and sport? And why now? One possible explanation is because these were topics of common interest shared between us. From an interpersonal point of view, these contents were felt to be safe and facilitate the reconnection or re-attunement between therapist and patient after the resetting phenomenon (described below). These contents would have the effect of eradicating the anxiety associated with uncertainty and reestablish a familiar state of mind. In the absence of an organic, continuous, train of thought, J.L. used the relationship with the therapist to reset the mental apparatus. However, while it appeared to serve this function, it also suggested much more. The questions usually ignited a discussion between us and became the launching point for further analytic work, within which the other forms of repetition were also to be seen. It was as if once we were on safe ground, again the analytic work could recommence. In object relations parlance, the function of this form of repetition was to facilitate a transition from a paranoid schizoid position to a depressive position (Klein, 1940, 1946), a transcending of a paranoid and persecutory fear state, akin to being pursued by a predator, to a much calmer state of mind which allowed J.L.to recover his capacity to think. The dropping of content from J.L.'s consciousness, in these resetting moments, induced a state of confused trepidative fear in him. Out of this chaos of confusion, a "selected fact" (Bion, 1962, 1963; Freud, 1912) emerged – the fixed repetitive narrative such as "did you watch any sport over the weekend?" or "have you seen any good movies lately?". Asking me a question also allowed J.L. to be in control and determine future direction of the narrative. It also provided the possibility of J.L. relocating the "good" therapist/me and to experience refuge from the "bad" therapist/me who might have, in J.L.'s unconscious fantasy, been responsible for this frightening confused state. Not only was communication reestablished in this interaction, but new links to different material usually presented themselves alongside the repeated narrative content.

An example of this linking to new, or different, material can be seen after one such resetting moment which took place in the first three months of the therapy with J.L., outlined below.

(After enquiring about the painting on the consulting room wall)
P: Do you remember last week we took a picture of the painting here in the room and sent it to your phone? You said you wanted to paint it.
J: I haven't painted it yet.
P: Were you able to get the photograph?
J: oh yeah.
P: I wasn't sure you could get it.
J: Oh yeah I did.. it's good cause it's a nice picture.
P: who's your key worker at the moment with Headway now that C is off?

J: M.

P: I'll try and get in touch with her about setting up an email address for you
   Silence (3mins)

J: did you watch any of the football?

P: No but I saw some of the highlights.

J: players just want the money.

P: Mmm ... its disappointing for you is it?

J: In a sense, it is as if, if you don't pay me enough money I'm not going to
   play for you.

P: So it's not about playing for the club.

J: Whoever pays them the most money they'll play for and you end up sitting
   on the bench like Tevez.

P: Does it feel like that sometimes for you... sitting on the bench?

J: Oh yeah and waiting to see what happens next...

P: And there's something about people doing things for money not really for
   the love of it?

J: Oh yeah.

P: Maybe around your care?

J: I don't know if it's the same.

P: I think it might feel like that ... sometimes when we have discussed your
   insulin and when it comes, what time it comes, it might feel like that
   then people don't really care and that if they did they would have it in
   time.

J: Oh yeah I know I see ... they'd make sure to have it in time.

P: That's what is really annoying not so much the fact that it doesn't come on
   time, which is annoying too, but the fact that people don't care enough
   to have it there on time.

J: like I said I've stopped worrying about it at this point in my life if the
   insulin is there in the morning I eat my breakfast if it's not I don't eat
   my breakfast.

P: It's like you've given up on the hope that things will change.

J: Yeah.

P: it feels pointless?

J: Can't teach an old dog new tricks... that sort of way *(silence 4mins)*... so
   have you been to the cinema lately

P: No I haven't have you?

J: Last thing I went to see was cars in 3D

P: when was that?

J: I don't know ...

P: it's out a while that film.

J: Yeah.

P: Did you enjoy it?

J: It was ok it was a cartoon... I prefer not the action ones but The Rock you
   know that movie? Where there is a story behind it.

P: I haven't seen that what is it about?

J: Sean Connery is in it it's about Alcatraz and Connery is an ex prisoner.

P: I think I have seen that a long time ago I can't remember the details.

J: some criminals take it over and want to launch missiles from there.... He's a good actor Connery and Nicholas Cage is in it he's the FBI agent who is supposed to look after Connery while he breaks in to Alcatraz and takes him with him ..... The great train robbery is on tonight I think on RTE 1.

In considering, further, the question why these repetitive phenomena should occur at the times they did, a possible hypothesis presents itself. That, emotionally, this repeated action of asking the therapist a question relating to a familiar topic of mutual interest provides access to an emotionally safe place in the therapeutic relationship, thus providing a means for J.L. to regulate his emotional experiences of loss and confusion which accompany the disorientation of an organic, or sometimes psychogenic, shutting down of the train of thought as an ego-protective maneuver.

The utilization of this fixed regulatory form of repetition is seen in the vignette just presented. After significant silences in both instances, which it is difficult to say whether there is a defensive shutting down or whether it is owing to the organic resetting of the mind because of his brain injury, J.L. restarts the conversation with a question. These are questions he has asked before and will ask again in similar situations. It is interesting to note where the questions lead to. In the first instance, issues of care, and in particular the perceived authenticity of the care received in the residential unit, arise out of his disappointment with the Man Utd teams' level of commitment to the club – do they really have loyalty and passion for the club? Or are they simply doing it for the money? A link arises in the therapist's mind in relation to previous issues discussed by J.L. in previous sessions about his dissatisfaction and annoyance at the quality of care he receives in connection with certain aspects of his diabetes management, and the staff of the residential unit, and how this can lack consistency – if they really cared and were really loyal to J.L. and not only doing it for the money, they would make sure his insulin arrived on time. The therapist then offers this putative link to J.L., which he partially takes in.

It is likely in the second instance that the silence is a defensive maneuver against feeling too much painful emotion in connection with the powerlessness J.L. experiences about the timing of the arrival of his insulin medication. Again, the function of the fixed repetitive content that follows seems to be to reconnect with the therapist and to restart the work – after a dropping of content. The material that emerges is darker in nature and speaks to feelings of being trapped and fantasies about escape – clearly J.L.'s unconscious mind is generating scenarios that may offer a solution to his

5.1.2 Epistemological repetition

This is the repetition of explicit content that was variable and context dependent. This type of repetition often emerged triggered by external situations experienced by the patient as puzzling. These contents were – amazingly, given his diagnosis of profound amnesia – brought repeatedly by J.L. to sessions in order to make sense out of confusion. Theoretically speaking, this form of repetition appeared to represent an epistemophilic drive, since it facilitated the transition from confusion to understanding, or from what might also be considered as part object to whole-object mental representation. This type of repetition can also be understood as a function of the transference–countertransference relationship between the patient and the therapist. Another category of repeating in order to work through a difficult experience is the set of repetitive material concerned with establishing objective facts about events occurring outside the therapeutic setting. These "knowledge repetitions" were variable, context dependent, and triggered by external events and situations, and therefore relate to episodic and semantic memory systems (Tulving, 1972, 2002; Tulving & Markowitsch, 1998). They occurred consistently across the duration of the treatment, and their function appeared to be related to meaning making – for example, the working through of a rigid but confusing understanding of an event. This has significance psychoanalytically for the area of Freudian metapsychology and post-Freudian relational theory and praxis. It is consistent with what Freud tells us in relation to the function of repetition and the aim of psychoanalysis. The aim of psychoanalytic therapy is to "...to fill in gaps in memory..." (Freud 1914). From a relational perspective, Bion (1959) held the view that thinking evolved to deal with thoughts, and psychoanalytic therapy was a means to facilitate thinking. Difficulties, for Bion, occurred where the demands placed on the mind outpaced the capacity for the mind to think. This is expressed well in his idea that it can take two minds to think a person's most disturbing thoughts. Bion's theory is underpinned by the premise that thinking is driven by the human need to know the truth (Bion, 1959). Humans are inherently aware that "a failure to adequately grasp the truth of reality" (Bion, 1959) results in an inability to learn from experience and grow psychologically. This is also what he termed the epistemophilic drive, a yearning after understanding. This process is illustrated in the following clinical vignette, where J.L. transforms his understanding of an event, and in doing so comes to a realisation of a new reality. In this interaction J.L.'s internal mental representation of an experience undergoes a transformation, form a part object representation to a more comprehensive whole object representation. Arguably, the medium for this internal psychological transformation is the evolving transference relationship between J.L. and I.

During the latter end of the fifth session with J.L., the following narrative emerged in the process.

J: Here do you know what they call that pedestrian bridge that crosses the
      Liffey down there?
P: The Ha'penny Bridge?
J: No, no, no, not the Ha'penny Bridge... It's a new pedestrian bridge.
P: That, that's not a pedestrian bridge... traffic can go across that bridge.
J: No, no, it's not big enough for cars.

The topic became quite alive for J.L. as he really tried, quite hard, to process
the discrepancy between his memory of the bridge and my own knowledge
of this external object. As he tried to make sense of his experience, he first
defended his own internal representation of the bridge. J.L.'s main mode of
doing this was to attack and challenge my version of the bridge. This can be
understood as a narcissistic defense against the realistic possibility that his
version may be incorrect and the ensuing devastating psychological consequences of acknowledging this fact; that is, his subjective experience of self
and world was highly unreliable.

   The retention of this narrative and train of thought for the remainder of the
session was also indicative of a shift in the intrapersonal dynamic between
J.L. and myself. It signaled a transformation in J.L.'s capacity not only to
challenge me but to explore what kind of a person I was and what kind of a
mind I possessed. It also signified the development of the transference relationship, albeit a tentative one, as evidenced by the tone of the interaction. In
this phase of the treatment, J.L.'s responses to my offerings in relation to an
alternative reality regarding the bridge – that is, it carried traffic – were rigid,
narcissistically defensive, somewhat omnipotent, and tinged with sadism.

J: It's just a little pedestrian (bridge), it's only about from here to the wall
      apart wide. I'm telling you, no cars can cross it.
J: You couldn't have, it's not big enough for a car... or a bike (laughs).
J: There's a little foot bridge across there. There's no way a car could cross it.
J: No, well there's no way you saw cars on this bridge anyway I can tell you
      that much, there's no way you drove over it either. Nah, it's just a little
      pedestrian bridge.
J: Come in next week and tell me you drove across it, and I'll give you a
      thousand euros, ten thousand euros, a million euros! (both laugh). You
      wouldn't even get your car up on to it. Something Mr. Bean would try
      now, to cross over it in his car, wouldn't work.

It is interesting to note here that while the topic had been retained and discussed, the dynamic of the relationship had become one, possibly through
projective mechanisms (Klein, 1946), where I was now the one who did not
know, was wrong, and by implication had become a stupid and unreliable
source of information, and subsequently an object of derision. This perhaps
is how J.L. often felt about himself.

Astonishingly, given the presence of profound amnesia, J.L. reintroduced the topic of the bridge once more, four weeks after its initial appearance in the therapy. Three sessions had elapsed, and now in session nine, J.L., unprompted, asks, "You didn't find out the name of that bridge across the Liffey, no?... You know, I was just saying to you last week about that bridge, but I didn't know what it was called". I informed J.L. that it is the James Joyce Bridge and reminded him that, in a previous session, there was some confusion as to whether or not it was a pedestrian bridge.

J: Yeah no it's just a footbridge. I'm adamant it's just a footbridge. You're adamant it wasn't; it was a traffic bridge. It's not it's just a footbridge. I know it's just a footbridge, you can only walk across it. Did you go and check it out?
P: I did.
J: And can you only go and walk across it?
P: No, you can drive across it.
J: No you can't drive across it. No way you could drive across it... It's only about a metre and a half wide.
J: Mm hmm, I'm just trying to think how you get a car across the freakin' thing. I'm trying to think now if I'm wrong, but I'm not. I'm dead right. It's only footpaths only for walkers.

The repetition of this material is significant for several reasons. First, it is quite astounding, given J.L.'s neuropsychological profile of profound memory impairment, that the opposing views from a session four weeks earlier should be retained and reemerge in such detail. Second, it represents an acknowledgement, from J.L., that there are two minds in the room, both capable of independent thinking with the capacity to arrive at different viewpoints. This in turn is a tacit acceptance by J.L. that his perception of the event may not be an entirely accurate one. The memory of the contradictory details opens the way for the potential for developing a more accurate representation of reality: "I'm just trying to think how you get a car across the freakin' thing? I'm trying to think now if I'm wrong...". The window of tolerating uncertainty, and the concomitant potential for change, closes quickly and certainty returns: "but I'm not. I'm dead right. It's only footpaths only for walkers". In this final line of the vignette, the transformative function of the repetition can be seen in operation – with a move from certainty to uncertainty and back to certainty again.

The subject of the bridge is introduced by J.L. once more, and again unprompted, at the beginning of the next session, that is, session ten.

J: How are you?
P: I'm good. How are you?

J: Fine. Okay, I went and checked that bridge out. You're right. There's two walkways across the sides of it.

P: What do you think happened there?

J: I don't know how the hell I got that...

P: So it was confusing for you?

J: Mm-hmm (40 second pause) Did you watch any football over the weekend?...

A few minutes later, J.L. spontaneously started to discuss the movie *A Few Good Men*, quoting the famous Jack Nicholson's line:

J: The truth? You can't handle the truth.

P: I recognise the line

J: Mm-hmm

P: Hmm. The truth is hard to handle.

J: Yup.

P: I wonder, is there something in why that comes up here... that particular film and that particular line? You know truth is hard to handle, you know, maybe some parts of what's happened to you? Your memory? It's hard to acknowledge at times?

J: I Don't know...

After a two-minute silence, J.L. attacks me with a riddle, which I am unable to solve. I feel stupid and persecuted by this attack. He relieves my anxiety, and confused state, by teaching me the answer, thus becoming the one who knows in the presence of one who does not.[2]

In the fourth week, which is the third consecutive week, of discussing the episode of the bridge, an even greater transformation in how the bridge experience was represented became evident. This transformation was characterized by a change in the transference relationship between J.L. and me – where the style of relating had developed from a closed and defensive position to an open and more flexible one. This more open style of relating, signified by J.L.'s increased capacity to take in information, facilitated the development of J.L.'s mental representation of the bridge from an incomplete part-object representation to a more comprehensive whole-object representation.

J: So I went down to look at that bridge

P: Did you yeah?

J: Yeah. Okay I'm wrong. Ha. But you can see over from both sides of it though...

P: Umhum, yeah

J: ...That it's attached to the bigger bridge.

P: It is very important to you the bridge, and how the bridge was remembered, and how it was brought in here. Because I think it's probably one of the few things that we've engaged in and had a strong disagreement about…

J: Umhum…

P: …that was very important for you to try and figure it out, when I had one opinion and…

J: …I had another.

P: You had another yeah. There was something very confusing about that. And I think that's why it stayed in your mind, because of the connection that was there between you and I.

J: The differences…

The nature of the epistemological repetition outlined above is evocative of much of the classical and contemporary research in psychoanalytic theory and current neuropsychoanalytic research (Freud, 1914; Klein, 1946; Moore et al., 2017). The pediatrician and psychoanalyst D.W. Winnicott (1969), in a seminal paper on the use of an object, in which he discusses his ideas about how the relationship between patient and analyst develops, describes a process whereby the patient first needs to use the analyst before they can relate fully to them. He theorized that in order for the patient to arrive at a realistic representation of self and analyst, the patient must first destroy the analyst, that is, destroy the approximated and hypothesized initial representation of the analyst. This virtual initial representation is one that is, to a large extent, usually flawed and fuelled by projective mechanisms, as determined by the unique matrix of the transference–countertransference relationship between the analyst and the patient. In other words, the patient (and to some extent the analyst also) is, in what is known, in psychoanalytic terms, as a part-object mode of relating to the analyst. According to Winnicott, in order for the patient to achieve a more accurate representation of reality, they must first destroy the initial representation, if the analyst, and the therapy, can withstand the accompanying attacks, only then will the patient have a chance of developing a reasonably accurate representation of reality.

This process, which incidentally is a core tenet of post-Freudian relational theory, can be clearly seen in the vignettes presented here. J.L. tests and probes my mind in a tentative and cautious manner at first. He then, gradually over time, becomes less defensive and moves from a closed narcissistic position of relating to an increasingly more open and fluid interchange with me. Along the way his hypothesized part-object representation of me is chipped away at, by J.L.'s sadistic attacks, until after a time a capacity to use me as a meaningful object is arrived at.

From a relational perspective, this process can only occur, according to Bion (1965), in a therapeutic relationship that is containing, or in a Winnicottian sense, a relationship that first "holds" the patient. For Bion, thinking develops in order to deal with thoughts; it is the pressure of thoughts that propel J.L. to search for a way to think about them. This is to use the therapist's mind by proxy, as his own mental apparatus is not functioning well enough to perform this task. Gradually, across the sessions, in a process that has its origins long before the issue of the bridge erupts on the scene, and through the development of a positive transference relationship, a good pairing if you will, the therapeutic dynamics of the relationship evolve through transferential and countertransferential projective mechanisms. It is in this intrapsychic space, created from the therapeutic dynamics, that a potential matrix is formed. One that is felt to be able to contain the disturbing thoughts that cannot be thought alone – emerging thoughts that pressure the mind to think, such as hate, feelings of stupidity, confusion, and persecution. Interestingly, at the same time, anecdotally, J.L.'s key workers and carers report a concomitant decrease in angry outbursts and improvement in general well-being. From a Freudian perspective, J.L. could perform some remembering and no longer needed to act in order to remember.

From a neuropsychological perspective, it is difficult to determine what had transpired. J.L.'s brain injury, according to the neuropsychological evaluation, had impaired his ability to lay down and retrieve episodic memories. One possible explanation is that in the absence of the functional component of the "meaning-making" system responsible for encoding and retrieving information, J.L. sought out a means of making sense of the bridge experience in his therapist. J.L. used the therapist's functioning component to bypass his own damaged unit, thus allowing him to achieve a more realistic representation of the episode. This is supported by contemporary research in the neuropsychoanalytic literature. The process of using the other person (therapist) to compensate for neuropsychological deficits is well documented – for a detailed review of this phenomenon, see the neurorehabilitation research work of Christian Salas (2012). The work of Giles Yeates (2013) in the area of relational neuropsychology also demonstrates how relationships can help to modulate cognitive impairments in persons who have experienced a brain injury.

The experience of confronting the therapist was survived by J.L. This was underscored by the developing positive transference relationship, an unconscious understanding that it was safe to explore difficult issues with the therapist, without which it was unlikely that the rigidity of the distorted memory of the bridge would have subsided. Crucially, in terms of clinical practice, the affective experience of a good therapeutic relationship needed to take place first. Even more crucially, this does not mean that both parties in the relationship have to like each other or "get on" necessarily, but have a good enough relationship that can withstand difficult feelings such as hate and stupidity. From a Winnicottian perspective (Winnicott, 1945, 1949, 1986), J.L. was afforded an opportunity to "be" and experience himself authentically, which in turn provided the potential space for him to think creatively.

5.1.3 Implicit repetition

This is the repetition of deep unconscious transference themes in the session content connected to material in the patient's premorbid characterological structure. These implicit repetitions differ from the first and second types of repetition in terms of phenomenology and function. Phenomenologically, they manifest as implicit underlying themes, contained in a wide range of spontaneously reported topics, not referred to explicitly in the content. Speculatively, the function of these implicit repetitions may serve to facilitate the expression of split-off/projected, or yet to be fully integrated, very early internal object and object relationships as a means of relieving and working through associated unconscious psychic tension. These deep psychic phenomena while influencing present-day dynamics and interactions do not constitute a response to them nor are they generated by them. Themes such as omnipotence, destructive impulses, hate, being cared for, self-care (or lack thereof), frustration, despair, envy, regret, and guilt were present. Interestingly, while these unconscious aspects of mental functioning have been forgotten explicitly, they are being expressed, repeated, and worked through implicitly psychoanalytically in the therapy process. This type of repetition refers to the repeating of unconscious transference themes that possess a clear relevance to current events in J.L.'s life at the time, which were not expressed explicitly in the therapeutic process. These implicit repetitions are, in all likelihood, also related to premorbid and early object relational dynamics; however, the details of which can only be speculated upon and inferred from notes taken at intake to the rehabilitation services. Importantly, for clinical practice, the implicit repetition of "here-and-now" emotional events appear to serve one principal function, that is, to express, relieve (and re-live), and work through unconscious conflicts. These were, in fact, unresolved emotional experiences, remembered affectively, but not cognitively. Unable to achieve cognitive consciousness, these affective memories appear to have been diverted and redirected into the content of J.L.'s in a free-associative and spontaneous fashion. The implicit repetitive themes that emerged from J.L.'s free associations included omnipotence, destructive impulses, being cared for, self-care (or lack thereof), frustration, despair, envy, regret, and guilt.

J: ... The amount of grass that is confiscated, and people getting fined and all that going to jail and everything ludicrous. Some guy was caught with two big suitcases full of grass trying to get it back... Crazy, you know what I mean? No clothes. No nothing else in the suitcases just grass how he expected to get them through I don't know... ... It was ridiculous two thousand pounds he had paid, and he reckons he would have made three hundred thousand pounds from it... Now he's serving time in a Caribbean jail.

P: … I'm just thinking about what comes in to the session today. The excess
    alcohol.. The excessive use of alcohol, the huge amounts of marijuana
    and the consequences of engaging with that… The cops are involved,
    there is punishment, and somebody ends up in jail.. I am just thinking
    about that in terms of your own experience of alcohol and marijuana
    use and your diabetes and the subsequent brain injury?
J: Yep.
P: And how that might feel the same. That you are being punished for that.
J: Being stuck in jail.

The similarities between the plight of the protagonist in J.L.'s material and
the plight of J.L. himself are striking. In the section of narrative which
preceded this vignette, J.L. spoke to me about out-of-control drinking by
bachelor parties who visit the Caribbean in order to smoke marijuana. One
individual ends up getting in way over their head, resulting in their deten-
tion and subsequent incarceration. This is what appears to have happened
also to J.L. His out-of-control drinking and cannabis misuse resulted in the
exacerbation of complications leading eventually to a brain injury. It also
resulted in the loss of freedom and the prison like regime J.L. now found
himself in, where he was monitored around the clock. Freedom and a great
desire to leave the residential unit, and move in to independent or semi-
independent living arrangements, were ever-present recurrent themes across
the duration of the therapy. The restrictions and limitations placed on his
autonomy were the source of J.L.'s many disputes and altercations with staff
and other residents, but primarily the staff he had most contact with and
who were responsible for his care.

Many of the movies J.L. discussed contained the topics of imprisonment
and freedom as central themes; indeed, *Escape from Alcatraz*, *Return to Alcatraz*, and *The Great Escape* appeared to be J.L.'s favorites. While these
themes were alive and current for J.L., he never explicitly confronted the
contribution of his own actions to the situation in which he now found himself. Arguably, this would be too disturbing for J.L. to acknowledge. It is
difficult to see, with such a high level of preserved executive functioning,
that J.L. was incapable of making these links cognitively. It is most likely a
defensive not-thinking about them. Nevertheless, the unconscious fantasy
of being responsible for his brain injury through out-of-control drinking
and drug misuse and the ensuing serious consequences permeates the free
associations of the session.

Given J.L.'s profound amnesia, it is unlikely he was capable of generating episodic memories that could allow for the reflective processing of past,
present, and wished-for experiences in an integrated way. This is a crucial,
and necessary, stage without which the linking of past events with current
dilemmas cannot take place. Again, impairment of this vital element of the
functional system, involved in meaning making, does not stop the system

from working completely, but it does seem to result in a distorted final outcome. The inability to generate episodic memories which can be used to cognitively understand the self in relation to actions and consequences fully prevents J.L. from learning from his experiences, and to therefore adapt sufficiently to his new circumstances. Clearly, a psychoanalytic level of input can assist in bridging this shortfall, in a way that contemporary cognitive and behavioural approaches cannot.

Further implicit repetition can be seen in the penultimate and final sessions with J.L. where endings and unconscious mourning are the covert themes.

The following clinical vignette is an excerpt from J.L.'s final session with me. Previous sessions had been spent focusing on the difficult topic of termination. This was a long and arduous process, owing to J.L.'s inability to remember "cognitively" that we were approaching the ending of the therapy. The decision to end, unusually for a psychoanalytic therapy, was solely mine. This was an extremely difficult decision to arrive at and was the culmination of several external pressures, mainly financial and logistical in nature. Typically, in psychoanalytic treatments, termination of the therapy is something that is negotiated jointly between the therapist and the patient. Clearly, J.L. was capable of, and arguably would have benefitted from, continuing the treatment. Indeed, in the here and now of the sessions, he expressed a desire to continue and regret at the idea of not being able to continue. The difficult ending was compounded even further by the fact that J.L. was unable to consciously remember the fact that the therapy was ending, leaving the task of carrying this knowledge to me alone. Under the circumstances and with J.L.'s memory deficit, you would think that this process was much more difficult for the therapist in such a situation – consciously – but as will be seen J.L. too struggled with this topic, albeit implicitly and in a way that he himself was not aware of.

J: The Cliffs of Moher... I used to kick the ball out over the cliffs, and the ball would come straight back to you. I never lost a ball over the cliffs .... Ahh yeah everybody used to walk down the cliffs from the cottage we were staying in... I always wanted to run and jump off, to get pushed back by the wind, but I was never allowed to. It always amazed me you could kick a ball as hard as you could out over the sea and it would just come floating back... They parasail off it now, they go parasailing off there.

This was a poignant exchange from J.L. in the context of the termination phase of the treatment not being explicitly remembered, even more so that it should occur in the final session. It is important to note that in previous sessions, building up to this point, the issue of ending and how this might be for J.L. had been discussed many times. J.L. had verbalized on these occasions that he was going to "miss the sessions" and not "know what to do" with the time where the sessions used to be. J.L. was capable, when prompted, of acknowledging the loss of the therapeutic space but not capable of retaining that experience cognitively. It is clear, however, that J.L. was capable of retaining the emotional experience, the feeling of losing something important, while at the same time not knowing what that "something important" was. This was the affective memory which had reworked, and rerouted its way into J.L.'s free associative material.

The working through of important emotional experience in an alternative non-declarative domain is not a new idea in psychoanalysis. This particular implicit repetition is reminiscent of Freud's (1920) Fort-Da scenario, wherein an 18-month-old child processes the experience of being separated from his mother by designing a game of "gone and there" with a toy reel. The little boy masters his experience of loss by throwing the reel into his cot, where it disappears from sight, and subsequently retrieving it again. Freud proposes that the wish of controlling the separation is satisfied through the game under the aegis of the pleasure principle. This same mechanism is evident in J.L.'s psychical processes where he fantasizes about getting rid of the ball and retrieving it.

Multiple episodes of loss in J.L.'s life are represented and re-presented in this fantasy – bereavements, loss of social and family relationships, loss of self through brain injury, the subsequent loss of independence, losing the capacity to remember, and now the loss of the therapy and our now long-standing relationship. These loses require processing in the service of mastery. Similar to Freud's (1895) idea of the multiply determined symptom, the fantasy generated in J.L.'s narrative about kicking a football off of a cliff, only for it to be blown back, contains the symbolic elements of loss and retrieval. Arguably, this illustrates an unconscious mechanism for achieving psychical and emotional homeostasis – simultaneously satisfying the needs to both experience and master the multiple losses of many objects in an expedient and energy efficient manner, while at the same time disregarding any need to attend to the external realities pertaining to them.

6 Discussion

Working from a psychoanalytically oriented frame of reference allowed the therapist to access emergent layers of meaning to the repetitions. This information facilitated the understanding and integration of difficult experiences for the patient and appeared to be a function of the developing transference–countertransference relationship between the patient and the therapist and to facilitate the development of this relationship.

The topic of memory holds a key position in the history of psychoanalytic thought. An example of this is Freud's (1895) early conceptualization of pathogenic experience, in which he posited the repressions of traumatic memory as the cause of hysteria. While Freud revised his theories of the mind frequently over time, he always retained this genetic perspective, that is, the core belief that the past exists in the present in complicated and powerfully influential forms. This, of course, is also the cornerstone of the concept of transference, and subsequently countertransference (Heimann, 1949). The phenomena can also be thought of as reliving (relieving) of complex experiences not consciously remembered, in other words acting out. Many contemporary dilemmas within psychoanalysis, and indeed psychology, center on facets of memory. These puzzling dilemmas are reproduced here in the vignettes demonstrating the different iterations of repetition to be found in the sessions with J.L. Attempting to identify and investigate these processes in action in profoundly amnesic persons such as J.L. can teach us much about the structure and process relating to the psychoanalytic model of the unconscious mind.

Early on in the development of Freud's thinking (1900), he viewed perception and memory as separate systems within the mental apparatus. Moreover, he thought of memory – what he termed "mnemic traces" – as structural alterations to these systems, which were linked through association. The majority of these associations remain unconscious or preconscious. The preconscious memories, which have already been symbolized, can become conscious by receiving enough cathexis; that is, the common material becomes especially salient to an external cue. A clinical correlate of this phenomenon can be seen in the repetitive themes J.L. produces in the session, where some symbolized and quasi-symbolized memories are made available to further symbolization.

In a later revision of his views on therapeutic action, while writing about technique (1914), Freud develops the concept of unconscious wishes being expressed through repetition or enactment within the transference relationship. Freud conceptualized this repetition in the transference relationship as a "new edition" or "facsimile" of impulses or fantasies belonging to an early object relationship, for Freud object choice is always a re-finding of an object. In this way of thinking, the repetitive phenomena encountered in J.L.'s treatment are no different to the phenomena Freud was meeting and thinking about in his early clinical work and theoretical formulating. This suggests that psychoanalytic treatment for individuals with profound memory problems can indeed be particularly effective as the model pays great attention to the unsymbolized and pre-symbolic themes that run through the narrative of therapy with this population. Indeed, many psychoanalytic theorists and practitioners see psychoanalytic work taking place at the border between the preconscious and unconscious systems of the psyche.

The work with J.L., where therapeutic gain appears to take place in the absence of cognitive recall, also supports more recent theorizing in the field. In these more recent conceptualizations (Fonagy, 1999; Stern 1994), it has been argued that the active agent in psychoanalytic therapy is not necessarily the conscious recall or symbolization of partially remembered of unconscious experiences, but rather the modification of mental models of object relationships or in other words the updating of implicit knowledge concerning ways of being with others. This can clearly be seen to be in effect between J.L. and I where the lines of communication between us become more fluid and less concrete over time. This updated way of being together facilitates knowledge and affect transfer, and the transformation of the same over time.

As previously mentioned, repetition phenomena are at the core of psychoanalytic theory and practice. Patients repeat symptoms and inhibitions, in an attempt to master the accompanying tension produced, a means of binding the tension and eliminating the ensuing excitation. These repetitions can also be thought of as a failure to integrate traumatic encounters in the world, whether the traumatic event is a physical trauma, separation, loss, or puzzling episode. Freud (1920) held the view that many of these repetitions operated beyond what he had previously termed as the "pleasure principle". This was also the progenitor of the concept Freud termed the "death drive" (Freud, 1920), an aggressive drive that propels all living matter towards an inorganic state, which emerged from the clinical phenomenon the compulsion to repeat. This drive is also reminiscent of cognitive neuroscientist Karl Friston's (2003, 2005, 2010) Bayesian model of the brain/mind as an error prediction system. This idea has been ingeniously reinterpreted psychoanalytically by Mark Solms (2013), where he correlates Freud's ideas around repetition and what he termed the "Nirvana principle" with Friston's ideas of Bayesian error prediction models. A mechanism which can clearly be seen at work in what I have termed the "epistemophilic repetitions" observed in the work with J.L.

At the core of each repetition phenomenon is the development of transference–countertransference relationship between the patient and the therapist. This is a unique layer of the interpersonal relationship only accessible through the application of a psychoanalytic mode of practice. It is a process where hate, sadism and stupidity in the countertransference, use of narcissistic defenses, can come alive and available to understanding, and in doing so dissipate the concomitant tension accruing in the psychical system owing to the conflicts and paradoxes generated by them. In the post-Freudian relational (Bion, 1962; Klein, 1946; Winnicott, 1986) way of viewing therapy, this approach facilitates the evolution of part-object representations to whole-object mental representations.

7 Conclusion

In depth single case studies such as the work with J.L. presented in this chapter highlight the need for awareness of the presence of different forms of repetition, each with its particular phenomenology and functionality. These repetitions are relevant to the understanding of unconscious processes in amnesic patients and the often-overlooked presence of complex mental operations existent in such presentations. An awareness of the differing modes and levels of repetition provides therapists working in the area of brain injury with greater opportunities for creating understanding with patients. Paying greater attention to unconscious processes, particularly affective transference dynamics, and not just manifest cognitive content, is an important aspect of psychotherapeutic technique for all clinical presentations but perhaps especially so for persons who present with a brain injury. Moreover, attention to, and awareness of, the importance of the developing transference dynamics may be a prerequisite for rehabilitation in psychotherapeutic work. It is important to note that awareness of, and therefore insight from, these psychoanalytic concepts is only possible through long-term psychotherapy, with a psychotherapist who has been trained psychoanalytically and preferably undergone their own psychoanalytic psychotherapy process.

Furthermore, the area of clinical psychoanalytic practice with individuals presenting with profound amnesia is a rich and fertile arena within which to test and fine-tune our psychoanalytic theories. As can be seen in the work with J.L. presented in this chapter, which is only a small subset of the many clinical psychoanalytic phenomena observed, the art and science of clinical psychoanalytic practice is relevant to and greatly enriched from the therapeutic treatment of this population. This is a population who greatly deserve to have access to an empirically valid and evidence-based psychological treatment, such as psychoanalytic psychotherapy, which appears to be better suited methodologically than more cognitively oriented models to this population's needs.

Acknowledgments

I am especially indebted to Sarah Crowe, Divya Mukhopadhyay, Clare Cullen, and M.Sc. Principles of Clinical Neuropsychology students at Bangor University, for all their hard work in assisting in the transcription of the clinical material included in this chapter.

Notes

1   This chapter is based on the research conducted by Paul Moore, Christian Salas, and Oliver Turnbull, which was presented by Paul Moore in a talk entitled "Forgetting, Repeating, and Working Through", on the 11th of July 2015 at the 16th International Neuropsychoanalysis Congress "Plasticity and Repetition" in Amsterdam. The presentation was part of the research symposium "A neurobiological basis of interpersonal functioning: transference and countertransference as neuropsychoanalytic phenomena" convened by Xavier Jimenez. This presentation was derived from previously published preliminary observational research with the same patient. For further information on this case, please refer to the research paper "Observations on Working Psychoanalytically with a Profoundly Amnesic Patient" (Moore et al., 2017).

2   Interestingly, the above vignettes contain examples of each class of repetition discussed in the chapter.

References

Aggleton, J.P. & Brown, M.W. (1999). Episodic memory, amnesia, and the hippocampal–anterior thalamic axis. *Behavioral and Brain Sciences*, 22(3): 425–444.

Baddeley, A., Eysenck, M.W. & Anderson, M.C. (2014). *Memory* (2nd edn). Hoboken: Taylor and Francis.

Bion, W. (1959). Attacks on linking. *International Journal of Psychoanalysis*, 40: 308–464.

Bion, W. (1962). *Learning from Experience*. London: Heinemann.

Bion, W. (1963). *Elements of Psycho-analysis*. London: Heinemann.

Bion, W. (1965). *Transformations*. London: Heinemann.

Boston Change Process Study Group (2008). Forms of relational meaning: Issues in the relations between implicit and reflective domains. *Psychoanalytic Dialogues*, 18: 125–148.

Charles, M. (2005). Patterns: Basic units of emotional memory. *Psychoanalytic Inquiry*, 25(4): 484–505.

Cheng, S., Werning, M. & Suddendorf, T. (2016). Dissociating memory traces and scenario construction in mental time travel. *Neuroscience & Biobehavioral Reviews*, 60: 82–89.

Claparede, E. (1911). Recognition and "me"ness. In *Organization and Pathology of Thought: Selected Sources*, ed. D. Rapaport. New York: Columbia University Press, 1951, pp. 58–75. [Reprinted from Archives de Psychologies11 (1911): 79–90.]

Clyman, R. (1991). The procedural organization of emotions: A contribution from cognitive science to the psychoanalytic theory of therapeutic action. *Journal of the American Psychoanalytic Association*, 39: 349–382.

Damasio, A., Damasio, H., & Tranel, D. (2013). Persistence of feelings and sentience after bilateral damage of the insula. *Cerebral Cortex*, 23(4), 833–846.

Delis, D.C., Kaplan, E. & Kramer, J.H. (2001). *Delis-Kaplan Executive Function System: Examiners Manual*. San Antonio: Psychological Corporation.

Feinstein, J., Duff, M.C. & Tranel, D. (2010). Sustained experience of emotion after loss of memory in patients with amnesia. *PNAS*, 107(17): 7674–7679.

Fonagy, P. (1999). Memory and therapeutic action. *The International Journal of Psycho-Analysis*, 80(2): 215.

Fonagy, P. & Target, M. (2004). Relationships to bad objects. *Psychoanalytic Dialogues*, 14(6): 733–741.

Fosshage, J. (2005). The explicit and implicit domains in psychoanalytic change. *Psychoanalytic Enquiry*, 25(4): 516–539.

Freud, S. (1895). Project for a scientific psychology. In *The Standard Edition of the Complete Psychological Works of Sigmund Freud, Volume I (1886–1899): Pre-Psycho-Analytic Publications and Unpublished Drafts* (pp. 281–391).

Freud, S. (1900) in Strachey, J. (ed.) (1953). *The Standard Edition of the Complete Psychological Works of Sigmund Freud. The Interpretation of Dreams (Second Part) and On Dreams*. i–iv. The Hogarth Press and the Institute of Psycho-analysis, London.

Freud, S. (1912). The dynamics of transference. *Classics in Psychoanalytic Techniques*. ed. R. Langs. London: Hogarth Press. pp. 3–9.

Freud, S. (1914). *Further Recommendations in the Technique of Psychoanalysis: Recollection, Repetition, and Working through, in Collected Papers*, (1959) vol. 2. New York: Basic Books, pp. 366–376.

Freud, S. (1920). *Beyond the Pleasure Principle*. Translated and Newly Edited by James Strachey. New York: Liveright, 1950.

Friston, K. (2003). Learning and inference in the brain. *Neural Networks*, 16(9): 1325–1352.

Friston, K. (2005). A theory of cortical responses. *Philosophical Transactions of the Royal Society B: Biological Sciences*, 360(1456): 815–836.

Friston, K. (2010). The free-energy principle: A unified brain theory?. *Nature Reviews Neuroscience*, 11(2): 127.

Genovese, C. (1990). Narcissistic repetition and primary creativity in the analytical situation. *Rivista Psicoanal.*, 36(4): 1082–1110.

Hassabis, D., Kumaran, D., Vann, S.D. & Maguire, E.A. (2007). Patients with hippocampal amnesia cannot imagine new experiences. *Proceedings of the National Academy Science of the United States of America*, 104: 1726–1731.

Heimann, P. (1949). On Countertransference. In *About Children and Children-No-Longer: Collected Papers*, ed. M. Tonnesmann. London, Routledge, 1989, pp. 73–79.

Hengst, J.A., Duff, M.C. & Dettmer, A. (2010). Rethinking repetition in therapy: Repeated engagement as the social ground of learning. *Aphasiology*, 24(6–8): 887–901.

Joseph, B. (1960). Some characteristics of the psychopathic personality. *International Journal of Psychoanalysis*, 41: 526–531.

Klein, M. (1940). Mourning and its relation to manic-depressive states. *International Journal of Psychoanalysis*, 21: 125–153.

Klein, M. (1946). Notes on some Schizoid mechanisms. *International Journal of Psychoanalysis*, 27: 99–110.

Klein, S.B., Loftus, J. & Kihlstrom, J.F. (2002). Memory and temporal experience: The effects of episodic memory loss on an amnesic patient's ability to remember the past and imagine the future. *Socical Cognitive*, 20: 353–379.

Luria, A.R. (1973). *The Working Brain: An Introduction to Neuropsychology* (p. 43). New York: Basic Books.

Mahr, J.B. & Csibra, G. (2018). Why do we remember? The communicative function of episodic memory. *Behavioral and Brain Sciences*, *41*, 1–42.

Milner, B., Corkin, S. & Teuber, H.L. (1968). Further analysis of the hippocampal amnesic syndrome: 14-year follow-up study of H.M. *Neuropsychologia*, 6(3): 215–234.

Moore, P.A., Salas, C.E., Dockree, S. & Turnbull, O.H. (2017). Observations on working psychoanalytically with a profoundly amnesic patient. *Frontiers in Psychology*, 8: 1418.

Osterrieth, P. & Rey, A. (1944). Le test de copie d'une figurecomplex. [The test for copying a complex figure]. *Archives de Psychologie*, 30, 205–221.

Rey, A. (1964). *L'examen Clinique en Psychologie*, Paris: Presses Universetaries de France.

Sacks, O. (1995). "The Last Hippie". *An Anthropologist on Mars*. New York: Vintage, pp. 42–107.

Salas, C.E. (2012). Surviving catastrophic reaction after brain injury: The use of self-regulation and self-other regulation. *Neuropsychoanalysis*, *14*(1): 77–92.

Schacter, D. (1992). Implicit knowledge: New perspectives on unconscious processes. *Proceedings of the National Academy of Sciences*, 89: 11113–11117.

Scoville, W.B. & Milner, B. (1957). Loss of recent memory after bilateral hippocampal lesions. *Journal of Neurology, Neurosurgery, and Psychiatry*, 20(1): 11.

Solms, M. (2013). The conscious id. *Neuropsychoanalysis*, 15(1): 5–19.

Squire, L.R. & Zola, S.M. (1997). Amnesia, memory and brain systems. *Philosophical Transactions of the Royal Society of London. Series B, Biological Sciences*, 352(1362): 1663–1673. doi:10.1098/rstb.1997.0148

Squire, L.R. & Zola, S.M. (1998). Episodic memory, semantic memory, and amnesia. *Hippocampus*, 8(3): 205–211.

Stern, D.N. (1994). One way to build a clinically relevant baby. *Infant Mental Health Journal*, 15(1): 9–25.

Tranel, D. & Damasio, A.R. (1990). Covert learning of emotional valence in patient Boswell. *Journal of Clinical Psychology and Experimental Neuropsychology*, 12: 27.

Tranel, D. & Damasio, A.R. (1993). The covert learning of affective valence does not require structures in hippocampal system or amygdala. *Journal of Cognitive Neuroscience*. doi:10.1162/jocn.1993.5.1.79

Tulving, E. (1972). Episodic and semantic memory. *Organization of Memory*, 1: 381–403.

Tulving, E. (1985). Memory and consciousness. *Canadian Psychology/Psychologie Canadienne*, 26(1): 1.

Tulving, E. (2002). Episodic memory: From mind to brain. *Annual Review of Psychology*, 53(1): 1–25.

Tulving, E. & Markowitsch, H.J. (1998). Episodic and declarative memory: Role of the hippocampus. *Hippocampus*, 8(3): 198–204.

Turnbull, O.H. & Evans, C.E.Y. (2006). Preserved complex emotion-based learning in amnesia. *Neuropsychologia*, 44: 300–306.

Wechsler, D. (1998a). *WAIS-III UK Administration and Scoring Manual*. London: Psychological Corporation.

Wechsler, D. (1998b). *WMS-III^{UK} Administration and Scoring Manual*. London: Psychological Corporation.

Wechsler, D. (2001). *Wechsler Test of Adult Reading - UK Adaptation (WTAR—UK)*. San Antonio: The Psychological Corporation.

Wilson, B.A. & Wearing, D., 1995. Prisoner of consciousness: A state of just awakening following herpes simplex encephalitis. In R. Campbell & M. A. Conway (Eds.), *Broken memories: Case studies in memory impairment* (pp. 14–30). Oxford: Blackwell Publishing

Winnicott, D.W. (1945). Primitive emotional development. *International Journal of Psychoanalysis*, 26: 137–143.

Winnicott, D.W. (1949). Hate in the counter-transference. *International Journal of Psychoanalysis*, 30: 69–74.

Winnicott, D.W. (1969). The use of an object. *International Journal of Psychoanalysis*, 50: 711–716.

Winnicott, D.W. (1986). Holding and interpretation. *International Journal of Psychoanalysis Library*, 115: 1–194. London: The Hogarth Press and the Institute of Psycho-Analysis.

Yeates, G. (2013). Towards the neuropsychological foundations of couples therapy following acquired brain injury (ABI): A review of empirical evidence and relevant concepts. *Neurodisability and Psychotherapy*, 1(1): 108–150.

Zellner, M.R. (2014). Preliminary steps toward a neurobiology of the repetition compulsion. *Modern Psychoanalysis*, 39(1): 1–25.

Chapter 10

Working with narcissism in psychotherapy with people with dementia

Richard Cheston

I Dementia

Dementia is an umbrella term used to describe a group of illnesses that reduce the ability of the brain to function. The most common of these illnesses is Alzheimer's disease, which, in the initial stages, is characterised by difficulties in establishing new, verbal memories, and by a gradual loss of fluency. However, the clinical signs and symptoms experienced by people with dementia vary widely: memory and perceptual impairments are characteristic of vascular dementia, while visual hallucinations, fluctuating cognition and movement problems, are common in dementia with Lewy bodies. Nevertheless, regardless of the exact presentation of symptoms, all forms of dementia are characterised by common factors: the illness is progressive, so that it gradually affects all areas of cognitive and behavioural functioning, and, at present, it is incurable.

In the UK, recent estimates suggest that there are between 670,000 and 800,000 people living with dementia (Matthews et al., 2013). This figure represents around 7% of the population who are aged over 65 and includes about 15,000 people from black or minority ethnic groups. Dementia primarily occurs in those aged over 65, with the incidence of dementia roughly doubling every six to seven years. Thus, while most people who have dementia are older, there were thought to be over 42,000 people with young-onset dementia (under the age of 65 years) in the UK in 2013. Although people with Alzheimer's disease can be prescribed medications such as Donepezil or Aricept, the impact of these drugs is limited, and while they may slow the rate at which people decline for a brief period, dementia cannot be cured.

2 Narcissism in people with dementia

Narcissism is typically referred to as existing on a spectrum or continuum ranging from people who display a few narcissistic traits to others who would meet the diagnostic criteria for a narcissistic personality disorder (McBride, 2008). Narcissists oscillate between states of high, often, grandiose levels of outward or explicit self-esteem and fragile states of shame, anguished depression and dysregulated affect in which their interior or implicit self is experienced as empty (Dimaggio et al., 2002; Horowitz, 1989; Young & Flanagan, 1998). Consequently, narcissists have a need for admiration or validation as well as a deep sense of entitlement, even though their achievements do not merit this. At the same time, however, narcissists are unable to deal with criticism, and their own hidden feelings of insecurity and shame are projected into others. Consequently, narcissists are themselves highly critical of others and attacking of those who challenge or undermine their external self.

The causes of narcissism are likely to be complex with multiple components (Paris, 2014), but have been associated with parenting styles that both overemphasise the child's specialness and yet involve excessive criticism with fears and failures being harshly responded to (Symington, 1993). During their childhood, a narcissist learns to see themselves and the world through a dual lens: both that they are special and that failure is intolerable. To experience failure or to acknowledge a fall from the special position risks being experienced as profoundly shameful – in which the self is threatened by feelings of worthlessness, failure, rejection and vulnerability. Consequently, the narcissistic child may hide their low self-esteem by developing a superficial sense of perfection and behaviour that shows a need for constant admiration – this is a false self (Modell, 1975).

Narcissists often struggle to recognise or to understand other people's emotions, and as well as disdaining those people that they feel are inferior to them, they typically have little compunction in abusing or exploiting any positions of power that appear (Kernberg, 1975). The relationship between the narcissist and those who are close to them, therefore, is often complex, as the narcissist's behaviour forces others into a position whereby they either allow themselves to be crushed and dominated or rebel in order to regain some control. When a narcissist feels that their importance has been brought into question, such insults to the self may lead to narcissistic rage. For Kohut (1972), narcissistic rage is related both to revenge and to the narcissists' need for total control or the world around them, including the wish to restore a sense of safety and to eliminate the threat to their self-esteem. For those around the narcissist, then, much of their behaviour may be motivated by the need to avoid puncturing the fragile bubble of the narcissist's self-esteem, and thus triggering their rage.

Given that a central feature of narcissism concerns the need of an individual to position themselves as perfect, and thus to reject any suggestion of fault or failure, it is not surprising that the association between narcissism and cognitive impairment, including dementia, has recently been explored (e.g. Poletti & Bonuccelli, 2011). In a prospective cohort study of 452 participants, narcissistic vulnerability traits were significantly associated with increased risk of Alzheimer's disease (Serrani, 2015). It has also been suggested that narcissism may influence adaptation to traumatic brain injury, typically being associated with poorer recovery (Barak, 2017). In these instances, brain injury serves as a severe narcissistic insult, which threatens self-worth and triggers distress. In particular, individuals with a history of pre-morbid narcissistic problems may have intensified problems in accepting and coping with the effects of brain injury (Klonoff & Lage, 1991).

3 Dementia and psychotherapy

Psychotherapy can often play an important role in helping patients adjust to a broad range of life-limiting and life-ending illnesses. The emphasis within psychotherapy on helping clients to resolve emotional threats, to take greater control over their lives and to find strategies to "live well" means that psychotherapy also potentially has much to offer within dementia care. Given the combination of powerful emotional responses to dementia (Aminzadeh, Byszewski, Molnar & Eisner, 2007) and the desire of most people to know about their illness (Ouimet, Dendukuri, Dion, Beizile & Elie, 2004), it is perhaps unsurprising therefore that psychotherapeutic approaches with people affected by dementia are becoming increasingly common. In a recent review of psychotherapy with people with dementia, Ada Ivanecka and I were able to identify 26 papers that had used controlled trials or repeated measured designs (Cheston & Ivanecka, 2016). We found that these papers described a broad mix of therapeutic modalities, lengths and settings, including two studies using psychodynamic interpersonal therapy (Burns et al., 2005; Carreira et al., 2008). In addition, a number of case studies and other reports of psychodynamic therapy exist (e.g. Balfour, 2014; Davenhill, 2007; Sinason, 1992).

At the same time, however, there are many challenges to adapting psychotherapy for this client group: not only is there the impact of the neurological impairment, but the emotional weight of a diagnosis and the residual social difficulties in talking about dementia can all make it difficult for clinicians to find ways to engage meaningfully with people affected by dementia. These barriers are likely to be further exacerbated by the lack of specialist support provided to people after they have received a diagnosis (Watts, Cheston, Moniz-Cook, Burley & Guss, 2014). The reality, then, is that while the role of psychotherapy is increasingly recognised, most people who are diagnosed with dementia will not be routinely offered access to any form of counselling, let alone psychodynamic therapy.

4 Threat, dementia and psychotherapy

Dementia represents a significant, potential threat to self not only because it is an incurable illness that involves a progressive decline ending ultimately in death but also because it is characterised by increasing dependency, the potential loss of identity and challenges to meaning and purpose. For these reasons, worries about developing dementia are one of the most significant fears of growing old (Kessler, Bowen, Baer, Froelich & Wahl, 2012). A potential role for psychotherapy with people with dementia, then, is to help people to engage with their experiences of dementia – and in particular with the psychological threat that dementia represents. For many people, the initial task is to find a way of putting a form of words to their experiences (Shotter & Gergen, 1989). One aspect of this use of language to frame their experiences comes in the use of terms such as "dementia" or "Alzheimer's Disease" (Cheston, 2013). While ostensibly this is a simple task, in practice it is often much harder. For instance, one study of awareness in people with dementia found that over a third of the 64 participants did not use a diagnostic label to refer to their symptoms (Clare, Quinn, Jones & Woods, 2016).

One way to think of this is to draw a parallel with the way in which many of the characters in JK Rowling's Harry Potter stories are too terrified of Lord Voldemort, the central villain, to refer to him directly and instead resort to euphemisms such as "he-who-must-not-be-named" or "the Dark Lord". Elsewhere I have argued that one reason for this reluctance to put a name or label to the illness of dementia arises from a fear that to do so will lead to a loss of internal control (Cheston, 2015). Many people with dementia describe facing just such a dilemma: either to engage with the emotional threat of dementia (and risk an escalation of their distress) or to avoid exploring those experiences (and risk the loss of control that arises from pushing away such knowledge). Within psychotherapy, expressions of this choice have been referred to as markers of a "fear-of-loss-of-control" (Honos-Webb, Lani &Stiles, 1999; Honos-Webb, Surko &Stiles, 1998). Amongst the different fears that further expression of the problematic material may lead to are fears of going mad, being excluded or rejected or being defeated. All of these concerns relate, fundamentally, to a fear of loss of control. For people with dementia, then, beginning to explore and put a name to their illness can be problematic. As one man in a psychotherapy group explained:

> Mr B: I find I've, I've got a great deal of moral uplift by coming here
>   Meeting you, listening to the way you do it
>   And I don't see the problem now
>   it frightened me, the problem of declining memory,
>   until I came here
>   and now I'm not frightened
>   (...)
>   _It frightened me_
>   _because I thought, well, I'm going mad, I'm going crazy_
>   What am I going to be like in another five years?
>   But now I realize that everybody is getting this problem
>   (quoted in Watkins et al., 2006)

The way in which this existential threat is experienced by people who are living with dementia is likely to differ. For narcissists, the increasing difficulties in carrying out the many different tasks that are part and parcel of everyday living may present specific challenges. In particular, these changes may be experienced in terms of a loss of control over not only their cognitive functioning but also in terms of a changing relationship with the social world. To admit to no longer being able to carry out simple tasks because of the diminishment of dementia is likely to be intolerable because such failures threaten the narcissist's heightened sense of their own self-worth. Similarly, even to acknowledge the diagnosis of dementia would threaten the fragile nature of their self-concept. I will now look at a case example of working with a woman with strong narcissistic tendencies to illustrate the potential impact of marital psychotherapy in easing adjustment and enhancing resilience.

5 Anna King: the need to be right even when you're wrong

Anna King was a 78-year-old retired medical secretary when she was referred to the memory clinic. She had four children and five grandchildren, and it had been her family who had persuaded her that she first talked to her General Practitioner (GP) about her memory difficulties. Anna had suffered a small stroke ten years before she was referred, but this did not cause significant memory difficulties. Anna's husband and two of her daughters confirmed that they had noticed her becoming more forgetful over the past few years – she could be muddled with facts and could not always recall what they had told her. They felt her problems were exaggerated if she was anxious or outside her usual routine.

After Anna's initial appointment at the memory clinic in September 2013, she was referred for a CT scan. She returned to the memory clinic in November to learn the results of the assessment and was told that the most likely diagnosis was one of mild cognitive impairment, as although there were some cognitive changes, these did not appear to be impacting significantly on her daily activities. Anna's scores on the assessment tool used in our clinic are shown in Table 10.1.

When Anna returned in 2014 for an annual follow-up appointment, her family emphasised that her cognitive impairments were having more of an impact on her ability to carry out normal daily activities. As her scores on the cognitive assessment tool had also deteriorated, Anna's diagnosis was altered to one of "memory impairment, probable early Alzheimer's Disease", and she was offered donepezil. A year later, in September 2015, Anna's cognitive and functional difficulties had remained stable, but her doctor at the memory clinic felt that it might be helpful for Anna and Philip, her husband, to work with a psychotherapist and referred her to me. According to the referral letter:

Table 10.1 Anna's cognitive and emotional assessment from 2013 to 2015

Test	Subtest	September 2013	November 2013	November 2014	September 2015
ACE-III	Orientation (max 18)	16*	15**	13**	15**
	Memory (max 26)	13**	11**	11**	6**
	Fluency (max 14)	11	12	9*	9*
	Language (max 26)	24	26	26	26
	Visuo-spatial (max 16)	14	13*	9**	11**
	Total (100)	78	77	68	67
Clock Drawing (max 5)		5	5	2	2
Picture Naming (max 10)		10	10	10	10
Geriatric Depression Scale (max 15)		3			
National Adult Reading Test		107			
Bristol Activities of Daily Living (max 60)			7	4	3

* Less than 5th percentile; ** less than 1st percentile.
max, maximum.

> Anna and Philip are both frustrated about her forgetfulness. She has varying levels of insight and sometimes gets stuck on the same thing in a conversation but is anxious about the diagnosis and is finding it hard to accept. Philip admits to having his own difficulties in adjusting to the situation ... He finds he now over-reacts when Anna gets muddled and forgetful with things.

I met Anna and Philip for the first time in October. Anna, herself, did not feel that she needed any help – or at any rate, no more help than any woman of her age, with a large family, would need. She joked that her family name was King – King by name and King by nature. Her description of her life positioned her as an independent and self-reliant woman. She told me that "I know that I can push to the back of my mind things that don't matter or which are irrelevant". There was also some sense of a slightly self-knowing and self-mocking narcissism when she told me "I can't be wrong, I have to be right – just like my father ... I don't like to be wrong. Ever!! (with emphasis)"; then she caught my eye, winked and laughed. Later, when describing the way in which her adult children had insisted that she come to the memory clinic, she said that they thought she was "doolally". Similarly, at the end of our session, when I told her that she could leave her tea cup, she joked that

I would think her a terrible woman to make a mess like this and not clear it up. She then apologised for taking my time up and added that she was sure I would go home and tell my wife that a stupid woman had wasted my time today.

I was struck by Anna's difficulties in acknowledging personal weakness and change. Her perceptions of me seemed to be coloured by defensive projections of her own unwanted self-traits onto others. If Philip gently suggested that she had made an error because of her memory, then Anna responded either by blaming him or by dismissing his concerns. Anna's response to her dementia therefore seemed to include a number of what Hotchkiss has described as the seven deadly sins of narcissism. First, she used elements of magical thinking to frame herself as a perfect, whilst projecting the shame of failure into others (Hotchkiss, 2008). Then, when her cognitive impairments were mentioned, she responded by reflating her sense of self-importance and diminishing or minimising Philip. At the same time, other elements of narcissism including arrogance, envy and bullying exploitation seemed to be minimal or absent.

During their childhood, a narcissist learns to see themselves and the world through a dual lens: both that they are special and that failure is intolerable. To experience failure or to acknowledge a fall from the special position risks being experienced as profoundly shameful – in which the self is threatened by feelings of worthlessness, failure, rejection and vulnerability. So Anna described a father who was punitive and critical: demanding and egotistical. It was from her father that Anna had learnt the phrases that she so often repeated during our sessions: "king by name, king by nature" and "always right, even when I'm wrong". For her father, his specialness was a matter of family pride – and Anna critically described how her siblings had deviated from this template of specialness.

At the same time, Anna's childhood involved a struggle with disability. She had been born with one leg significantly shorter than another and spoke both of courses of treatment in hospital and of the long time that she had spent wearing a leg brace or calliper. However, she emphasised that unlike her sister, she had never let disability stand in her way – she had always excelled. In this sense, Anna seems to have hidden her low self-esteem by developing a false self – a superficial sense of perfection and behaviour that also demanded admiration from others and especially from Philip.

A central aspect of narcissism, then, concerns the way in which the person relates to failure. As her Alzheimer's disease progressed, so the neurological impairment inherent in the illness reduced the range of daily activities that Anna could engage in: at first tasks like using the phone or keeping appointments were compromised, but steadily skills that were even more fundamental to her well-being, including driving their car or cooking, became threatened. Anna responded to the potential narcissistic injury to herself through a multi-layered strategy: first she claimed that she had chosen not to engage in these tasks, because she knew that Philip liked to do them; then she asserted that she still did all the jobs that she wanted to, and that nothing of significance had changed; finally, she rejected any implication from Philip's description of her life that could be taken as suggesting that she experienced problems.

In therapeutic terms, my aim was to find a way of helping Anna and Philip to talk together about those changes that had taken place. For Philip, it seemed important to be able to have a conversation with Anna in which she could, at least occasionally, acknowledge his role and her neediness. However, I was unsure whether this would be a useful strategy for Anna, who was engaged in warding off her diagnosis – not only did she insist that there was nothing wrong with her, but she avoided talking about her Alzheimer's disease. In our third session, therefore, I tentatively offered a reformulation to them both: I suggested that both Anna and Philip were being asked to address a painful issue – one of how their life had changed as they grew older. For some people growing old meant having a hip replacement, while for others it meant that their memory was worse. I said that this often led people to be angry with themselves for not being able to do all that they wanted to do, and that sometimes this anger spilled out. One way through this was to be able to forgive oneself for growing old.

The analogy between memory loss and needing a hip operation appealed to Anna – because these changes were more likely with age, even if they were not inevitable. We agreed to meet on a monthly basis to talk about how ageing had affected them both. In talking about how change affects people, so Anna found it helpful to reflect on her parents contrasting approaches to life: while she identified with her father's independent self-reliance, her experiences of her mother were of a more compassionate and forgiving person. Anna recalled how as a child she had hated the way in which her disability meant that her independence was constricted. It was her mother's compassion and tenderness at this time that touched her now.

The narcissistic defence, then, against failure and its implication of a shameful self of weakness, is to develop a false self of omnipotence. The artificiality of this false self may be experienced as something of a role, played out for public consumption. At times, Anna was able to position herself within a slightly self-knowing, self-mocking persona. If she felt safe within the sessions, for instance when her difficulties around living were constructed in a gentle way that did not directly confront her, then she tended to end discussion by delivering what was clearly something of a familiar catchphrase – "as you know, darling, I'm always right, even when I'm wrong".

A year into our work together, Anna reflected that as children, she and her brother and sister had been aware of her father's impossibility – that his determination to insist that he was right, even when he was wrong, was, in effect, more a reflection of his acting than of reality. She said her mother would come into the kitchen and "give one of those looks and say 'he's at it again'". I asked if it was like that with you and Philip, and Anna smiled while Philip gently laughed. This connection opened discussions up in two ways. First, Anna asserted that she would lose herself if she stopped arguing and asked Philip, "what sort of person would you prefer – someone who had character, who answered back and did things, or someone who just sat there, doing nothing except watch the TV all day". In turn, this led Philip to say that "it would be nice, even just once, if you could admit that you change your mind".

It also allowed us to think again about Anna's experiences of the memory clinic. She had found the assessment "embarrassing". I suggested that other people told me that they found being assessed made them feel stupid – to which Anna agreed that was what she had felt too. Shortly after this, Anna allowed Philip to talk about a cognitive stimulation therapy (CST) group that Anna attended as being for people with Alzheimer's disease. In response, Anna said to me: "it's a good thing for you, that there's people like me with this condition, otherwise you'd be out of a job". Later in this session, Anna again repeated the phrase "with my condition". When I reminded Philip and Anna of his remark about hoping that she might admit that she changed her mind, Anna then joked that she often said he should buy her a camera, so that she could play it back to him and prove that he was wrong. Philip replied, laughingly, that she would blame him and refuse to accept it. Anna joined in the joke and said that she would say he had bought the wrong camera.

5.1 Oscillating ambivalence

Although Anna rarely initiated a discussion about her dementia and did not use the terms "Alzheimer's disease" or "dementia" to refer to herself, nevertheless she continued to allow Philip or myself to do so without contradicting us or rejecting these labels. As our work progressed, then, she moved away from consistently rejecting any suggestion that her memory was less than perfect towards a more nuanced position. If her memory and other failures were empathically positioned within a broader context of ageing, then Anna would often allow herself to be framed as having dementia. At these times, she also became more accepting of her difficulties. She asserted that she still did things that she felt were important, such as cooking, but what she now thought was important had changed and had become more focussed. Anna said she was able to let things go now in a way that she wouldn't have done when she was younger. As the sessions progressed, so Anna also acknowledged how she had lost confidence in herself and found it increasingly difficult to go out. She said she was aware of becoming more introverted and now wanting to stay at home even when Philip encouraged her to go out. During one session, I asked Anna what the worst thing about having Alzheimer's disease was for her. She told me that it was the thought that she might become stupid, and when I asked her to tell me more about this, she replied that she meant it was being dependent, inactive and being looked after – the horror of not being able to do crosswords and puzzles, or of being like her cousin who was lying in bed and not being able to look after herself. This freeing up of her defences against change meant that Anna began to consider the future, and that she had decided to see a solicitor and to create a Power of Attorney. She felt strongly that if, in the future, she was unwell, then she did not want to be resuscitated as she would not want to be weak and cared for.

At other times, however, if the therapeutic dialogue had been more threatening, then Anna responded more bluntly to the narcissistic injury thrust on her by the dementia. At these times, she firmly claimed there was nothing wrong with her brain – that nothing had happened to change her or her memory. There was a clearer glimpse of her anger and the rage that both she and Philip mentioned – of how the TV remote control would be thrown across the sitting room or how furious she could become if she could not have her way.

Stiles has suggested that this movement between different positions or voices is a common element of therapy in people without cognitive impairments, especially when problematic material has been incompletely processed or assimilated (Stiles et al., 1990). This process of oscillating between approaching and retreating from the problematic diagnosis of dementia also occurs in people with dementia (Robinson, Clare & Evans, 2005). Indeed, it may be more pronounced for people with dementia precisely because their cognitive impairment makes it harder for people to hold onto therapeutic changes and gains. Thus, elsewhere this movement between dominant and problematic voices has identified in both couples (Lishman, Cheston & Smithson, 2016; Snow, Cheston & Smart, 2015) talking about their diagnosis and within-group psychotherapy (Cheston, Jones & Gilliard, 2004; Watkins, Cheston, Jones & Gilliard, 2006). Anna, then, continued to alternate between a dominant, false narcissistic self in which she voiced her omnipotence and a more problematic voice of change. In this latter position, she talked about her defences at one remove from them, rather than talking from within them.

5.2 Supporting a joint understanding

A central role of the therapeutic work was to offer support to Philip by seeing them together and by facilitating a joint dialogue about their life. The narcissist's behaviour forces others to either take the role of being crushed and dominated or rebel in order to regain some control. Throughout our work, Philip had a patient and enormously tolerant ability to manage Anna's grandiosity. For him, our monthly therapeutic contact allowed him an opportunity to talk about and to make sense of what was happening. He spoke about rediscovering Anna – that her dementia hadn't made her a different person; it hadn't changed how she was, just made her more intense. In one session, Philip said that he had seen a TV programme about dementia in which a woman said that "the condition doesn't define who you are". This, Philip said, described Anna perfectly – she was still the same woman she had always been, and while her dementia was just another obstacle in her life, it didn't define her.

Working jointly with the person with dementia and their partner has a number of potential therapeutic advantages: it facilitates communication, enhances empathy, and prompts the recall of problematic experiences. Working with Anna and Philip together allowed us to discuss Philip's dilemma when Anna forgot something: it seemed that either he drew her attention to this (and risked being blamed by her for it) or he did nothing (and risk being blamed when things went wrong). During one session, Philip described himself as an enabler, standing in the background and tactfully suggesting ideas rather than insisting on them. In response, Anna said that without Philip's help she might have ended up like her sister – not going out – staying on her own and getting worse, helpless and weak.

5.3 Reflection

It has been argued that an apparent lack of awareness amongst people affected by Alzheimer's disease may act as a form of emotional regulation (e.g. Clare, 2002; Clare et al., 2011). This warding off of awareness may allow people to retain a psychological balance in the face of the significant existential threat that dementia represents (Cheston, Christopher & Ismail, 2015). Consequently, narcissism has a dual role to play for people with dementia: a healthy level of narcissistic regard can enable people to resiliently acknowledge their dementia without being overwhelmed by this existential threat. However, when high levels of narcissistic defences lead to the creation of a false self that is unable to acknowledge even the slightest degree of cognitive impairment, then this can create difficulties both for the person themselves and for those around them. While Anna clearly fell back on her false self in which she continued to articulate a dominant voice of always being in the right, as we worked together, there were also clear indications that she was beginning to articulate some of the more problematic elements of dementia. In particular, she was clearly pained by the way in which her dementia made her feel stupid. At first, she could only articulate this indirectly, by projecting this fear into others. However, increasingly over the course of our work together, she began to acknowledge this more directly.

Nevertheless, in Stiles' terms, Anna continued to alternate between warding off her dementia and a vague awareness of it. One obvious impact of dementia is the difficulty in laying down new memories that it creates for people. Within the context of psychotherapy, this may translate itself into problems in holding onto insights, recalling significant events or implementing new strategies. Consequently, while a series of studies (Cheston, 1998; Cheston & Ivanecka, 2016) have shown that therapeutic change is possible for at least some people with dementia, it may well become harder for clients to hold onto new insights and ways of understanding themselves and their relationship to their dementia that is achieved within therapy.

Working with Philip has enabled him to develop his own narratives about Anna and her narcissism. In one session, he described how they were participating in a research study looking at quality of life of people with dementia. When Anna had been asked about the impact of dementia on her life, she continually joked and insisted again to the researcher that everything was well for her. Philip described how he felt that this jokiness was a defensive act – that it was too threatening for Anna to talk about her dementia. In doing this, he drew an analogy between Anna's difficulties in accepting the truth and Donald Trump. Just as Trump was always boasting and talking about fake news, so Anna, too, had her "alternative truths".

6 Summary

The reality of current dementia care is that while there has been significant progress in improving awareness of dementia symptoms and in achieving higher and more timely levels of diagnosis, there is often little recognition of the emotional challenge of dementia. Yet dementia acts as an existential threat onto which we project our worst fears: it is as if for each person who receives a diagnosis of dementia, the illness acts in the same way as Room 101 within George Orwell's *1984* – in which Big Brother's thought police confront prisoners with their worst nightmare, fear or phobia. Thus, for Anna, the worst aspect of dementia seemed to be the prospect of shame that comes with thoughts of being made "stupid". Consequently, as people with dementia begin to articulate the feared nature of the illness, so their levels of affect are likely to rise. For many people, this is experienced as signifying a potential loss of control – embodied in feelings of panic or distress as they move closer to their fears. Thus, as we help people to adjust to their dementia, so we may also begin to work with people who are frightened of a loss of emotional control.

The potential for psychotherapy in supporting this process of adjustment is considerable. However, the availability of therapy is still very limited, even if research in this area is steadily increasing and now stretches across most of the main therapeutic modalities (Cheston & Ivanecka, 2016). While the nature of the cognitive deficits inherent in dementia presents challenges, these do not in and of themselves mean that psychotherapy is impossible. Thus, the relative preservation of the amygdala compared to the hippocampus means that while it may be difficult to establish new memories, it may nevertheless still be possible to use therapy to help clients to emotionally process threatening material (Evans-Roberts & Turnbull, 2011). Moreover, in determining the capacity of a person to adapt to their dementia, so the social and personal resources that individuals have available to them are as important as the level and nature of the cognitive impairment in dementia. Where the personal resources available to people are thin, as is the case for those people who habitually fall back on narcissistic defences, then psychotherapy can play an important role in sustaining and enhancing their resilience. Given the significant potential for dementia to threaten the fragile bubble of self-importance that narcissists surround themselves with, psychotherapy can have both direct and indirect effects. Therapy can directly influence the ability of people to adjust to the illness, by enabling them to accommodate the problematic, threatening elements of dementia within a dominant, self-narrative of superiority. In addition, where a carer is also involved in the therapeutic process, then building a more sustainable discourse around dementia can also have indirect benefits.

References

Aminzadeh, F., Byszewski, A., Molnar, F. J., & Eisner, M. (2007). Emotional impact of dementia diagnosis: Exploring persons with dementia and caregivers' perspectives. *Aging and Mental Health, 11*(3), 281–290.

Balfour, A. (2014). Developing therapeutic couple work in dementia care: The living together with dementia project. *Psychoanalytic Psychotherapy, 28*(3), 304–320. https://doi.org/10.1080/02668734.2014.934524.

Barak, O. (2017). The impact of early childhood narcissistic injury on rehabilitation prognosis following mild traumatic brain injury in adulthood. *Neuropsychoanalysis, 19*(1), 1–25.

Burns, A., Guthrie, E., Marino-Francis, F., Busby, C., Morris, J., Russell, E., Margison, F., Lennon, S., & Byrne, J. (2005). Brief psychotherapy in Alzheimer's disease. *British Journal of Psychiatry, 187*, 143–147.

Carreira, K., Miller, M. D., Frank, E., Houck, P., Morse, J. Q., Dew, M. A., Butters, M. A., & Reynolds, C. F. (2008). A controlled evaluation of monthly maintenance interpersonal psychotherapy in late-life depression with varying levels of cognitive function. *International Journal of Geriatric Psychiatry, 23*(11), 1110–1113.

Cheston, R. (1998). Psychotherapy and dementia: a review of the literature. *British Journal of Medical Psychology, 71*, 211–231.

Cheston, R. (2013). Dementia as a problematic experience: Using the Assimilation Model as a framework for psychotherapeutic work with people with dementia, *Neurodisability and Psychotherapy, 1*(1), 70–95.

Cheston, R. (2015). The role of the fear-of-loss-of-control marker within the accounts of people affected by dementia about their illness: implications for psychotherapy, *Quaderni di Psicoterapia Cognitiva, 37*, 45–66. http://dx.doi.org/10.3280/qpc2015-037003.

Cheston, R., Christopher, G., & Ismail, S. (2015). Dementia as an existential threat: The importance of self-esteem, social connectedness and meaning in life, *Science Progress, 98*(4), 416–419. http://dx.doi.org/10.3184/003685015X14467423210693

Cheston, R., & Ivanecka, A. (2016). Individual and group psychotherapy with people affected by dementia: A systematic review of the literature, *International Journal of Geriatric Psychiatry, 32*(1), 3–31.

Cheston, R., Jones, K., & Gilliard, J. (2004). "Falling into a hole": Narrative and emotional change in a psychotherapy group for people with dementia, *Dementia: The International Journal of Social Research and Policy, 3*(1), 95–103.

Clare, L. (2002). Developing awareness about awareness in early-stage dementia the role of psychosocial factors. *Dementia, 1*(3), 295–312.

Clare, L., Marková, I. S., Roth, I., & Morris, R. G. (2011). Awareness in Alzheimer's disease and associated dementias: Theoretical framework and clinical implications. *Aging and Mental Health, 15*(8), 936–944.

Clare, L., Quinn, C., Jones, I. R., & Woods, R. T. (2016). "I don't think of it as an illness": Illness representations in mild to moderate dementia, *Journal of Alzheimer's Disease, 51*, 139–150. http://dx.doi.org/10.3233/JAD-150794.

Davenhill, R. (2007). *Looking into later life: A psychoanalytic approach to depression and dementia in old age.* London: Karnac Books.

Dimaggio, G., Semerari, A., Falcone, M., Nicolo`, G., Carcione, A., & Procacci, M. (2002). Metacognition, states of mind, cognitive biases and interpersonal cycles. Proposal for an integrated narcissism model. *Journal of Psychotherapy Integration, 12*(4), 421–451.

Evans-Roberts, C. E., & Turnbull, O. H. (2011). Remembering relationships: Preserved emotion-based learning in Alzheimer's disease. *Experimental Aging Research, 37*(1), 1–16.

Honos-Webb, L., Lani, J. A., & Stiles, W. B. (1999). Discovering markers of assimilation stages: The fear of losing control marker. *Journal of Clinical Psychology, 55*, 1441–1452.

Honos-Webb, L., Surko, M., & Stiles, W. B. (1998). *Manual for rating assimilation in psychotherapy: February 1998 version.* Unpublished manuscript. Department of Psychology, Miami University, Oxford, Ohio.

Horowitz, M. J. (1989). Clinical phenomenology of narcissistic pathology. *Psychiatric Clinic of North America, 12*, 531–539.

Hotchkiss, S. (2008). *Why is it always about you? The seven deadly sins of narcissism.* New York: Simon and Schuster.

Kernberg, O. (1975). *Borderline conditions and phatological narcissism.* New York: Jason Aronson.

Kessler, E., Bowen, C. E., Baer, M., Froelich, L., & Wahl, H. (2012). Dementia worry: A psychological examination of an unexplored phenomenon. *European Journal of Ageing, 9*(4), 275–284.

Klonoff, P. S., & Lage, G. A. (1991). Narcissistic injury in patients with traumatic brain injury. *The Journal of Head Trauma Rehabilitation, 6*(4), 11–21.

Kohut, H. (1972). Thoughts on narcissism and narcissistic rage. *Psychoanalytic Study of the Child, 27*(1), 360–400.

Lishman, E., Cheston, R., & Smithson, J. (2016). The paradox of Dementia: meaning making before and after receiving a diagnosis of dementia. *Dementia: The International Journal of Social Research and Policy, 15*(2), 181–203. http://dx.doi.org/10.1177/1471301214520781

Matthews, F. E., Arthur, A., Barnes, L. E., Bond, J., Jagger, C., Robinson, L., & Brayne, C. (2013). A two-decade comparison of prevalence of dementia in individuals aged 65 years and older from three geographical areas of England: Results of the cognitive function and ageing study I and II. *The Lancet, 382*(9902), 1405–1412.

McBride, K. (2008). *Will I ever be good enough? Healing the daughters of narcissistic mothers.* New York: Simon and Schuster.

Modell, A. H. (1975). A narcissistic defence against affects and the illusion of self-sufficiency. *The International Journal of Psychoanalysis, 56,* 275.

Ouimet, M. A., Dendukuri, N., Dion, D., Beizile, E., & Elie, M. (2004). Disclosure of Alzheimer's disease. Senior citizens' opinions. *Canadian Family Physician, 50*(12), 1671–1677

Paris, J. (2014). Modernity and narcissistic personality disorder. *Personality Disorders: Theory, Research, and Treatment, 5*(2), 220.

Poletti, M., & Bonuccelli, U. (2011). From narcissistic personality disorder to fronto-temporal dementia: A case report. *Behavioural Neurology, 24*(2), 173–176.

Robinson, L., Clare, L., & Evans, K. (2005). Making sense of dementia and adjusting to loss: Psychological reactions to a diagnosis of dementia in couples. *Aging and Mental Health, 9*(4), 337–347.

Serrani, D. (2015). Narcissism vulnerability as risk factor for Alzheimer's disease-a prospective study. *Austin Journal of Clinical Neurology, 2,* 1057.

Shotter, J., & Gergen, K. (1989). *Texts of identity.* London: Sage.

Sinason, V. (1992). *Mental handicap and the human condition: New approaches from the Tavistock.* London: Free Association Books.

Snow, K., Cheston, R., & Smart, C. (2015). 'Making sense' of dementia: Exploring the use of the MAPED to understand how couples process a dementia diagnosis, *Dementia: The International Journal of Social Research and Policy, 15*(6), 1515–1533. http://dx.doi.org/10.1177/1471301214564447

Stiles, W. B., Elliott, R., Llewelyn, S. P., Firth-Cozens, J. A., Margison, F. R., Shapiro, D. A., & Hardy, G. (1990). Assimilation of problematic experiences by clients in psychotherapy. *Psychotherapy, 27*(3), 411–420.

Symington, N. (1993). *Narcissism: A new theory.* London: Karnac Books.

Watkins, B., Cheston, R., Jones, K., & Gilliard, J. (2006). "Coming out with Alzheimer's disease": Changes in insight during a psychotherapy group for people with dementia. *Aging and Mental Health, 10*(2), 1–11.

Watts, S., Cheston, R., Moniz-Cook, E., Burley, C., & Guss, R. (2014). Post-diagnostic support for people living with dementia, in R Guss et al (on behalf of the Faculty of the Psychology of Older People, and in collaboration of people living with dementia and the Dementia Workstream Expert Reference Group). *Clinical Psychology in the Early Stage Dementia Care Pathway.* London: British Psychological Society.

Young, J. E., & Flanagan, C. (1998). Schema-focused therapy for Narcissistic Patients, In E. F. Ronninggstam (Ed.), *Disorders of narcissism: Diagnostic, clinical, and empirical implications* (pp. 239–267). New York: American Psychiatric Press.

Chapter 11

The role of language as a symbolic function to regulate emotion

Neurorehabilitation and psychodynamic treatment of a child with Landau-Kleffner syndrome

Manuel Fernández-Alcántara, Juan Francisco Navas, Francisco Cruz-Quintana, Christian Salas and Carolina Laynez-Rubio

1 Introduction

Psychoanalytic research outlines the relevance of early infant experiences on the constitution of the psychic apparatus and the genesis of neurosis and symptoms. Although Freud's initial work was focused on adults, he explored childhood experiences via the analysis of patients' dialogue and included these findings when defining some of his core theoretical concepts. After Freud, numerous psychoanalysts have specifically developed theoretical frameworks and interventions for children, while using a variety of techniques.

The same pattern can be found in the field of clinical neuropsychoanalysis, which has mainly studied adult patients suffering from acquired brain injury (ABI). Kaplan-Solms and Solms (2000) reported 12 cases of adults with lesions to different cortical areas. However, they did not describe any clinical cases of children. This is surprising since, in contrast with the study of adults, the study of children with ABI can offer important insight into how damage to specific brain structures can arrest or derail the normal development of certain mental abilities and neuropsychological domains (Eslinger, Flaherty-Craig, & Benton, 2004).

Neurological development in children has specific characteristics that need to be considered. During this period, the brain is more plastic, and some cognitive functions, such as language, attention and executive function, have not fully developed (Diamond, 2013). These neuropsychological functions are distributed in different networks along the brain and have different curves of development (Shonkoff et al., 2012). The developmental process is sensible to the influence of physical injury (e.g. ABI) and other risk factors (e.g. parenting styles, perinatal circumstances or socioeconomic status), which can influence both physical and psychological well-being (Bradley & Corwyn, 2002; Shonkoff, 2011). Considering these characteristics, neuropsychological interventions with children demand a different approach, such as the use of adapted assessment tools and therapeutic techniques (e.g. symbolic game).

In addition, the in-depth study of clinical cases of children with ABI from a neuropsychoanalytic perspective may shed light upon the functions of the mental apparatus affected by the brain lesion and the subjective state of the patient, as well as the necessary modifications associated with the psychoanalytic and neurorehabilitation treatment (Salas, Casassus, & Turnbull, 2017). Moreover, there is an important gap in the literature in neuropsychoanalysis regarding the report of clinical cases of children with ABI. For example, as far as we know, in the journal *Neuropsychoanalysis* we did not find any report with children, although there were experiences with adolescents (Kovacs, Stock, & Bernert, 2011) and also some reports in the Neuropsychoanalysis (NPSA) congresses (i.e. Akimoto et al., 2014).

The objective of the present chapter is to describe the assessment and intervention of a child diagnosed with LKS, using a neuropsychoanalytic approach, combined with neurorehabilitation treatment. The psychodynamic Lacanian treatment including initial interviews and the different phases of the treatment, the neuropsychological assessment and the neurorehabilitation treatment are fully described, along with the psychodynamic hypotheses that guide the entire intervention.

2 Landau-Kleffner epileptic syndrome: definition and clinical profile

LKS, also named acquired epileptic aphasia, is a rare neurodevelopmental disorder that appears in childhood. In 1957, Landau and Kleffner described it for the first time in a sample of six children with previously normal language acquisition, who developed an acquired aphasia. The etiology of LKS is still unknown, with most cases having a spontaneous origin without a defined cause (Caraballo et al., 2014; Duran, Guimaraes, Medeiros, & Guerreiro, 2009). In a recent review by Stefanatos (2011), the main features of LKS have been described as (1) a specific age of onset (around five years old), (2) normal premorbid development, (3) language impairment (i.e. aphasia), (4) epileptiform electroencephalographic (EEG) abnormalities, (5) behavioral disturbances and (6) altered cognitive functioning.

Aphasia, which is the main symptom in children with LKS, is characterized by a verbal auditory agnosia, a deficit where children cannot give a semantic meaning to environmental sounds or spoken language (Kuriakose, Lang, Boyer, Lee, & Lancioni, 2012). Importantly, auditory agnosia may also appear along with expressive aphasia (Caraballo et al., 2014), thus including articulatory difficulties, paraphasias, perseverative expressions, jargon, dysnomia, syntactic simplification and alterations in voice quality (Landau & Kleffner, 1957; Stefanatos, 2011).

Regarding epileptiform EEG abnormalities, the available evidence suggests that EEG alterations tend to appear in the temporal lobes – mainly unilaterally – and are directly associated with the language deficits observed in this population (Caraballo et al., 2014; Duran et al., 2009). The presence of seizures is also common (70–85% of children diagnosed with LKS) and can be easily controlled through medication (Caraballo et al., 2014). Studies using fMRI in this population are not common, and up until now, the results are not consistent. However, it has been noted that a decreased metabolism in the temporal lobes and volume reduction in superior temporal structures in both hemispheres can be observed in children with LKS (Ramanathan, Ahluwalia, & Sharma, 2012; Takeoka et al., 2004).

The behavioral disturbances, and their probably related altered cognitive functioning, observed in children with LKS are impulsivity, distractibility, cognitive rigidity, hyperactivity and aggressive behaviors (Caraballo et al., 2014). Interestingly, some studies have suggested that children with LKS can present symptoms that are often related to the autism spectrum disorder (ASD), such as difficulties in the processing of social information, lack of eye-gaze contact, social isolation and repetitive behaviors (Ballaban-Gil & Tuchman, 2000). These similarities may be related to the areas of the brain with abnormal electric activity. Additionally, research is pointing to the possibility that some children diagnosed with ASD, who have previous symptoms involving the loss of language and seizures, may have a non-diagnosed LKS (Deonna & Roulet-Perez, 2010). In fact, the term "epileptiform autistic regression" includes children who present language impairment, problems to socialize and to communicate and cognitive deficits (Mulas, Hernández, & Morant, 2001).

The subjective experience of children diagnosed with LKS and their families deserves some consideration. A recent case study of a 21-year-old young adult used a qualitative methodology to explore the main problems and challenges faced by these patients (Wairungu, 2015). Parents, medical staff and teachers identified intense feelings of anxiety and frustration related to the appearance of aggressive (verbal and nonverbal) behaviors. Parents also reported economic, social and support issues, which are in line with existing evidence found in parents of children who have been diagnosed with other types of disability (Fernández-Alcántara et al., 2013, 2015, 2016).

Rehabilitation in LKS is an under-investigated topic. Some clinical cases (Sieratzki, Calvert, Brammer, David, & Woll, 2001) have suggested the value of using alternative communication methods (nonverbal communication) that are not directly based on language (e.g. use of visual material at school), as well as the potential benefit of employing intensive speech therapy and behavioral strategies to manage disrupting behaviors (e.g. using reinforcers, response cost or overcorrection) (Kuriakose et al., 2012).

3 Case description

R is a boy who was six years old when he arrived for a consultation. He began to show epileptic seizures when he was four years old. Previously, he had no significant health problems and his biopsychological development occurred without difficulties. At that time, R was diagnosed with partial epilepsy. Nevertheless, the pharmacological treatment (the antiepileptic medication Depakine®) employed to manage the symptoms failed, and R's symptomatology worsened, while his EEG records were deteriorating progressively.

During the next two years, R showed a steep decline in language and motor abilities. He gradually lost his capacity to speak, to play and to perform previously learned routines (e.g. getting dressed, brushing his teeth), and his interaction with the environment (family and school peers) was drastically reduced. Therefore, he was severely impaired in his everyday functioning, and he became a burden to his family. The magnitude of such impairment made his mother quit her job in order to take care of him. R's mother was the only person capable of soothing him during the epileptic seizures. R also lived with his father and a ten-year-old brother. R's father worked most of the time and appeared rather disengaged from R's care.

The diagnosis of LKS was given two years after the onset of symptoms. The pharmacological treatment was modified by adding Clobazan® and ACTH®, and he was referred for psychological assessment and treatment to the Unit of Clinical Psychology and Neuropsychology, at San Cecilio Clinical Hospital in Granada, Spain.

3.1 Initial interviews

R's mother held him up and helped him walk when they attended the first session. His movements were unstable and disorganized. Although signs of tiredness in his mother were observable, she spoke to him with patience and with warm affection. She told the analyst (CLR) that she had witnessed during the previous two years a physical and psychological deterioration in R. During that time, she felt as if she did not receive a proper explanation of the cause of her son's illness, nor clear information of the ineffectiveness of the previous treatments. Nevertheless, the new pharmacological treatment seemed to have reduced R's epileptic seizures, but she did not observe a significant improvement in most of his impairments (e.g. R could not speak, had difficulties with sphincter control and could not eat by himself), and his behavior had become even more problematic (e.g. outbursts of anger or squeals without identifiable purpose).

After the first interview, three assessment sessions were scheduled. During these, the analyst observed the following pattern of behaviors: R could not speak with intelligible words; he did not focus his attention on any specific thing/task; he moved from one side of the room to the other, throwing objects and toys he found in his way without touching or manipulating them in detail; he did not show any sign of understanding instructions from the analyst, neither looking at her nor even paying attention to her – except during situations when he got angry. In those episodes of rage, R reacted with bursts of laughter and hitting the analyst or his mother, while observing their reactions. During these recurring events – unlike in other situations – R was more able to control his actions and physical movements. His behavior was not influenced by the presence or absence of his mother, although he seemed a little bit calmer when she was with him.

From the initial interviews, and based on clinical observations, the analyst identified a series of symptoms and impairments in different domains:

1   *Language*: R could only emit screams and non-articulated sounds. He reacted to the different tones of voices but did not understand the verbal content of the message. He was not able to follow simple orders.
2   *Psychomotricity*: The main symptom was hyperkinesia. R could not tolerate to remain in a closed room/environment and tended to move restlessly. He became anxious when such hyperkinetic activity was limited. Nevertheless, R needed his mother's hand in order to walk without falling. A series of stereotyped movements were also identified, such as balancing and hand clapping.
3   *Symbolic play*: All manifestations of symbolic play were absent. R touched, threw or hit objects and toys, but he did not explore them or gave them a functional use. In addition, he did not imitate the analyst behavior or initiate any kind of play interaction during the sessions.
4   *Social relationships*: He had problems with eye gaze (R did not look at other people, with the exception of the angry episodes described above), and he could become aggressive in most social interactions. These issues, along with the other impairments, had contributed to his social isolation, even with his brother.

Considering the clinical profile of R, the analyst concluded the existence of an acquired aphasia with autistic regression and significant neuropsychological deficits that needed an in-depth assessment.

4 Psychodynamic hypothesis

Based on the initial observations, the following hypotheses were formulated at the beginning of the psychodynamic treatment:

1   The brain damage experienced by R, which was reflected on his EEG, affected his bodily organization and sense of identity. Following Freud (1923), we consider that the *I* (*ego*) is primarily based on a bodily experience. If the unconscious image of the body is not well established

or there are problems with it, corporal and emotional symptoms may appear (Dolto, 2014; Nasio, 2007).

2   R's aggressive behavior was (a) an expression of his intense anxiety and (b) a form of establishing a connection with the world (Lacan, 1948) (when he behaved aggressively, he looked at the therapist and laughed). This is important, because R had been isolated from his world due to his motor and speech problems.

3   The aggressive behavior was considered as the result of a mark, a trace of the traumatic experience of losing his abilities and, at the same time, his way to interact with the environment. On the other hand, observing and laughing at others during an aggressive episode could have been the repetition of a traumatic experience (Freud, 1914). This repetition was used as a way to control his anxiety by projecting it outside/externally. Watching other people suffering (due to his behavior) could transform the unpleasant feeling into something pleasant as in the Freudian Fort-Da (Freud, 1920).

4   These aggressive episodes could be considered as the main expression of R's subjectivity. This fact seems to indicate the possibility of an analytic work and of establishing a transference relationship. It was expected that therapy could facilitate the reconstruction of R's identity and regulation of his drives (*trieb*).

Given the Lacanian approach used for the analytic treatment, the clinical hypotheses were considered as possible questions related to the conceptual and clinical perspectives of the analyst. Lacan (1964) named "desire of the analyst" as the motivations and questions that guide the interventions of the analyst, beyond trying to do "the good" for the patient, or the analyst's own feelings and emotions. When working with patients with important language impairments, or when there is no demand (like in autistic structures), the classical analytic setting requires adjustments. In this case, the desire of the analyst became an active instrument to set the transference. In addition, and following Lacan's works on aggression (Lacan, 1948), the aggressive responses of R were considered as his only emotional connection with the environment and a potential vehicle to establish the analytic transference.

5 Treatment

First, an initial psychodynamic treatment was implemented to develop the transference and social bond. Second, the psychodynamic treatment was complemented with a neuropsychological rehabilitation, based on a previous neuropsychological assessment performed when R's initial main symptoms decreased.

The psychodynamic treatment considered two types of interventions – that were implemented at the same time – by means of which the analyst put herself in the place of R and gave him both words and an object to direct his aggressive drive. Both strategies aimed at establishing the transference between R and the analyst (Lacan, 1958).

1   *Naming and interpreting R's actions/behaviors and emotions in order to symbolize them* (Freedman & Russell, 2003). Examples of these interventions were: "It seems that you're angry because you were able to speak before and now you can't say what you want" and "You can also say and do things". The goal of these interventions was to facilitate emotion regulation through the use of language (from a symbolic perspective), making the analyst present by means of the verbalization of R's subjective experience. The rationale behind this technique was that the verbal expression of his feelings could help him to separate from them and not get dragged into behaving in this particular way.
2   *Proposing an activity/game to redirect and elaborate the aggressive drive.* The objective of this intervention was to introduce a specific object or game that could be used as a mediator and a container of R's feelings.

5.1 Psychodynamic treatment from month 1 to 12: verbalizing anger

The beginning of treatment sessions was extremely difficult as R constantly wanted to leave the room. He did not respond to the analyst's questions in any way and was often irritated and angry. Although there were many toys and games in the room, none of them captured his attention, and he picked them up and threw them immediately. When R behaved angrily, the analyst interpreted his behavior: "It seems that you're angry because you were able to speak before and now you can't say what you want". R did not respond to this intervention. However, the objective of such an interpretation was to verbalize his subjective experience.

A game based on the construction–destruction of blocks was proposed to R: the analyst built towers and then teared them down. Initially, R participated in the game by tearing down the tower. Surprisingly, he uttered sounds and grunts of satisfaction. A similar approach was used in order to verbalize R's subjective experience: "You like to destroy, to tear down. Where is the tower? Who tore it down? What have you done?", "Do you want to play again?". The first observed effects of these interventions were that R began to pay attention and focus on the activity of tearing down the tower.

As the treatment moved forward, R began to enjoy the game of the tower. He looked for it when he went into the consultation room, and he was able to focus on it for long periods of time (he could spend the whole session playing repeatedly this game). In the ninth month of interventions, the game became more complex. R began to build towers that were progressively taller and his behavior changed with the game. He delayed the act of tearing down the tower, and sounds and grunts changed into interjections ("uy") and words ("yes", "no", "almost"), which were intertwined with looks and laughs directed to the analyst. The analyst interpreted this behavior: "It nearly fell, you almost tore it down!" or "What happened? Where is the tower?". The game continued for the next 15 sessions, and the language of R gradually improved. He began to use well-constructed and articulated sentences ("almost down" or "it's about to fall"), which seemed to indicate that he was recovering previous learned grammatical structures.

Progressively, by the end of the treatment sessions R began to say "No" – a verbalization that was accompanied by the refusal of leaving the room. The analyst understood this as an expression of intense interest for the game and a difficulty to emotionally tolerate its ending. She started symbolizing the idea that activities could end and continue in another moment: "We will continue playing next week", she said. Although it did not seem that R initially understood such interpretations, little by little he seemed more able to tolerate the end of the sessions and to leave the room voluntarily, while complaining. The analyst also began to offer R reminders (5 or 10 minutes before), when the end of the session was close, so he could prepare himself for such transition.

A variant of the tower game was introduced by the analyst. The game involved a doll that R placed on chair at the top of the tower. R tried to balance the doll while repeating phrases such as "The chair...almost down" and "they fall, bother". The analyst offered the following interpretation: "You like to do difficult things". R replied to this by saying, "Difficult, yes, it does not fall". An interesting question here is, why did R introduce a chair and a doll in the game? We could hypothesize that perhaps R projected himself on the doll, in order to portray a problem caused by the LKS: the loss of balance. Perhaps by balancing the doll at the top of the tower, he was actively controlling such loss. The analyst offered this interpretation to R ("If the doll fell from the chair, he's going to get hurt" or "The doll is afraid of falling...He could stand still!"), but apparently it had no emotional impact on him. R continued to make general comments about the tower such as "Uy, almost down", "it's difficult" and "it seems that it's going to fall", without elaborating the personal meaning of the game. Nevertheless, he tolerated the introduction of another person in the tower game, namely, an interesting change in the relationship with the analyst. At this time, R was able to enounce phrases in first person ("I can") and phrases oriented to the other ("Look, it does not fall" or "Did you see? It has fallen").

From a theoretical point of view, it is possible to consider that R projected himself not only into the doll but also into the tower itself. The mechanism of projection indicates that the imaginary order is being established. For Lacan, the three orders (imaginary, symbolic and real) are the ones that structure human subjectivity. This could be considered as a milestone in R's development, because he could not manifest this register in his emotional interactions or linguistic expressions. In other words, the game could be understood as a representation of R's anguish of his falling and disintegration as well as a reflection of his subjective experience of physical impairments. It can be argued that R used the game to face both the physical (motor impairment) and psychological (anxiety and mental disorganization) consequences of the traumatic event. By maintaining a physical and psychological equilibrium, R was able to re-organize his self-image and identity (Maleval, 2011).

These interventions were the beginning of the establishment of a solid relation of transference between R and the analyst. The position of the analyst was similar to those cases of autism, in the sense that she acted as *partenaire* (partner), becoming an alive and bearable object to help the child develop his own language and subjective position (Grollier, 2015). This point of inflexion in the treatment may be explained following the Freudian logic of the Fort-Da (Freud, 1920). The child transforms the unpleasant feeling into a pleasant one using an object (e.g. the tower). The tower could be considered as a transitional object (Winnicott, 1982) that serves to master the anguish. The continuous repetitions of a pair of signifiers that represent the presence–absence (tower–no tower) which become signified by words (interpretations by the analyst) allow the symbolization and the representation (Slimobich et al., 2002). As a consequence, the disorganized hyperkinetic and aggressive behavior decreased, along with an improvement of the language and social bond.

This subjective movement can also be explained by the Freudian distinction between "word-representation" and "thing-representation" (Freud, 1915). Thing-representations are related to impressions from the Unconscious, the primary process and the *trieb*. When these representations are activated, they can provoke the subject into directly acting the same unconscious repetitive behavior, without any possibility of symbolic regulation (Bernardi, 1978). Therefore, thing-representations will be directly associated with the *jouissance* of the Subject (see Dimitriadis, 2017, for a recent review). On the contrary, as R began to use word-representations (related to the use of this initial pair of signifiers), the anxiety and emotions associated with the representation can be symbolized (Luria, 1978).

5.2 Neuropsychological assessment: beyond language impairments

The neuropsychological assessment took place one year after R was diagnosed with LKS, as the severe impairments of R did not allow us to do it before. This assessment was performed by means of modified tasks from standardized tests or *ex professo* tasks, due to the aggressive behavior in response to instructions or changes in his activities. Considering R's cognitive difficulties and behavioral problems, the assessment required almost three months.

It was conducted following a flexible battery approach, in order to assess the main brain functions, but with task selected based on the idiosyncratic characteristics of the patient (for a more detailed explanation of this approach, see Kreutzer, Caplan, & DeLuca, 2011). The starting point for R's assessment was his preferred game (the game of the towers) and other activities that did not generate negative emotional reactions. Besides, alternative games were gradually introduced trying to widen/expand the features of the assessment.

The first two sessions were aimed at establishing a positive relationship between R and the examiner (JFN) and just consisted in building and destroying towers in the same way that he used to do. Every single attempt from the examiner to introduce any change in the game produced intense negative reactions from R. From the third session, aggressive responses to any intervention decreased, allowing a better involvement of the examiner in the game. Likewise, although R continued having a certain resistance to changes in what he liked to do, alternative activities were tolerated during short periods of time in every session. Thus, the assessment was aimed at determining R's level of impairment in (1) language comprehension and visuo-perceptual abilities, (2) visual and verbal memory and (3) executive functions.

5.2.1 Language comprehension and visuo-perceptual abilities

These areas were jointly assessed using a modified version of the Token Test (De Renzi & Vignolo, 1962). Thus, a new game was proposed by the examiner to R: to just touch or manipulate the blocks of his towers. R has to follow several verbal instructions, such us "touch the green block" or "put the green block over the yellow one". The examiner increased the level of difficulty in the instructions until R committed several consecutive failures. It was observed that R was able to identify objects and follow simple instructions, yet he failed following instructions with complex adverbs, such as "instead" (e.g. "instead of touching the blue block, touch the red one").

5.2.2 Visual and verbal memory

The assessment of verbal memory span was performed using a "running errands" task, in which R had to repeat messages with different levels of complexity to his mother (e.g. "you have to bring a cup tomorrow"), who was waiting in an adjacent room. After that, the examiner checked what information he gave to his mother. When three elements were introduced in the message (e.g. a cup, a car and a pen), intrusions or elements with no relation with errands appeared.

Visual memory span was assessed by asking R to remember the location of objects (e.g. car toys) that were hidden in front of him. R failed locating four cars. He often tried to locate them in places where previously other cars had been hidden or in new locations that had not been used before.

5.2.3 Executive functioning

5.2.3.I VISUAL WORKING MEMORY

This function was assessed using a modified version of the Corsi Test (Kessels, Van Zandvoort, Postma, Kappelle, & De Haan, 2000). By means of pictorial material that R was capable of identifying (i.e. children's books drawings), the examiner asked him to touch the elements in a reverse way of what he had previously done. R performed three consecutive mistakes when he had to manage four elements.

5.2.3.2 INHIBITION

The capacity to inhibit impulse responses was assessed through a classic go/no-go task (Torralva, Roca, Gleichgerrcht, López, & Manes, 2009). To discard the influence of language difficulties, comprehension of the instructions was checked by practicing three consecutive go trials, "when I hit the table once, you hit it too", and three no-go trials, "when I hit it twice, you do not". R performed this practice with no mistakes. However, during the task (go/go/no-go/go/no-go/no-go/no-go/go/go/no-go), R failed specifically in the no-go trials, namely, in the times that R should inhibit the motor response. He always hit the table.

5.2.3.3 COGNITIVE FLEXIBILITY

A variant of the Wisconsin Sorting Card Test (Grant & Berg, 1948) was used to assess this function. A first step to reach this assessment was the inclusion of a card game, in which a deck (i.e. cards with geometric-colored pictures) was split in half, and both participants have to show at the same time one of their cards. If the cards were exactly the same, they had to compete to catch a wooden totem, located in the middle of the table, and the winner got one point. This game became one of R's preferred games.

The assessment of cognitive flexibility was performed with an alternative of this game. Thus, the examiner drew a card and R had to match that card following a prefixed rule but unknown to him (i.e. first, match it by color until he reached ten hits, and after that, match it by shape). When he chose well, the therapist said, "yes", and they had to compete between them in order to catch the totem. When he failed, the therapist asked him to try again. R needed 16 attempts to reach ten successes. When the rule changed (and the correct answer became to match the cards by shape), R achieved just three hits in 25 attempts; namely, he chose perseveringly to match the cards by color. The task was interrupted because of the negative emotional responses triggered by these failures.

It is relevant to keep in mind the limitations of this assessment protocol. For instance, as we employed modified or *ex professo* tasks, it was not possible to compare R's performance with a normative sample. There were many factors that prevented a systematic application of the assessment (e.g. emotional reactions). In addition, the lack of information regarding R's premorbid cognitive functioning – beyond R parents' description of a normal development before the epileptic seizures – made extremely difficult to estimate the level of cognitive deterioration generated by the LKS.

However, the information obtained by this neuropsychological exploration had a relevant clinical value. It allowed the identification of the most markedly impaired areas of cognitive functioning, and thus helped to design the neurorehabilitation interventions. Other than the language problems – typically observed in children with LKS – and from moderate to high impairments in memory and visuo-perceptual ability, inhibitory failures and cognitive inflexibility were the main features of R's neuropsychological functioning. These impairments could underlie, on the one hand, the observed pattern of uncontrolled emotional reactions and, on the other hand, the extreme adherence/perseverance to certain routines (e.g. to play the same game constantly without changes, namely, to build and to shoot down towers) and the difficulty to understand the reversibility of certain facts (e.g. activities can end and can continue in other times).

5.3 From month 15 to 24: neuropsychological rehabilitation, improving inhibition and flexibility

Neuropsychological rehabilitation began after the fifteenth month of treatment (performed by JFN). It was implemented in parallel to the psychodynamic treatment (one session per week) and was based on the findings from the neuropsychological assessment and the evolution observed during psychotherapy. By considering the relevance of deficits in inhibition and flexibility, the rehabilitation efforts tackled specifically these areas.

Inhibition was trained through different games suggested by the therapist, once R accepted him and his involvement in the dynamic of clinical sessions (this process was gradual during the three previous months; see Section 5.3). One of the games consisted in passing a balloon. In the first trials during the first session, R exploded with joy by shouting, hitting the balloon with excessive strength and dropping it to the ground, squirming and laughing. In that moment, the therapist stopped the game and verbalized R's emotional state, confronting at the same time with the consequences that his behavior produced: "It seems that you like it very much, but you have forgotten to speak. Now, I do not understand what I have to do". The game started again when R said with words what he wanted: "like playing". The therapist repeated the same message – that is, to interpret what happened to R and what the therapist was going to do in those moments – every time such emotional burst happened. At the end of the first session, R repeated in every single time verbalizations such as "I like" or "Glad I am".

In the second session, a new rule was introduced: if the therapist was not able to reach the balloon, because R hit it with excessive strength, R had to pick it up. The first time that it happened, R grunted and shouted. The therapist interpreted these states and pointed out that he could speak and he would be glad to know what was happening to him. Then, R answered with a monosyllable: "no", "wrong". The game did not resume until R had caught the balloon. In this session, most of the times R hit the balloon with excessive strength and the delay to pick it up was high, during around two to three minutes. In those moments, the therapist was still putting into words the negative emotional states of R (e.g. R's grunts and shouts). It was not until the fifth session when the game became more fluid, showing an important decrease in the application of strength to the balloon and a in the frequent negative emotional reactions to failures, along with an increase in R's verbalizations during the game.

Another example of a game aimed at training inhibition was a modification of the card game used to assess flexibility. The competition for a wooden totem when the pair of cards showed were similar in their color (for a more detailed explanation of this game, see Section 5.2.3.3) – it is worth noting that in a second stage, this game was also used to develop flexibility. The component of inhibition in this game was introduced through a rule which penalized (losing one point) commission errors, that is, to catch the totem when the cards showed were not similar. During the first three sessions, these commission errors were highly frequent, and every single time R lost a point, he burst into anger. The therapist took advantage of those moments to verbalize R's emotional states. R began to inhibit to a greater extent the preponderant response of catching the totem during the fourth session. It was only after the 13th session that R obtained a total positive score. Although R improved in his capacity to inhibit such behavior, the motor response was triggered most of the time (i.e. he began the movement with his arm although at the end he retracted to catch it).

Once the capacity to inhibit motor responses had increased, another variation was included to train flexibility. The criterion to match cards could change; that is, sometimes cards should be matched by color, while other times by shape. The modifications of the rule were always announced and its frequency increased during the following sessions. Perseverative errors decreased progressively, although in the 20th session (the last session specifically focused in neurorehabilitation) they still happened with certain frequency. It is important to note that the motor tendency to catch the totem never disappeared completely.

5.4 From month 24 to present date: psychodynamic treatment

Two years into the treatment, the game of the tower was still central in R's sessions. However, R began to spontaneously add variations to the game (further than those suggested by the therapist in previous stages), such as lining up cars and moving them around the tower while describing what was happening: "The yellow one (car) did not fall. Now the white car...almost". R played the same game over and over again, with little modifications. Sometimes the tower could stand in one piece, sometimes it fell.

After certain time, R began to refer to cars as if they had animated properties; they could look at places, they were boring and they enjoyed specific positions on the line, among other things. Thus, cars became characters in R's narrative, a narrative often concerned about cars' movements, interactions and feelings. More interestingly, R began to use comments that relatives had addressed to him, as scripts of the interactions that occurred between cars. For example, R was usually being told that he was boring because he always made the same drawings, sang the same songs or had the same stereotypies. In consequence, "boring" was a recurrent characteristic of cars:

R: The ambulance is boring, it always does the same thing...Do you see? Does it want to be first?

R: The yellow car is looking at the taxi...It's looking to you now...it's looking to me, do you see how is looking at me? It is so boring (the car)!

A: Why is that car looking at me?

R: This car is boring. Tell him to not to look to yourself.

A: Now the car can't see me, because I've changed my place.

R: It's looking at you, do you see?

R: It (the car) wants to go first, always want to go first, this white ambulance is boring, always the same.

A: The ambulance is not always the first; there are other cars that can be first.

R: It doesn't want; it always wants to be the first.

R: The taxi is tired of the yellow car; it (the yellow car) is boring.

A: Maybe he wants to be his friend.

R: But it's boring. Now is going to drive near the tower. Almost down!

A: If it doesn't care, it can tear the tower down. If the tower falls it will lose.

R: He's not careful, almost down! Look! It is going to tear it down!

R: The yellow car is looking at the green car. It doesn't stop. Do you see? They (the cars) are looking at me. Leave me. It doesn't stop. They are also looking at you (to the analyst)...the white ambulance is really boring.

A: They look, but they do not talk, they can't speak. You and I can speak, we could ask and tell what is happening, but the cars can't do it.

R: Yes, I can speak. He's looking at me... bother!

Compared to games developed in earlier phases of the treatment, where R only repeatedly represented the falling and reconstruction of an object (the tower), we can identify here a more elaborated form of symbolic play. Now, the child is both the narrator and the audience, and the transitional object (the tower) works as a symbolic element that organizes the performance; all the scenes take place around it. In other words, the game has evolved from a presence–absence duality (Fort-Da) to a more elaborated and symbolic interaction. It is possible to hypothesize that the use of the Fort-Da allowed R to turn unpleasant feelings into pleasant ones and to introduce a basic structure of language (a pair of signifiers: tower–no tower). Using these two signifiers R slowly began, as a Subject of the language (in Lacanian terms), to tell stories and to develop a narrative about the cars – and himself.

The last fragment (F5), however, deserves to be considered apart because of how it introduces interactional elements (gaze). In R's narrative, cars are looking at each other, at the analyst and himself. It seems like a network of gazes that introduce the narrator and the audience in the scene. The presence or appearance of R in the scene (as a Subject) is only made when the cars are looking at him (Lacan, 1956, 1964). When speaking about Subject in Lacan, we are referring to the Subject of the Unconscious, which is not equivalent to the ego. This entity is an effect of the language and is essentially divided (Evans, 1996), being an indirect effect of the signifier (see the classic definition of Subject proposed by Lacan: "the subject is that which one signifier represents to another signifier", cited in Fink, 1995). At this moment R appeared able to interact with the analyst, answer her questions and verbalize his subjective experience instead of discharging through aggressive behavior: "No, it has not ended. A little bit...Uff! You're boring!".

At this point of the treatment, R had significantly improved at school. He had a diary that helped him to know the date and remember his activities. Teachers reported that R was able to quickly learn concepts as well as showing progress in reading and writing. Improvement in language skills was also reported by teachers despite still presenting minor deficits in verbal fluency. Considering such progress R's parents and teachers decided to include him in an ordinary school within a specific education classroom. This decision was supported by the analyst and the neuro-pediatrician of the hospital, because it would allow R to share time and space with other children allowing him to further improve language skills and establishing new emotional relationships.

5.5 Present moment

Three years after beginning the interviews R continues attending psychodynamic treatment (with CLR). There are sessions when he wants to go back to his previous games (the tower and the cars), but he quickly gets bored. The analyst continues interpreting his behavior: "Now you're older, the time passes and you're not the same than before". R answers with irritation: "Of course, you believe that you know everything, but you don't". R often moves away from old games and explores logic stories, memory games or board games. At school R appears to be able to tolerate the presence of other children, although he still lacks appropriate social skills to fluidly interact with his peers, often needing an adult to mediate such interactions. For example, R can easily participate in games and activities directed by an adult, but have more difficulties when he speaks with children of his own age. Currently R is working in small groups (with four to six children) to develop his social skills. The aggressive and violent behavior has disappeared, although he sometimes reacts with anger (that he expresses verbally: "Let me alone"). The hyperkinesia has also been reduced, showing only some mannerisms and repetitive behavior when he feels anguish. R is particularly sensible to situations when he loses in a game or when he becomes frustrated by an activity. Academically, R can read and write and has learned how to make the basic algebraic operations and his working memory capacity has augmented.

6 Discussion

We have presented how an integrative intervention, including Lacanian psychodynamic treatment and neuropsychological rehabilitation, may be useful in the case of LKS. In addition, we have outlined several mechanisms and theoretical aspects that may be useful in the study of early acquired brain damage and in the understanding of psychic functions.

During the course of treatment, initially R's motor symptoms improved quickly after the modification of the medication. Through the psychodynamic treatment and neuropsychological rehabilitation, there was an improvement in his language and behavior, and executive functions were also increased. By the end of the treatment, R was capable to read and utter complex sentences. This change may be a reflection of the plasticity and the reorganization of the brain networks after therapy and rehabilitation, as well as an indicator of the role of language in the regulation of affects and emotions (Luria, 1961). This clinical case outlines important topics regarding the interventions with children following ABI and the role that psychoanalysis plays in helping to develop a subjective discourse in order to control and modify behavior, promoting emotional regulation strategies and outlining the role of repetition in the clinical setting. We will briefly discuss these topics mainly from Lacan's and Luria's perspectives.

6.1 Structure and development of language as regulator of behavior

The case presented highlights on the importance of language in two main aspects: language as a way to regulate behavior (Luria, 1961) and language considered as a symbolic place that the child has in the discourse and the thoughts of his parents (Mannoni, 1996).

Regarding language as a symbolic place, even when the child doesn't speak, or due to cerebral damage the fluency or understanding is impaired, as in the case of R he's already part of the language (Slimobich et al., 2002). The existence of cerebral damage, which impedes the articulation of words, is not associated with a lack on the subjective experience or inner world of the child. In that sense, we can state that although someone can't speak, he is already subjected to the language (Lacan, 1964). This is clearly represented in his aggressive responses that were the entrance to his subjective world and to the development of transference. During the treatment, interpretations were given to R to try to symbolize these bodily sensations, so he can create a distance between the feeling and himself.

The interventions that the analyst did with R were based on games, specially useful in the cases when the discourse of the child is not developed or he/she has difficulties to express through spoken language (Akimoto et al., 2014; Hirao et al., 2008; Suri, 2012). In psychoanalysis the game, defined as one of the earliest practices of the psychical apparatus and a way of expression of the unconscious drives (Freud, 1920), has been widely used when working with children (Winnicott, 1982). The games that children play are of vital importance to their subjective constitution and to elaborate their identity. Games are a discourse that expresses the children's problems and anxieties and thus can be interpreted (Mannoni, 1996). This discourse needs someone that can read it, a position that in the psychoanalytic context is occupied by the analyst (Slimobich et al., 2002). The analyst is the one that will signify and symbolize (Freedman & Russell, 2003) the experience of the child during the game, helping him to find a proper and subjective meaning of his traumatic experience.

At the beginning of the treatment, R could only emit grunts and shouts. From this perspective, these were already signifiers that the analyst could use to help him in the development of the language. Following Lacan (1958), just an opposition of signifiers, on the logic of the presence–absence, is needed to work with the symbolic and imaginary aspects of the unconscious. This model is based on the Fort-Da discovered by Freud (1920), which represents an unconscious activity that the child performs to overcome and master his anguish: the child plays with a coil, making it appearing and disappearing, while emitting two words, Fort and Da (appear and disappear). In this fragment, the child becomes an active Subject, while the coil is assumed the role of a transitional object (representing the mother).

The whole process is illustrated through the case of R. At the beginning of the psychodynamic treatment, playing with the towers (construction–deconstruction) was a simple game that progressively increased its complexity and emotional involvement. During the game, the analyst gave him his place ("you can talk") as a Subject.

We need to consider the role of R's impairments, deduced from the neuropsychological assessment, in the temporal (left hemisphere) and frontal regions of the brain. Examining the areas affected and R's behavior, we could hypothesize the existence of a relation between language and emotion-regulation systems. Children use language to speak about what they feel, which allows a discharge of the drive (in the sense that words can bind affect) and, at the same time, modify what is felt. As we have outlined in Section 1, the development of the language is an important function for the psychical apparatus to convert object into word-representations (Bernardi, 1978; Freud, 1915), and in the cases where expressive language can't cover this operation, emotions are difficult to regulate and to symbolize.

The importance of language as a way to regulate behavior is also supported by the clinical work of Luria. In his works about aphasia, importantly influenced by Vygotsky's theory, he showed the relationship between language process and thinking (Luria, 1978). Luria identified the interrelationship between frontal lobe damage and alterations in expressive and comprehensive language, in line with the findings in the current clinical case. A distinction between (1) naming an object and (2) making a narrative (which requires intentions and planning, involving executive functions) was made (Luria 1976, 1978). Making a narrative with emotional content about oneself requires, in addition, the existence of a Subject (in a Lacanian sense).

Later on, Luria described the interaction between the motor and emotional functions (Vocate, 1987). He hypothesized the existence of a functional barrier that will keep emotions from being directly transferred to the motor system. The existence of this barrier, which was created through socialization, will allow the child to inhibit and to direct his/her emotions and impulses. This primary mechanism to regulate behavior is based on speech, conceived as a symbolic system, which will mediate between emotion and motor response. This process is progressive, being initially the excitatory/impulsive aspects of speech more intense, while gradually the inhibitory or significant aspects of spoken language gain predominance (Vocate, 1987).

Vygotsky's studies have indicated how language could directly regulate cognition, emotion and behavior in children. Along the development, the child acquires, through the process of internalization, an inner speech that can be defined as "the subjective experience of language in the absence of overt and audible articulation" (Alderson-Day & Fernyhough, 2015, p. 1). This speech had its origin in the Other (external speech) and the child integrates it in a process that begins by enunciating and articulating it speaking aloud (egocentric or private speech), until he doesn't need to do it, achieving inner speech (Jones, 2009). Luria indicates four moments of the development of speech (Vocate, 1987): (1) when speech has no influence in the child, (2) when external speech has an initial effect on actions, (3) when external speech has an inhibitory effect and (4) when the external changes into inner speech with the development of verbal principles that will help to guide behavior. In the case of R, who had lost his language when he was four years old, it is possible that the internalization of the language was affected, subsequently producing problems to regulate his emotions and behaviors. The psychodynamic interpretations and the use of the pair of signifiers (presence-absence) can also be viewed, from this neuropsychological perspective, as a way to stimulate R's own inner speech. In the beginning, it is the analyst who introduces the desire and the language, as it is usually done in the treatment of children with autism (Grollier, 2015), and later R can assimilate and integrate the interpretations making them as a way of communicating his subjectivity.

Finally, through the development of language during treatment, R not only finds a tool to speak about himself and his desire but also acquires, following Luria's words (1961), the potentiality to organize his perception and his memory and to draw conclusions about the external world and his connections with significant others (social bond). The effects of the initial games with R seem to suggest this fact, especially because he was more attentive and focused on the emotional interaction with the analyst.

6.2 Emotion regulation

We have previously stated that language is all-important in emotional regulation. Additionally, current research with adult patients suffering from brain lesions on the left hemisphere is pointing to the importance of other modes of managing emotional states, such as external regulation. It includes how other people, often closed ones, to the patient (self-other regulation) can help him regulate emotional states (Salas et al., 2014; Salas, Gross, Rafal, Viñas-Guasch, & Turnbull, 2013). From this perspective, we identified in R a difficulty to generalize and to flexibly manipulate verbal representations in order to articulate – and regulate – emotional experience (Salas, 2012).

The interventions on R considered these two types of emotion regulation: internal and external. Internal regulation was addressed through interpreting R's games, expecting that he will progressively use his own words to do it. External regulation was mainly focused on parents, by suggesting a change of school in R to improve his social bonds. It is interesting to note that, although his family felt alarmed and anguished due to his aggressive behavior, on the therapeutic setting this symptom was the door to work with the unconscious representations and the possibility of emotional regulation.

The persistence of frontal symptomatology (mainly des-inhibition) following intense emotional episodes seems to signal the vulnerability of prefrontal cortex during childhood (Diamond, 2013). This impulsivity and des-inhibition were addressed through game and neurorehabilitation techniques. The repetitive game of R, where he built and tore down a tower, was slowly modified and a pause was introduced (pauses that were essential, for instance, to play the totem game). The possibility of waiting, in contrast to a quickly satisfaction of the drive, was associated with a regulation of his emotional state. R began to play with the time, to make a dummy (e.g. he began to laugh before tearing the tower down). This fact indicates that internal regulation mechanisms related to the symbolic (versus those associated with the impulsivity) are being introduced (Lacan, 1964; Luria, 1961). The drive doesn't need to be instantly satisfied; it can wait for some time.

6.3 Repetition

Observing the games performed by R we could differentiate between the moments where he acted impulsively (just with the objective of destroying) and the moments where he systematically demolish something that was made by the analyst. This introduces the issue of repetition as a clinical tool in psychodynamic interventions (Fernández-Alcántara, Navas, & Cruz-Quintana, 2015). Tearing the tower down repetitively with intention and emotion (looking at the analyst and laughing) is a way to establish social bonds, beyond the pure discharge of the drive. This change was possible through the transferential relationship with the analyst that allowed R to extend his internal world, establishing better emotional relationships with others.

The concept of repetition was first defined by Freud as the reappearance of a number of symptoms in the analytic setting (Freud, 1914). However, repetition can also be considered as a tool that guides psychodynamic treatment. For example, it is possible that in cases of acquired brain damage, when defense mechanisms (e.g. repression) cannot function adequately (Turnbull, Fotopoulou, & Solms, 2014), the drives may be expressed directly through a repetition, without the mediation of any symbolic resources.

The analyst can use the moments of repetition to introduce, progressively, something new. Lacan (1956) considered repetition as a psychological process that never happens the same way, so there are small differences in each event that is repeated. In the current case, minor (but constant) changes were proposed to R while playing. These modifications in the game supposed an improvement in cognitive flexibility and the functionality of cognitive faculties such as spatial orientation, language, memory and functionality of the prefrontal lobe.

We should also consider that repetition is associated with the death drive (Freud, 1920). The experiences that are repeated are pointing to the real, to the aspects that are not signified and can't be symbolized (Lacan, 1953). The analyst can identify those repetitions in the game of the child, which are representing a particular mode of *jouissance*. From this perspective the clinical intervention will address its transformation into other types of drive satisfaction that do not generate such an intense suffering.

The current clinical case has important limitations that need to be considered. First, although we have used neuropsychological instruments to assess the main domains, no retests were performed. In addition, due to the important modifications, we can't compare R's results with normative data.

Second, due to the design of the study, we are not able to disentangle if R's improvements are directly related to the psychoanalytic treatment or to the neuropsychological intervention. We decided to integrate both approaches, using a multicomponent intervention, as is usually done in other cases of ABI (Prigatano & Salas, 2017).

6.4 Conclusion

In conclusion, the psychoanalytic treatment intertwined with the neuropsychological rehabilitation and the pharmacological treatment was effective to address the main symptoms of R. The use of interpretations helped R to develop an emotional language about his own inner and subjective world leading to a better emotional regulation. In addition, the neurorehabilitation, considering the psychodynamic approach, allowed working on inhibition and flexibility, improving these two core functions. Finally, this chapter outlines the necessity of integrating the neurorehabilitation approach with the subjective and emotional aspects from the psychodynamic treatment.

References

Akimoto, M., Kishimoto, N., Hirao, K., Narita, K., Yama, M. Kubota, Y. & Kato, T. (2014). *Psychotherapy for an elderly woman with anosognosia – images of trauma expressed in sandplay and Baumtest.* Paper presented at the 15th International Neuropsychoanalysis Congress, New York.

Alderson-Day, B. & Fernyhough, C. (2015). Inner speech: Development, cognitive functions, inner speech: Development, cognitive functions, phenomenology, and neurobiology. *Psychological Bulletin, 141*(5), 931. doi: 10.1037/bul0000021

Ballaban-Gil, K. & Tuchman, R. (2000). Epilepsy and epileptiform EEG: Association with autism and language disorders. *Mental Retardation and Developmental Disabilities Research Reviews, 6*(4), 300–308. doi:10.1002/1098-2779(2000)6:4<300::AID-MRDD9>3.0.CO;2-R

Bernardi, R. (1978). Representación de palabra y representación de cosa en la concepción freudiana del inconsciente. *Revista Uruguaya de Psicoanálisis, 57.*

Bradley, R.H. & Corwyn, R.F. (2002). Socioeconomic status and child development. *Annual Review of Psychology, 53*, 371–399.

Caraballo, R. H., Cejas, N., Chamorro, N., Kaltenmeier, M. C., Fortini, S. & Soprano, A. M. (2014). Landau-Kleffner syndrome: A study of 29 patients. *Seizure, 23*(2), 98–104. doi:10.1016/j.seizure.2013.09.016

Deonna, T. & Roulet-Perez, E. (2010). Early-onset acquired epileptic aphasia (Landau-Kleffner syndrome, LKS) and regressive autistic disorders with epileptic EEG abnormalities: The continuing debate. *Brain and Development, 32*(9), 746–752. doi:10.1016/j.braindev.2010.06.011

De Renzi, A. & Vignolo, L. A. (1962). Token test: A sensitive test to detect receptive disturbances in aphasics. *Brain, 85*, 665–678.

Diamond, A. (2013). Executive functions. *Annual Review of Psychology, 64*, 135–168. doi:10.1146/annurev-psych-113011-143750

Dimitriadis, Y. (2017). The psychoanalytic concept of jouissance and the kindling hypothesis. *Frontiers in Psychology, 8,* 1593.

Dolto, F. (2014). *L'image inconsciente du corps.* Paris: Le Seuil.

Duran, M. H. C., Guimaraes, C. A., Medeiros, L. L. & Guerreiro, M. M. (2009). Landau-Kleffner syndrome: Long-term follow-up. *Brain and Development, 31*(1), 58–63. doi:10.1016/j.braindev.2008.09.007

Eslinger, P. J., Flaherty-Craig, C. V. & Benton, A. L. (2004). Developmental outcomes after early prefrontal cortex damage. *Brain and Cognition, 55*(1), 84–103. doi:10.1016/S0278-2626(03)00281-1

Evans, D. (1996). *An introductory dictionary of lacanian psychoanalysis.* London: Routledge.

Fernández-Alcántara, M., García-Caro, M. P., Berrocal-Castellano, M., Benítez, A., Robles-Vizcaíno, C. & Laynez-Rubio, C. (2013). Experiencias y cambios en los padres de niños con parálisis cerebral infantil: Estudio cualitativo. *Anales Del Sistema Sanitario de Navarra, 36*(1), 9–20.

Fernández-Alcántara, M., García-Caro, M. P., Laynez-Rubio, C., Pérez-Marfil, M. N., Martí-García, C., Benítez-Feliponi, Á., ... Cruz-Quintana, F. (2015). Feelings of loss in parents of children with infantile cerebral palsy. *Disability and Health Journal, 8*(1), 93–101. doi:10.1016/j.dhjo.2014.06.003

Fernández-Alcántara, M., García-Caro, M. P., Pérez-Marfil, M. N., Hueso-Montoro, C., Laynez-Rubio, C. & Cruz-Quintana, F. (2016). Feelings of loss and grief in parents of children diagnosed with autism spectrum disorder (ASD). *Research in Developmental Disabilities, 55,* 312–321. doi:10.1016/j.ridd.2016.05.007

Fernández-Alcántara, M., Navas, J.F. & Cruz-Quintana, F. (2015). *Use of repetition as a tool in clinical populations: A neuropsychoanalytic perspective.* Symposium presented in the 16th International Neuropsychoanalysis Congress, Amsterdam.

Fink, B. (1995). *The Lacanian subject: Between language and jouissance.* Princeton: Princeton University Press.

Freedman, N. & Russell, J. (2003). Symbolization of the analytic discourse. *Psychoanalysis and Contemporary Thought, 26*(1), 39–87.

Freud, S. (1914). *Recuerdo, repetición y elaboración.* Barcelona: Biblioteca Nueva.

Freud, S. (1915). *Lo inconsciente.* Barcelona: Biblioteca Nueva.

Freud, S. (1920). *Más allá del principio del placer.* Barcelona: Biblioteca Nueva.

Freud, S. (1923). *El yo y el ello.* Barcelona: Biblioteca Nueva.

Grant, D. A. & Berg, E. (1948). A behavioral analysis of degree of reinforcement and ease of shifting to new responses in a Weigl-type card-sorting problem. *Journal of Experimental Psychology, 38,* 404.

Grollier, M. (2015). Autisme, langage et partenaire. *L'Évolution Psychiatrique, 80*(3), 554–568.

Hirao, K., Naka, H., Narita, K., Futamura, M., Miyata, J., Tanaka, S., et al. (2008). *Self in conflict: Recovery from non-fluent aphasia through sandplay therapy.* Poster presentation at the 9th International Neuropsychoanalysis Congress, Montreal.

Jones, P. E. (2009). From "external speech" to "inner speech" in Vygotsky: A critical appraisal and fresh perspectives. *Language and Communication, 29*(2), 166–181. doi:10.1016/j.langcom.2008.12.003

Kaplan-Solms, K. & Solms, M. (2000). *Clinical studies in neuro-psychoanalysis: Introduction to a depth neuropsychology.* London: Karnac Books.

Kessels, R. P., Van Zandvoort, M. J., Postma, A., Kappelle, L. J. & De Haan, E. H. (2000). The Corsi block-tapping task: Standardization and normative data. *Applied Neuropsychology, 7*(4), 252–258.

Kovacs, Z., Stock, D. & Bernert, G. (2011). "You Are a Cannibal"—A case report: Psychoanalysis of an adolescent boy with bifrontal lesions (Part 1: The First Year). *Neuropsychoanalysis, 13*(1), 73–89.

Kreutzer, J. S., Caplan, B. & DeLuca, J. (2011). *Encyclopedia of clinical neuropsychology.* London: Springer.

Kuriakose, S., Lang, R., Boyer, K., Lee, A. & Lancioni, G. (2012). Rehabilitation issues in Landau-Kleffner syndrome. *Developmental Neurorehabilitation, 15*(5), 317–321. doi:10.3109/17518423.2012.701241

Lacan, J. (1948). *La agresividad en psicoanálisis.* En: Escritos II. México: Siglo XXI Editores.

Lacan, J. (1958). *La dirección de la cura y los principios de su poder.* En: Escritos I. México: Siglo XXI Editores.

Lacan, J. (1953). *Seminario de Jacques Lacan: libro 1: Los escritos técnicos de Freud.* Barcelona: Paidós.

Lacan, J. (1956). *Seminario de Jacques Lacan: libro 4. La relación de objeto.* Barcelona: Paidós.

Lacan, J. (1964). *Seminario de Jacques Lacan: libro 11: Los cuatro conceptos fundamentales del psicoanálisis.* Barcelona: Paidós.

Landau, W.M. & Kleffner, F.R. (1957). Syndrome of acquired aphasia with convulsive disorder in children. *Neurology, 7*, 523–530.

Luria, A. R. (1961). *The role of speech in the regulation of normal and abnormal behavior.* New York: Pergamon Press.

Luria, A. R. (1976). *The working brain: An introduction to neuropsychology.* New York: Basic Books.

Luria, A. R. (1978). *Cerebro y lenguaje: la afasia traumática, síndromes, exploraciones y tratamiento.* Barcelona: Fontanella.

Maleval, J.C. (2011). *El autista y su voz.* Madrid: Editorial Gredos.

Mannoni, M. (1996). *La primera entrevista con el psicoanalista.* Barcelona: Editorial Gedisa.

Mulas, F., Hernández, S. & Morant, A. (2001). Alteraciones neuropsicológicas en los niños epilépticos. *Revista de neurología clínica, 2*(1), 29–41.

Nasio, J. D. (2007). *Mon corps et ses images.* Paris: Payot & Rivages.

Prigatano, G. P. & Salas, C. E. (2017). Psychodynamic psychotherapy after severe traumatic brain injury. In T.M. McMillan & R.L. Wood (Eds). *Neurobehavioural disability and social handicap following traumatic brain injury* (pp. 188–201). Abingdon: Routledge.

Ramanathan, R. S., Ahluwalia, T. & Sharma, A. (2012). Landau-Kleffner syndrome-A rare experience. *Eastern Journal of Medicine, 17*(1), 36–39.

Salas, C. E. (2012). Surviving catastrophic reaction after brain injury: The use of self-regulation and self-other regulation. *Neuropsychoanalysis, 14*(1), 77–92. doi:1 0.1080/15294145.2012.10773691

Salas, C. E., Casassus, M. & Turnbull, O. H. (2017). A neuropsychoanalytic approach to case studies. *Clinical Social Work Journal, 45*(3), 201–214.

Salas, C. E., Gross, J. J., Rafal, R. D., Viñas-Guasch, N. & Turnbull, O. H. (2013). Concrete behaviour and reappraisal deficits after a left frontal stroke: a case study. *Neuropsychological Rehabilitation*, *23*(4), 467–500. doi:10.1080/09602011.2 013.784709

Salas, C. E., Radovic, D., Yuen, K. S. L., Yeates, G. N., Castro, O. & Turnbull, O. H. (2014). "Opening an emotional dimension in me": Changes in emotional reactivity and emotion regulation in a case of executive impairment after left fronto-parietal damage. *Bulletin of the Menninger Clinic*, *78*(4), 301–334. doi:10.1521/bumc.2014.78.4.301

Shonkoff, J.P. (2011). Protecting brains, not simply stimulating minds. *Science*, *333*, 982–983.

Shonkoff, J. P., Garner, A. S., Siegel, B. S., Dobbins, M. I., Earls, M. F., McGuinn, L., ... & Committee on Early Childhood, Adoption, and Dependent Care. (2012). The lifelong effects of early childhood adversity and toxic stress. *Pediatrics*, *129*(1), e232–e246.

Sieratzki, J. S., Calvert, G. A., Brammer, M., David, A. & Woll, B. (2001). Accessibility of spoken, written, and sign language in Landau Kleffner syndrome: A linguistic and functional MRI study Comprehension of English Lip reading. *Epileptic Disorders*, *2*, 79–89.

Slimobich, J.L., Gonzalez, R., Laynez, C., Grimberg, F., Reoyo, B. & Alonzo, M.L. (2002). *Lacan: la marca del leer*. Barcelona: Anthropos.

Stefanatos, G. (2011). Changing perspectives on Landau-Kleffner syndrome changing perspectives on Landau-Kleffner Syndrome. *The Clinical Neuropsychologist*, *256*(256), 963–988. doi:10.1080/13854046.2011.614779

Suri, R. (2012). Sandplay: An adjunctive therapy to working with dementia. *International Journal of Play Therapy*, *21*(3), 117–130. doi:10.1037/a0027733

Takeoka, M., Riviello, J. J., Duffy, F. H., Kim, F., Kennedy, D. N., Makris, N., ... & Holmes, G. L. (2004). Bilateral volume reduction of the superior temporal areas in Landau–Kleffner syndrome. *Neurology*, *63*, 1289–1292.

Torralva, T., Roca, M., Gleichgerrcht, E., López, P. & Manes, F. (2009). INECO Frontal Screening (IFS): A brief, sensitive, and specific tool to assess executive functions in dementia. *Journal of the International Neuropsychological Society*, *15*, 777–786.

Turnbull, O. H., Fotopoulou, A. & Solms, M. (2014). Anosognosia as motivated unawareness: The "defence" hypothesis revisited. *Cortex*, *61*, 18–29. doi:10.1016/j.cortex.2014.10.008

Vocate, D. R. (1987). *The theory of A.R. Luria: Functions of spoken language in the development of higher mental processes*. London: LEA.

Wairungu, G. (2015). *A case study of Landau Kleffner syndrome: A look at strategies, experiences, challenges, and perceptions of teachers, family and support personnel*. Pro-Quest Dissertations and Theses, 145. Retrieved from http://ezproxy.usherbrooke.ca/login?url=http://search.proquest.com/docview/1679462325?accountid=13835

Winnicott, D. W. (1982). *Realidad y juego*. Barcelona: Editorial Gedisa.

Chapter 12

The social reality of the self

Right perisylvian damage revisited

Sahba Besharati and Aikaterini Fotopoulou

I Introduction

Almost 20 years ago, Kaplan-Solms and Solms (2000) wrote a pioneering chapter on the clinical neuropsychoanalysis of right hemisphere syndrome, as part of their volume in *Clinical Studies in Neuro-Psychoanalysis*. Specifically, they dedicate a chapter to the presentation of five patients with damage to the areas of the brain surrounding the right sylvian fissure (the 'groove' in the brain that divides the frontal and parietal lobes from the temporal lobe, also known as lateral sulcus). Typically, such lesions are caused by a stroke, and they result in a set of different bodily and cognitive deficits, such as motor and sensory loss in the contralesional arm and leg and visuospatial deficits on that side of space. However, some patients also show a host of other aberrant presentations such as the denial of their paralysis (anosognosia for hemiplegia), an obsessive hatred of the paralysed arm (misoplegia) or even the delusional attribution of the affected body parts to other people, or the attribution of other people's body arts to the self (somatoparaphrenia). The main thesis of Kaplan-Solms and Solms was that such lesions can result in spatial integration deficits, which in turn undermine the cognitive foundations of the developmentally learned distinction between self and other. In the authors' psychoanalytic terms, what is lost after such lesions is the capacity for 'whole-object relationships', and therefore object instead of narcissistic love. The regression to the latter is characterised by drive diffusion and corresponding object splitting and related primitive defenses of introjection and projection. The sad reality of a sudden stroke and an unfamiliar, paralysed body has lost their independence as separate, whole objects. As a result, individuals cannot mourn the loss of their bodily integrity and independence in realistic ways, but are instead at the mercy of narcissistic defenses. Thus, any part or function of the body that is unconsciously perceived as incompatible with the demands of one's needs and wishes is treated as non-existent or as alien and unrelated to the self. Patients may therefore deny their paralysis, or they may form delusions about the ownership of their body parts, e.g. claiming that their paralysed arm belongs to a relative. At a superficial level, some of these patients can thus appear indifferent, emotionally detached and even joyful. In the relational, safe context of psychotherapy, however, this superficial facade breaks down, and deep feelings of loss, helplessness and dependency temporarily emerge from the ruins of splitting, introjective and projective defenses.

Kaplan-Solms and Solms (2000) cases are powerful examples of clinical neuropsychoanalysis, portraying the usefulness of psychotherapeutic approaches to brain injury, as well as revealing some of the metapsychological principles behind the unconscious manoeuvres of the mind. The metapsychological theory that the authors use is mostly inspired by Freudian and Kleinian considerations (indeed, this chapter seems to be the most object-relational and Kleinian chapter of the original volume). Nevertheless, given the centrality of narcissistic defences in many other psychoanalytic models, several other authors have since offered alternative psychoanalytic perspectives on this syndrome, such as more contemporary relational (Yeates, Henwood, Gracey & Evans, 2006) and Lacanian perspectives (Morin et al., 2003; Thibierge & Morin, 2013). There are also alternative Freudian perspectives on the syndrome (Prigatano & Weinstein, 1996), as well as a long interest in existential-phenomenological approaches (Fotopoulou, 2018; Malabou, 2015; Merleau-Ponty, 1945, 1960). Needless to say that despite ongoing research on this syndrome and advances in related neurocognitive theories on self and social awareness, the mainstream neurocognitive literature continues to be at best indifferent to such psychoanalytic and phenomenological hypotheses. Given our attempts for psychodynamic neuroscience (an approach that borrows inspiration from psychoanalytic theories but uses the methods of cognitive neuroscience to test them empirically, see Fotopoulou, 2012c), the more interdisciplinary versions of such hypotheses have made it to mainstream publications (e.g. Fotopoulou, 2010, 2014, 2015; Turnbull, Fotopoulou & Solms, 2014).

The present chapter cannot do justice to all these approaches and debates. Instead, trained in both the Kaplan-Solms and Solms neuropsychoanalytic tradition and mainstream neurocognitive approaches, we aim to revisit Kaplan-Solms and Solms' hypotheses and expand their interdisciplinary efforts in the light of more recent developments and new findings. Accordingly, this chapter attempts to revisit the hypotheses proposed by Kaplan-Solms and Solms in the light of novel, rich insights about mental and brain function, afforded in the field of neuroscience by new experimental and neuroimaging methodologies and in the field of psychotherapy by the opportunity to encounter and treat a much larger and varied cohort of right hemisphere patients. In the past 15 years, we have collaborated with nine different UK stroke units, encountering more than 60 severely anosognosic patients and more than 40 asomatognosic patients (see below for definition of these terms), in hyperacute, subacute and chronic stages, largely for the purposes of research and rehabilitation but in a minority of cases also for the sole purpose of psychotherapy (by KF). Thus, this chapter is an attempt to consolidate our theoretical assumptions and clinical experiences with empirical findings from our own and other labs. Although integration of experimental and neuroimaging methods to considerations of clinical phenomena entails some epistemological reductions and has met with resistance (Blass & Carmeli, 2007, 2015), we take the view that phenomena that cut across the mind and brain actually require interdisciplinary consideration and attempts at 'translation', even if in the process *the loss* of some of particularities of the science and some of the richness of the clinical encounter *would need to be tolerate*d (see Fotopoulou, 2012b; Yovell, Solms & Fotopoulou, 2015 for extensive discussion). As a way of disclaimer, we wish to emphasise at the onset that such interdisciplinary attempts do not aim to determine how patients with right-hemisphere stroke should be treated. This in our view would require a different, more applied tradition of research. Instead, our aim in this chapter is to translate and compare the 'models of the mind' put forward by psychoanalytic and neuroscientific theorists (see Fotopoulou, 2012b), not as an attempt to incorporate one in the other, but rather as an attempt to examine how both disciplines relate the phenomenon in question from their respective positions and in relation to each other.

2 The theoretical background

We will start by presenting the central question behind this syndrome and then presenting our theoretical position on this question. We will then proceed to unpack our answer and present the empirical findings supporting this position. We will use brief clinical examples of dialogue with right hemisphere patients to illustrate how their left-sided paralysis is experienced. All patients presented are adult, right-handed patients who suffered a stroke in the region of the right middle cerebral artery and were recruited in various research studies over the past 15 years. The interviews and observations were conducted by the authors (SB & KF) for research purposes.

2.1 The 100-year old-question of anosognosia

In 1914, Joseph Babinski, a talented pupil of Charcot in Paris who Sigmund Freud described as the "preferred pupil of the Maitre" (Clarac, Massion & Smith, 2008), presented a paper in which he introduced the neologism *anosognosia* (from the Greek, α = "without", νόσος = "disease", γνῶσις = "knowledge") to describe how some patients with left hemiplegia following a stroke were "unaware of or seem to be unaware of the existence of the paralysis which affects them" (Babinski, 1914, see translation by Langer & Levine, 2014, pp. 5–8). In the years since Babinski, anosognosia has since been at the focus of much medical and scientific research, including two dedicated volumes of collected essays (Prigatano, 2010; Prigatano & Schacter, 1991) and hundreds of scientific papers (see Jenkinson & Fotopoulou, 2014 for an edited collection marking the 100th anniversary of the syndrome's description). The term itself is now applied to other instances of unawareness of one's illness or deficits (e.g. in dementia or schizophrenia), but in this chapter we restrict ourselves to its classic use in the context of right hemisphere damage and left-sided paralysis. Hundreds of anosognosic patients have now been described who indeed seem to have lost the ability to update their beliefs about their bodily state and particularly their paralysis. Their beliefs about their body (e.g. I have no weakness since the stroke) no longer correspond to what the rest of their environment observes about the patients' bodies (e.g. their left side of the body is completely paralysed). Patients expect their paralysed arm and leg to be able to grasp their water glass, hug a friend and walk out of hospital and thus return back to their habitual lives. Furthermore, what is most striking is that although they get many opportunities to test the veridicality of their beliefs against experience and contrary social feedback, they still do not update their beliefs. The left arm does cannot pick up the glass, the hug is half and one cannot stand, let alone walk. Frequently everyday tasks cannot be completed, objects fall on the floor and break. Sadly, anosognosic patients also have higher incidents of falls than other patients in stroke wards. Patients appear to forget these incidents, to minimise their importance and relevance or to misattribute their causes to other people and events in ad hoc confabulations, or even in more fixed delusional beliefs (see Fotopoulou, 2010, for a detailed discussion of such differences). Indeed, in a subset of these patients, there are also concomitant body delusions (somatoparaphrenias; Gerstmann, 1942) affecting the sense of body ownership (the subjective feeling that our body is separate from the world and other bodies). Such patients may reject the ownership of one's limb (asomatognosia), misattribute it to others or vice versa (somatoparaphrenia proper), claim they have three or more limbs (supernumerary limbs), or treat the limb as though it was a separate person (personification; Critchley, 1955).

Behind this counterintuitive adherence to delusional beliefs about the motor abilities or the ownership of one's body lies a central question that scholars of the syndrome have asked for more than 100 years: Do these patients fail to learn from errors because they cannot or will not let go of their beliefs (e.g. related motor intentions, predictions, identifications, fantasies, motivations, wishes and hopes), or because they cannot observe that they have made an error (e.g. they have lost the ability to perceive or appreciate sensory, or other feedback). This question has been framed and debated in a number of ways in the past few decades, e.g. as 'psychogenic versus neurogenic', 'defense versus deficit', 'motivation versus cognition', 'top-down versus bottom-up', 'feedforward versus feedback', 'prediction versus prediction error', 'belief conservatism versus observational adequacy' and so on.

2.2 Previous attempts to answer the question of anosognosia

A classic example of how the above central question of anosognosia has been framed is the example of the role of motivation and psychogenesis versus cognition and neurogenesis in anosognosia. Babinski and his contemporaries portray a profound dualism in their thinking. For example, Babinski wonders whether anosognosia is motivated by self-esteem or whether it is 'real'. In a commentary in the same volume, M. Henry Meige wonders whether "Is it resignation, a wish to hide from himself or others a defect that afflicts him? It is possible, in certain cases; but in others one is faced with a true psychopathological problem" (see Langer & Levine, 2014, pp. 5–8). This alleged contrast between a psychological wish to be healthy leading to self- and other-deception, and a more 'real' neurological condition that deprives the person of knowledge into their abilities, is a contrast that many scholars and clinicians adhered to for most of the 20th century (Prigatano & Schacter, 1991). In fact, it is still common among some clinicians to insist that a distinction between 'denial' and 'anosognosia proper' may be useful (Prigatano, 2014), even if they would not adhere to dualism more generally.

However, in the past 15 years, a number of integrative perspectives have also emerged, linking emotion and motivation more directly to the brain damage seen in anosognosic patients (e.g. Fotopoulou et al., 2010; Turnbull, Fotopoulou & Solms, 2014). In such theories, anosognosia is neither a psychodynamic defense nor a pure neurological deficit. Instead, as we explain in further detail below, it is the outcome of a change in the dynamic balance between motivation and cognition, or in other terms, it is both a defense and a deficit.

Indeed, many other scholars have argued in recent years that neither pole of the above distinctions is sufficient to explain anosognosia (Frith, Blakemore & Wolpert, 2000; Marcel, Tegnér & Nimmo-Smith, 2004; Ramachandran, 1995; Vuilleumier, 2004). Instead, in order to account for the embodied (sensorimotor), emotional and delusional aspects of the syndrome, some scholars have proposed 'combination' theories of anosognosia. These accounts stress the necessary combination of bottom-up and top-down deficits and corresponding lesioned brain regions (Davies, Davies & Coltheart 2005; Levine, 1990; Levine, Calvanio & Rinn, 1991; Vuilleumier, 2004). For example, considering anosognosia in the more general context of delusional beliefs, Davies et al. (2005) proposed that anosognosic beliefs may be explained by a two-factor account used to explain other delusions; abnormal beliefs arise due to a first impairment in perception that prompts the abnormal belief and a second impairment that interferes with higher order, monitoring processes, thus allowing the abnormal perceptions to become abnormal beliefs. The scope of these 'combination' theories has clearly improved understanding on this syndrome. However, these theories have been for the most part 'additive'. Like more general so-called biopsychosocial models, these views do not tell us much more than the fact that different factors need to be added together for a more comprehensive understanding of a phenomenon. Moreover, reflecting the modular epistemology of cognitive neuropsychology (see Fotopoulou, 2014, for a critical review), these models treat the syndrome as caused by simultaneous damage to functionally independent lesion sites. For example, Vocat, Staub, Stroppini and Vuilleumier (2010) suggested that a combination of lesions with two or more brain areas within the insular, premotor, parietal and temporal cortex, or the white matter connections that link one or more of these areas with subcortical regions, may lead to different combinations of deficits in functions such as proprioception, spatial neglect and error monitoring, which in turn lead to anosognosia in different patients. While such 'combinations' of lesion sites and deficits are consistent with the multifaceted nature of the syndrome, what these accounts lack is a more precise account of the dynamic and hierarchical relation between relevant affected and unaffected areas and their functional role in body awareness.

3 A new answer to the question of anosognosia and our main thesis: self-awareness is socially mediated emotionally and cognitively

The advantage of neuropsychoanalytic theories, like the one put forward by Kaplan-Solms and Solms, is that they can also tell us how some of the above factors may relate to each other dynamically. In other terms, they assume a dynamic integration between these factors so that change in one domain will influence the other. This is a view of the brain that now most advanced neuroscientific theories also adhere to (e.g. Friston, 2010). In this case, Kaplan-Solms and Solms argued that deficits in spatial cognition caused by the right hemisphere damage have led patients to lose the capacity to represent their relation with their body as a 'whole object'. As a result, they have also lost the ability to accept one's disability as one's own and they instead employ primitive means for representing a fragmented body and for regulating the related negative emotions. Building upon these ideas as well as our empirical findings on this syndrome and recent dynamic neuroscientific theories of self-awareness (Fotopoulou, 2014, 2015; Friston, 2018), we propose that anosognosia is best explained as a disconnection between how one expects the body to feel in a first-person perspective (emotionally mine and under my control) and how one perceives the body in a third-person perspective, as it were from the outside, as in a mirror or in someone's else perspective. This difficulty in integrating current sensations and emotions **from the body** with their beliefs **about the body** corresponds to difficulties in the most abstract, metacognitive ('allocentric' and 'prospective') aspects of body awareness (Besharati et al., 2016), build on the socio-affective foundations of a second-person relation to the body during infancy (Fotopoulou & Tsakiris, 2017). Thus, self-awareness in anosognosia is subject to the influence of non-updated premorbid beliefs and emotions about the self (Fotopoulou, 2012a, 2014, 2015). We will explore below how the study of anosognosia from this theoretical standpoint reveals that there are at least three stances in self-awareness: a *first-person*, egocentric stance; an objectified, allocentric, *third person* stance and the developmentally important, intersubjective, *second-person* or interpersonal 'coincidence' stance. The rest of the sections are dedicated to unpacking this main thesis and presenting related clinical examples, as well as empirical evidence for this position. In all cases, we hope to demonstrate how the in-depth consideration of this syndrome can bring to light some layers of the human mind that are not typically observable without such a devastating brain injury. In addition, we hope to elucidate *that intersubjective (second person) encounters*, such as those between infants and good-enough caregivers, as well as patients and good-enough therapists, have a unique role in mental life; namely they can help us integrate first and third experiences of ourselves. Interactive, supportive states of interpersonal synchrony *facilitate the transition from egocentric to allocentric modes of mental functioning*, or in older, Freudian terms from the pleasure to the reality principle. As more modern, developmental perspectives have highlighted, this transition requires a period of playfulness, pretense and imperfect, second-person marked mirroring, operating on a principle which we have called the 'uncertainty principle' in previous writings (Fotopoulou, 2013, 2015). We will unpack all of these notions in the sections that follow.

4 Explanations and examples of anosognosia

Initial cognitive explanations of the syndrome proposed that patients with anosognosia may not be able to 'discover' their paralysis in their own, first-person experience because their brain lesions had prevented them from registering their motor failures (e.g. Levine, Calvanio & Rinn, 1991). For example, right hemisphere damage may impair one's arm sensation to the left, as well as one's ability to pay attention to the left side of space and the left part of one's body (a symptom called neglect that is also frequent after right hemisphere damage). Thus, it was considered plausible that patients may not be learning about their disability, because they do not get the feedback they need from sensation, including from vision. However, decades of work in neuropsychology has found that such deficits are not enough to cause anosognosia, in the sense that many patients have one or more of these deficits, but they are not anosognosic and vice versa (see Marcel, Tegnér & Nimmo-Smith, 2004, for an excellent study). Thus, progressively the idea of 'faulty feedback' was replaced with the idea of deficits in the comparison between feedforward and feedback signals.

Specifically, inspired by the popular idea in science and engineering in the 1990s (Wolpert, 1997) that a system monitors and corrects its own actions by comparing feedforward (anticipatory) and feedback signals, researchers argued that patients may fail to register the discrepancy between predicted and actual sensory feedback because of visuospatial neglect or other sensory deficits (Frith, Blakemore & Wolpert, 2000) or because of a deficit in the comparison mechanism itself (Berti et al., 2005). In other terms, patients may be confusing what they intended to do, with what actually happened, basing their awareness on the former despite large error signals in the latter. Indeed, we were able to show that patients did experience illusions of movement (see Case examples 1 and 2) as a result of a selective dominance of motor intentions over visual feedback, and this effect could not be explained by visual neglect. In other terms, when patients were intending to make a movement, but not when they were anticipating other people to move their own arms, their ability to imagine the anticipated action was confused with 'reality' (having actually executed the movement), and any feedback to the contrary was actively ignored rather than simply neglected (Fotopoulou et al., 2008).

We present examples below of an initial assessment conducted by the authors (SB & KF) for research purposes with two patients diagnosed with anosognosia to illustrate typical instances of first person, illusions of movement by the bedside, within one week from stroke. Both patients were female and in their 70s.

4.1 Case example 1: illusory movements

SB: Why are you in the hospital?

PATIENT: They say I had a stroke, but I don't remember anything about it.

SB: The doctors tell me you had a stroke, do you agree with them?

PATIENT: I don't know anything about strokes.

SB: What kind of symptoms have you noticed since you came to the hospital?

PATIENT: I haven't noticed anything really.

SB: Do you have any weakness anywhere?

PATIENT: Not really, I'm sure I can make a fist if I wanted to.

SB: Is your left arm causing you any trouble?

PATIENT: Not at all, no.

SB: [The examiner lifts the patient's left arm and moves it to the right hemispace]

THERE SEEMS TO BE SOME WEAKNESS IN YOU LEFT ARM, DO YOU AGREE?

PATIENT: No it's fine.

SB: Can you try and move your left arm for me?

PATIENT: Yes, I move it.

SB: But I didn't see your left arm move.

PATIENT: That's because you weren't paying attention, I just moved it now!

4.2 Case example 2: illusory movements against the lack of both visual and auditory feedback

SB: What symptoms have you noticed since the stroke? How does your body feel?

PATIENT: It feels alright.

SB: Do you have any weakness anywhere in your body?

PATIENT: No, no weakness.

SB: Is your left arm causing you any trouble?

PATIENT: No, of course not.

SB: Can you raise your left leg?

PATIENT: Yeah, sure I can.

SB: Can you please try and raise your left arm for me?

PATIENT: [Silence. The patient does not move.]

SB: Can you try and do it for me now?

PATIENT: [Patient uses right arm to move left arm]

SB: Did you do it?

PATIENT: Yes, you saw it move.

SB: Yes, but did it move on it's own?

PATIENT: Well, with the help of this [right] one [arm].

SB: Can you do it without the help of your right hand?

PATIENT: Yeah.

SB: Do you think you can clap your hands?

PATIENT: Yes, sure.

SB: Can you please show me?

PATIENT: [Uses right hand to lift left hand, then slaps the top of the left had to 'clap']

SB: Did you manage to clap your hands?

PATIENT: Yes, I did it. [The patient then winks at SB]

In both of these cases, the patients insist that they have executed a movement when in fact they are paralysed and unable to even raise their arms. Our lab and other labs have now verified the occurrence of these illusory experiences during carefully controlled experiments (e.g. Fotopoulou et al., 2008). According to influential, cognitive accounts, these illusions are sufficient to explain the syndrome, in the sense that this difficulty in monitoring motor errors against one's own sensorimotor predictions leads to a faulty (non-veridical) consciousness of movement, and this consciousness is responsible for all other delusional beliefs and emotional reactions observed in right hemisphere patients. As we will see below in greater detail, we have provided evidence to the contrary, arguing that such sensorimotor deficits are only a part of the syndrome's explanation.

Interestingly, during clinical 'confrontation' tasks (as in the examples above; interviewing during which the examiner asks a patient to demonstrate their beliefs), one can observe another feature of anosognosia that at face value can make an observer doubt the truthfulness of the patients' response – namely implicit or, tacit awareness, which in the cognitive literature is defined as "knowledge that is expressed in task performance unintentionally and with little or no phenomenal awareness" (Schacter, 1990, p. 157). Thus, while patients may explicitly deny their paralysis, they may be unconsciously processing some components of their deficits, including the emotional aspects. Indeed, in both examples one is unsure to the degree to which the patient 'knows' about the disability but nevertheless 'deceives' the examiner and maybe even themselves. Decades of clinical and more recently experimental work have established that these 'mixed messages' conveyed by the patients, such as the last patient who first moved the left arm with the help of the right arm and then winked at the examiner, or the first patient who claimed that the examiner is not paying attention, are actually not the result of deliberate deception by the patient but rather indications of the fact that our self-awareness is not unitary; these patients may have paradoxically unconscious knowledge of their deficits, despite their explicit denial. Below we present two, quite different between them, examples of what we think are indications of implicit awareness of one's deficits. Both patients were female, the first in the subacute (three weeks) and the second in the chronic stage (two years) since right-hemisphere stroke.

4.3 Case example 3: implicit awareness of paralysis

The patient underwent a physiotherapy session observed by junior trainees during a ward round who occasionally asked questions about her efforts and challenges. At the end of the session, the senior psychotherapist asked the patient if she now wanted to ask the trainees any questions. The patient, of very high and preserved intelligence, previously the director of a youth charity, asked the trainees several questions about their career plans and a five-minute-long pleasant discussion unfolded. After the trainees said their goodbyes and were preparing to leave the room, the patient who had not acknowledged her paralysis at all during the whole session, called out to them and said: 'Perhaps it would be useful to you to come and see me at a time when I'll be really ill and unable to move'.

4.4 Case example 4: misplaced loss

KF: Oh, I am sorry to see you upset about this memory [having a miscarriage while pregnant with thins about 30 years prior to this interview].

PATIENT: It is funny, you know. My sister was here the other day and she was very surprised to see me upset about this. She said that back then everyone thought I did not mind, I just got on with things, maybe I was even relieved a little, given that they were twins and all and my relationship with David [the father] was a mess. But now, when I think about it, oh the tears... the sorrow, I mean how can this happen to me? What did I do to deserve it? And yet back then...[patient falls silent]

Indeed, this facet of anosognosia for hemiplegia (AHP) has been commented upon by clinicians since the time of Babinski (see Jenkinson & Fotopoulou, 2014 for historical references), eliciting either suspicion of deceit or empathy for self-deceit (see Kaplan-Solms & Solms, 2000) to listeners and readers of such indications. One can say that even though what these patients express is not in accordance with the facts (I am not ill now, but I may be in the future) and it appears out of its correct cognitive context (my sorrow is not for my present loss, it is for my old, non-properly processed loss), it is *emotionally on target* (Kinsbourne, 2000). In recent decades, several case and group studies have now demonstrated that anosognosic patients may have implicit (unconscious) knowledge into their deficits that they cannot appreciate at an explicit, conscious level. For example, when patients are asked to perform an irrelevant cognitive task that includes neutral, emotionally negative and disability-related content, their performance to the cognitive task is particularly affected by the disability-related content, even though the content is unrelated to the task and patients themselves do not see its relevance to the self (Fotopoulou et al., 2010; Nardone, Ward, Fotopoulou & Turnbull, 2007). This is typically interpreted as an unconscious interference effect of content on performance, even though there is no explicit awareness of the self-relevance of the content (see also Cocchini, Beschin, Fotopoulou & Della Sala, 2010; Moro et al., 2011).

By contrast, other patients may be explicitly aware of their symptoms per se, but deny their emotional (usually referred to as anosodiaphoria; Babinski, 1914), or practical and 'future' significance (how it will affect life in the near future), or they may attribute their causes to other people (we will later call these faulty inferences about the causes of beliefs and experiences). Below we present two further examples, again quite different between them, but still alluding to the same difficulty in accepting the negative emotions associated with one's disability as either important or self-related. The first patient is male and in the acute phase (one week), and the second in the chronic stage (two years) since right-hemisphere stroke.

4.5 Case example 5: anosodiaphoria and lack of prospective awareness

KF: Why are you in the hospital?
PATIENT: I had a stroke, some days ago.
KF: What kind of symptoms have you noticed since you came to the hospital?
PATIENT: I have pain, here [points to left shoulder]. Ah, like that [touches it with the right hand], it hurts.

KF: I am sorry to hear that. Is there anything else that bothers you since the stroke?

PATIENT: Nothing that worries me.

KF: Nothing that worries you. Do you feel weakness anywhere?

PATIENT: No, I mean the left arm is sometimes weak but it does not worry me.

KF: The left arm. Can you move your left arm?

PATIENT: Yes, sometimes if the right hurts, I use the left to assist it.

KF: You use this arm [point to the left, patients follows her pointing], the left arm, to assist this arm [points and touches the patient's right arm], or I got it wrong?

PATIENT: No that's it. The left is not what it used to be but I can use it. It really helps when the right arm is tired, or something. [this is a reversal and minimisation of the true situation in which the left arm is completely paralysed]

KF: I see. So, you are not worried about losing the ability to move your left arm, even if you see some weakness.

PATIENT: oh, I know it will be alright. And it really does not bother me.

......

KF: Can you please try and raise your left arm for me now?

PATIENT: [Silence. The patient tries, lifts left shoulder, shows pain by expression]

KF: Did this hurt?

PATIENT: Yes. Here [points to shoulder].

KF: ok, lets not try this again then but did you manage to raise the arm you think?

PATIENT: No, not this time. Getting tired, now. But it is nothing that bother me.

KF: I understand....

4.6 Case example 6: misplaced anger

KF: It sounds like you are a bit upset today. Is that right?

PATIENT: Well, I am angry, or maybe disappointed. I mean how can they be so useless? How hard is it? My glasses were right here, on the left of the bed, and the card from my friend was next to it. Now, it is gone. Gone, forever, never to return, never to be fixed. They do not know what happened, they say. They just moved things to clean. They need to clean they say, well fine, but I need my letter. I mean, how am I supposed to function without my letters? And whose fault is it? Is it mine fault? No, what do I know? I was asleep. They came in, moved things again and now the letter is gone.

KF: I see, yes, you do sound very upset about it. Its sounds like an important letter?

PATIENT: Well, it is my friend. Of course, she writes frequently. I suppose it is important.

KF: Well, it sounds like it *feels* important to you.

PATIENT: Oh, yes it does and I am so angry at them. How can they take it away?

KF: It does sound like it feels important to you. I wonder if you feel the same about the stroke?

PATIENT: Well, you know, the stroke does not make things easy for me, sometimes I feel so desperate, but what really gets to me, is that they could help and they do not. The whole fear about me not been able to move is down to them, you know. That initial physiotherapist, I mean, she was helping me and it was better and then her friend came, and they then decided I cannot walk. Why? They are afraid, if I fall, I will sue and ask for compensation....

These apparent dissociations between how the body is experienced emotionally and cognitively, and 'who' is the agent or the owner of either can take even more extreme forms of delusional reduplication (splitting of the self, other people or places that lead to the corresponding beliefs of two, existing independent entities), as illustrated in the examples below. The first example is an interview with a male patient in the acute stage (two weeks), the second and third by chronic female patients (six months and two years) and the last by an acute female patient (two weeks).

4.7 Case example 7: two versions of events

SB: What happened to bring you here?

PATIENT: I have two versions. One, I was in the bathroom and I hit my head (all my troubles started in that bathroom). Two, I had a bit of a stroke.

SB: What kind of symptoms have you noticed since you came to the hospital?

PATIENT: I feel Okay. I mean, I know there are things I can't do. I have an age problem.

SB: Do you have any weakness anywhere?

PATIENT: Yes, my arm and leg, on the left side. They seem okay, but they might be dead.

SB: Are they causing you any trouble?

PATIENT: No, no trouble and no pain.

SB: Does it feel normal?

PATIENT: Not really, but it doesn't cause any trouble, as long as everything is near and I can reach it.

SB: Can you use it as well as you used to?

PATIENT: I can't, no.

SB: Are you fearful about losing the ability in your arm?

PATIENT: Yes, a little, but I feel it will come back.

SB: The doctors tell me there is some paralysis in your arm and leg. Do you agree?

PATIENT: I have never talked to a doctor about that. But he did say it will come alright.

SB: Do you think you can walk on your own?

PATIENT: I don't know, I haven't tried. I am a little tottery, but they won't let me anyway, they don't trust me.

4.8 Case example 8: two versions of my body

KF: Can you move your legs equally well since the stroke?

PATIENT: Yes, I can, I have no problems there. [Patient then spontaneously tries lifting her legs. She slightly lifted her left leg with her hands and commented] "Oh, yes, this one is a bit weaker".

KF: So, you cannot really move both legs well since the stroke?

PATIENT: Well I cannot move this one so easily because of the fall. They let me fall one day and I've hurt this side, otherwise it is ok. [Staff had indeed reported a fall in the preceding days].

KF: I see. And what about your hands, are they equally strong.

PATIENT: Well, this one [points to the left] is fine because I take it out at night to do things, but the other one [points to the right] gives me pain from time, to time.

KF: I see. So this arm [examiner lifts the left arm of the patient slightly] is ok, but...

PATIENT [INTERRUPTS]: This one [pointing to the left arm] is paralysed. I found it one morning in the bed and it has been stuck to me ever since. Useless, but it not mine. That is Peter's.

KF: Who is Peter?

PATIENT: My cousin. He came yesterday to visit. Didn't you see him?

KF: Oh, I am sorry, I was not here yesterday. But you say this arm [points to the patient's left arm] is his, and it is paralysed. But your own left arm is ok and you can move it?

PATIENT: Yes, I can. I do. Everyday.

4.9 Case example 9: two versions of space

KF: Good morning, how are you?

PATIENT: Not well, did they tell you?

KF: No, who, what happened?

PATIENT: Well, the girls [nursery staff]. I think I got into a bit of muddle today. I am still not sure. You see I woke up, looked outside and saw my darling [name of a village in Northumberland in north England, where the patient spent what appears to be a happy childhood]. I knew instantly it was that other one they made.

KF: the other one?

PATIENT: Yes, you know, I told you before how they have two [name of village], one here [we were in county Durham, south of Northumberland] and one up in Northumberland [the patient had indeed communicated various versions of this spatial reduplication to the examiner in past sessions].

KF: who do you mean by 'they'?

PATIENT: well, that is the thing. I suspect it is my nephew, you know, and his company, so much money and so much power. But then again, I do not know. Why? But the things they do. Did you know they also have two identical rooms in this building, or next building or wherever it is?

KF: No. Do they? How do you know?

PATIENT: They move me! There is a bridge, and they take me there, they move all my things and the room looks exactly the same, except I know it is not the same. I can feel it. It all feels wrong, I feel wrong and that is how I know they moved me again, it is not my room. Well, now I think they have two villages too.

KF: Oh, I see. Two identical villages?

PATIENT: Yes, although the girls say I am not making sense. I do get confused, you know, with the stroke and all.

KF: Yes, it must be very confusing not to know what is happening sometimes.

PATIENT: It is but I think it is them. Something to do with investments, it will help me they said. That way they are close to me. Well, I do not want it, I said. I do not like it here, I want to be up in [name of village]. Everything was beautiful, oh how beautiful.

4.10 Case example 10: two versions of reality

SB: You were telling me before, is this is not your arm? Whose arm is it?

PATIENT: Mathew's arm.

SB: Who is Mathew?

PATIENT: A friend of mine, I have known him a long time. [The patient had a former romantic partner with that name]

... some time later in the same conversation:

SB: and can you move your left arm?

PATIENT: I have been moving my left arm all day. I just can't seem to do it now. It just feels so heavy. I feel like I am lost in a dream and I can't get out of it. In the dream people have had accidents like strokes, but in reality everything is fine. I still feel the hand is more like his [Mathew's] than mine, but then when I pick it up, I know it is mine.

... some time later in the same conversation about her motor paralysis, the examiner asked:

SB: Does this this loss remind you of any other loses in your life?

PATIENT: I think you have to be a mother to know. My mother had a stroke, my brother as well. She did not have an easy life, a hard life. Now I feel like I have lost my life. I have lost my mind. Nothing feels real [starts to cry]. I still feel the loss of my mother. It never goes away that loss, my mother, the babies [previous miscarriages]. This all feels like a dream. I just don't know if it is a dream or reality.

The above brief examples illustrate the richness in the clinical variations of the presentation of anosognosia, even at the acute stage following stroke. Full descriptions of the clinical variability of this syndrome can be found elsewhere and fall beyond the scope of this chapter (see Besharati, Crucianelli & Fotopoulou, 2014; Marcel, Tegnér & Nimmo-Smith, 2004). However, the examples included here should be enough to illustrate the fact that a theory based only on sensorimotor deficits is not sufficient to account for the rich manifestations of AHP, as we further explain below with cross-reference to these examples.

5 Beyond the 'here-and-now' of experience: a difficulty in updating beliefs about the body

Indeed, it has long been apparent to us and other scholars that a strictly sensorimotor explanation is not sufficient to account for some of the delusional and emotional manifestations of the syndrome illustrated above, nor can it explain several other empirical findings in the literature (for discussion, see Fotopoulou, 2010; Ramachandran, 1995; Turnbull, Fotopoulou & Solms, 2014; Turnbull & Solms, 2007; Vuilleumier, 2004). For example, such theories cannot explain why some interventions, such as vestibular stimulation, can temporarily improve AHP (Cappa, Sterzi, Vallar & Bisiach, 1987; Ramachandran, 1995; Ronchi et al., 2013). We have also shown that mood induction can temporarily improve awareness (Besharati, Forkel, et al., 2014), supporting the psychotherapeutic observations of Kaplan-Solms and Solms (see above). Sensorimotor theories cannot also account for the non-unitary loss of motor awareness (i.e. why do some patients show implicit awareness into their deficits; see Case examples 3 and 4). Sensorimotor theories are valuable in explaining the illusion of moving (Fotopoulou et al., 2008; see Case examples 1 and 2), but patients do not simply claim that they have the phenomenal experience of moving as other non-anosognosic patients may claim (e.g. 'I have the impression that I am moving but I know it cannot be true because I know I am paralysed'). By contrast, patients with anosognosia ignore the wealth of contrary evidence and medical signs indicating that they are paralysed (e.g. their medical results, disabilities, occasional accidents and others' feedback; Case examples 3–10). This belief 'selectivity' is not the same as the one observed in other symptoms such as neglect, in the sense that patients with neglect can become aware of the fact that they have neglect after their errors are demonstrated to them. They then continue to do such errors in perception, but they are not surprised or in denial when these errors are pointed out to them again, as they have updated their more general beliefs about their perceptual abilities (an ability cognitive psychologists called 'metacognition', i.e. the cognitive evaluation of our own cognition; see below). In fact, the subset of patients who cannot become aware of their neglect would be diagnosed as anosognosic for these deficits. Moreover, as aforementioned, there is now also experimental evidence that patients with anosognosia maintain their denial even after they themselves had admitted their paralysis momentarily (e.g. Besharati, Forkel, et al., 2014). It appears that patients general beliefs about their body remain unaltered. What can be causing this failure to update one's abstract beliefs about the self beyond the 'here-and-now' of perception?

6 The subjective body: interoception and first-person experience

As we outlined above, while exteroceptive (sensations responsible for external perception such as vision and audition), prioprioceptive (sensations about the position of the body in space) and motor deficits may be important contributors to how the body is experienced from a first-person perspective in anosognosia, they are unlikely to be its primary or sufficient causes. By contrast, another facet of how individuals experience their own body subjectively, in the first person, may have a central role in anosognosia. Recent lesion mapping studies have indicated that grey areas such as the insula and limbic structures may be selectively associated with AHP (Fotopoulou et al., 2010; Karnath, Baier & Nägele, 2005; Moro et al., 2011; Vocat, Staub, Stroppini & Vuilleumier, 2010), and we have conducted a recent large study (174 patients) using advanced lesion mapping techniques that revealed a disconnection of these areas from frontoparietal sensorimotor attention and control networks Pacella et al., 2019). Previous functional neuroimaging studies have found that the functional role of these areas and their connections concerns interoception (Craig, 2009; Critchley et al., 2004). Interoception refers to the perception of the physiological condition of the body, involving modalities such as temperature, itch, pain, cardiac signals, respiration, hunger, thirst, pleasure from sensual touch and other bodily feelings relating to homeostasis (Craig, 2010; Critchley et al., 2004). It is distinct from the exteroceptive system, which refers to the classical sensory modalities for perceiving the external environment (e.g. vision, audition), as well as proprioceptive, vestibular and kinesthetic input informing about the movement and location of the body in space (Blanke & Metzinger, 2009; Craig, 2010; Critchley et al., 2004), as it is mediated by a separate specialised neuroanatomical system, linked to homeostasis and subjective, emotional core of the self (Craig, 2009; Critchley et al., 2004; Damasio 1994; Seth, 2013). Interoception informs the mind about *how* the body itself is doing in relation to certain inherited, homeostatic needs (e.g. one may be dehydrated or stung by an insect), while exteroception informs the organism about environmental changes in relation to such needs (there is a river ahead) but independently of the physiological state of the body itself. Thus, interoception is considered the basis of the sentient self, how we feel in the here-and-now of experience. From the point of view of modern neuroscientific theories, subjective feeling states arise from predictive inferences on the causes of interoceptive signals (Barrett & Simmons, 2015; Pezzulo, Rigoli & Friston, 2015; Seth, 2013; Seth, Suzuki & Critchley, 2012).

Accordingly, we have proposed that anosognosic and asomatognosic patients struggle to affectively *personalise* new sensorimotor information and related beliefs about the affected body parts because interoceptive and emotional signals about the current state of the body are weak or suppressed, or unable to update current predictions and expectations of how the affected body parts should *feel like* (Fotopoulou, 2015; Martinaud, Besharati, Jenkinson & Fotopoulou, 2017). In support of this hypothesis, a recent study (Romano, Gandola, Bottini & Maravita, 2014) has shown that right hemisphere patients who show somatoparahrenic beliefs about their affected body parts also show reduced physiological reactions to the threat of the same body parts, as measured by skin conductance responses. Moreover, given the higher position of such prior beliefs in the neurocognitive hierarchy (see Friston, 2013), such faulty inference may also 'explain away' contrary exteroceptive signals during instances of multisensory integration (see also Fotopoulou, 2015, for some more details on striatal lesions and their relevance to updating body beliefs in anosognosia). In words of one anosognosic patient, who also denied the ownership of his paralysed limbs: "But my eyes and my feelings don't agree, and I must believe my feelings. I know they [left arm and leg] look like mine, but I can feel they are not, and I can't believe my eyes" (C.W. Olsen, 1937, cited in Feinberg, 1997). Thus, it appears that as motor intentions may be confused with actually executed actions due to damage to frontoparietal networks of motor control (see above), so can interoceptive priors (*how I expect my body to feel*) can be confused with actual feelings of the body in the here-and-now (*how my body actually feels*) due to damage to brain areas processing and integrating (the salience of) interoceptive feelings about the body. Thus, patients may have illusory *feelings* of an intact body that they struggle to integrate with their current sad reality of their paralysis.

7 The objective body: taking a third-person perspective on the self

It further appears that some patients are well aware of what doctors and their relatives think about their current state, even if they do not feel it to be so or believe it or find it self-relevant. For example, one of our somatoparaphrenic patients described how she knew the nurses thought she was silly and talked as though she was an octopus with many legs and arms, but nevertheless she felt that she was right and they were wrong. Another anosognosic patient related: "Doctors tell me I cannot move. I do not mean to doubt them, if they are doctors, they know these things. But I also know myself. I know I can walk." Thus, the difficult of these patients is not necessarily that they cannot take the perspective of other people. Instead, we have found that although these patients, like other right hemisphere patients, have deficits in visuospatial perspective taking, these deficits were not specifically associated with the presence, nor the severity of anosognosic symptoms (Besharati et al., 2016). Instead, anosognosic patients know that from the perspective of other people their body appears paralysed, but their own subjectively experienced body is disconnected from such other, social perspectives on the body. Indeed, our group and others (e.g. Marcel, Tegnér & Nimmo-Smith, 2004) have demonstrated that when patients are given third-person perspectives (visual or mental) of their deficits (e.g. when they are given mirror feedback of their paralysed arm; Fotopoulou et al., 2011), their awareness of their body improves, but only temporarily (see Figure 12.1). In fact, we were quite surprised to observe that patients may suddenly have a recognition of their body parts in a mirror, despite vehemently denying its ownership for the past 30–40 days (Fotopoulou et al., 2011; Jenkinson, Haggard, Ferreira & Fotopoulou, 2013). Even more counterintuitively, this recognition was not

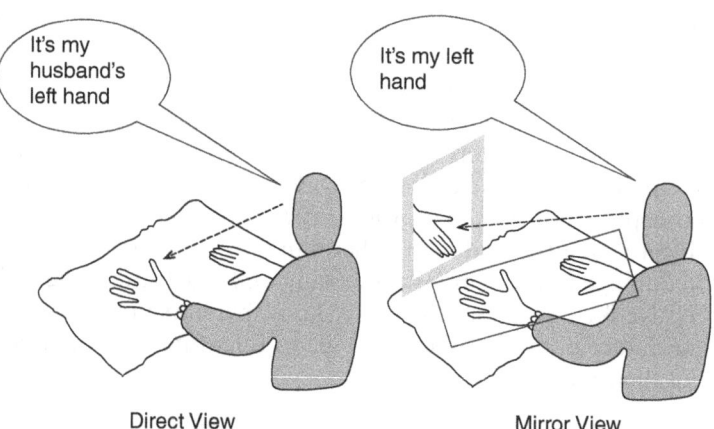

Direct View   Mirror View

Figure 12.1 Image showing how patients repeatedly change their beliefs about the ownership of the paralysed arm based on the visual perspective (first vs third) offered to them by direct versus mirror view, without any indication of a cognitive or an emotional integration between the two experiences (adapted from Fotopoulou et al., 2011).

experienced by the patient as a surprise. To put it bluntly, they did not thank us for 'finding' their lost arm after all this time, nor where they surprised when they lost it again a few seconds later. Indeed, patients' recognition of their own arm fluctuated every few seconds, without any apparent emotional reaction on their part. It appeared that the arm they saw in the mirror that they recognised as theirs and the arm that they experienced in front of them were actually two different arms, belonging to two different people despite their coincidence in time and space.

Following the insights of Kaplan-Solms and Solms (2000), we also made similar observations verbally, when we asked patients to tell us whether the arms they had 'in their mind' versus the arms that existed 'in reality' could move (for extensive clinical vignettes, see Fotopoulou et al., 2011; Jenkinson, Haggard, Ferreira & Fotopoulou, 2013). Patients tend to believe that the arms 'in their mind' can move, but when asked about the ones 'in reality', they either stayed silent and refused to answer or started to cry. It thus appears that perspective-taking difficulties per se are not the cause of anosognosia and related symptoms. Instead, patients are unable or unwilling *to integrate* social (third person) perspectives on body with their own subjective (first person) feelings and beliefs about their body. It is this understanding of anosognosia as *a disconnection syndrome* (failure to integrate), or the neurological equivalent of splitting, that psychoanalytic theory can best inform. Specifically, classic, Freudian metapsychology, as well as later more relational approaches in psychoanalysis, has offered insights about the developmental transition between early (narcissistic) stages of cognitive and emotional immaturity (when self and object are not integrated, but instead treated according to one's momentary, emotional needs) and more mature stages (when the self and other people can be experienced as integrated and as containing both positive and negative aspects). In accordance with Kaplan-Solms and Solms, but with added theoretical precision and empirical confirmation, we outline below that anosognosia can be best explained as *an integration deficit* that thus affects the latter more mature mode of psychic functioning that relies on the integration of first and third person perspectives on the self.

7.1 The cognitive integration of the subjective and objective body

In psychiatry and neuroscience, difficulties with self-awareness are typically described in the context of 'impaired clinical insight'. Moreover, in neuropsychiatry, clinical insight is not regarded as an all-or-nothing ability to accept one's illness, but rather as a set of processes about how one forms beliefs about the self (cognitive insight) that themselves rely on higher order cognitive abilities of other- and self-directed mentalisation, also known as social cognition (being able to see and judge oneself from the perspective of other people) and metacognition (the ability to evaluate our own cognition (Flavell, 1979; Fleming & Dolan, 2012), respectively). For example, one needs to infer the mental states of other people (other-directed mentalisation or social cognition) in the audience to interpret their reaction to one's own speech as a way to evaluate the success of the speech beyond their own, first-person experience of it. In the case of self-directed mentalisation or metacognition, one may have low confidence (defined as the degree of subjective uncertainty) in what they think they saw in a dark room or how well they performed a task when they did not receive any explicit feedback. Metacognition characterises the relation between this subjective uncertainty and accuracy, and in this sense, it affords a measure of insight into one's perception or beliefs. Some have claimed that the two abilities (self- and other-directed metacognition) are actually relying on the common core ability of social inference (self metacognition is simply the ability to see the self as another), a position that we return to later, but in the existing literature there is an ongoing debate regarding the relation between these two higher order abilities. Importantly, it has been shown that prospective metacognition (forecasting, knowing how well one will do in the future) is an even more higher order ability than retrospective metacognition (knowing how accurate one was on a given judgement), and similar dissociations between anticipatory and emergent awareness have been shown in anosognosia, with the former being more affected and harder to treat than the latter (Moro et al., 2011).

In previous publications, we have also introduced the term 'embodied mentalisation' (Besharati et al., 2016; Fotopoulou & Tsakiris, 2017) to ground such higher order concepts in their embodied and relational origins (as we will indeed explain below), as well as to highlight the role of such mentalisation in embodied, self-perception. The latter is also our aim here, with particular emphasis in explaining which neurocognitive mechanisms may support the transition from part-object to whole-object relating, as suggested by psychoanalysis. We unpack these notions below.

As outlined above, it seems that anosognosic patients cannot update their unconscious inferences and conscious beliefs about the body as they do not experience the current state of their body (which in neuroscientific terms should generate 'prediction errors' and lead patients to revised their predictions accordingly) as emotionally relevant to their more general sense of self, including their sense of (motor) agency and body ownership. However, a fundamental question remains. Patients seem unable to use other higher order knowledge, including with the help of social feedback, to update their beliefs, despite the fact that they themselves improve their awareness when sked to take a third-person perspective. This failure is not easy to explain on the basis of exteroceptive, proprioceptive or interoceptive deficits (i.e. lack of prediction errors about the external world or the inner body). Of course, patients' feelings that the paralysed body parts are of limited self-relevance partly explain why they would disregard social feedback for some time. As the aforementioned patient claimed, one has learned to trust one's feelings about the body over and above other sources of information. This is also consistent with the assumed hierarchy of the proposed model (brain areas thought of as subserving interoception and emotion are thought of as higher in the neurocognitive hierarchy than areas subserving exteroception; Friston, 2013). However, at the same time, it is not clear why other more reflective or higher order cognitive predictions about the self and others (e.g. 'my family and doctors would not lie to me about serious health issues') are not used to update one's beliefs, or at least generate some doubt (subjective uncertainty) about one's (duplicated) perception (see Case examples 7–10). In neuroscientific terms, why are more abstract, generative models about the self and others' beliefs not used to send predictions down the neurocognitive hierarchy and metacognitively correct faulty perceptual inferences. In psychoanalytic terms, why are such 'reality testing' processes not taking place?

We believe there are two interrelated answers to this question: one is cognitive that we will cover in this section and one is emotional that we will cover in Section 8. The first answer could be that these particular aspects of cognition are affected by the right hemisphere damage in question, and it is this damage that does not allow the integration between subjective, first-person and third-person perspectives on the self. In this section, we will try to describe the nature of this particular impairment as manifested in AHP and the nature of the presumed corresponding function in the undamaged brain. In previous writings, borrowing insights from Merleau-Ponty (1945/1962), one of us (KF) has called this aspect of body representation the 'impersonalised' body (Fotopoulou, 2015), to emphasise not only that it goes beyond our egocentric, first-person experience of the body but also that it does not relate to any particular social, third-person perceptive of the body. Rather it relates to the integration of all possible 'spaces', 'times' and 'social perspectives' on the body, so that the body can be represented as a 'whole-in-itself', irrespective of current embodied or social experiences of it. This level of integration of cognitions across space and time is best captured in the cognitive literature by notions regarding 'prospective metacognition' and 'allocentric' mentalisation (Frith & de Vignemont, 2005), as we outline below.

Our perception of the world, including our own body, is not only a matter of appearances. Indeed, my perception of the world is rarely confined to the characteristics of the input that reaches my sensory organs from my current, unique position and perspective in the world. Instead, my prior experiences of different possibilities and positions in the world define how I perceive the world in any given time and space. In other words, my perception of the world and my body appears to me to be about the 'here-and-now' of experience, but, in fact, my inferences about the causes of the 'here-and-now' of the world and myself are informed by my more broader expectations about the world and the self in any 'then and there'. A lemon on the table is not only the yellow, roundish thing I see from my perspective (the perception of colour and shape is, of course, already an inference), but the three-dimensional fruit whose acidity I can mentally taste and whose weight and action affordances my motor system simulates before I even move. Most perceptual experiences involve some degree of predictive, multisensory and sensorimotor integration, as well as our imaginative ability to integrate such features across space and time and person. Imagine that you see a child grabbing, cutting and tasting that lemon. Most people will have the intuition that they can feel the acidic taste on behalf of the child, and most importantly for present purposes, most people will interpret the subsequent facial expressions of the child on the basis of this intuition. Thus, even when we observe other people, we do not only perceive appearances. We do not see 'behaviours' in other people; we see intentions, wishes and more generally mental states. In other terms, we infer *the causes* of appearances in the world. When these appearances involve the physical world, we call these causes 'an object' such as lemon, which has given tastes and affordances. When these appearances involve the social world, we call these causes 'a mental state', or another person with a mind, not just a body. In this example, we will infer that the child's facial expression was caused by his experience of a sour taste perception, based on our 'integrated' perception of lemons as acidic and of children as capable of taste, rather than our own personal experience of that particular lemon or that particular child. We perceive the world as containing unique, whole-in-themselves objects and people despite the fact that our actual perception of them from a subjective point of view will always be limited to the constraints of our body in time and space, e.g. the position of our eyes on the head. This human ability to simultaneously perceive the world in an already organized and synthesised way, which entails many silent potential perspectives, and their corresponding action possibilities, suggest that our perception relies on integrating inferences and that such inferences about the physical world are deeply embedded in the social world (Fotopoulou & Tsakiris, 2017; see also section 8).

It turns out that this highly sophisticated (although somewhat 'hidden' from consciousness) ability to perceive the world beyond the 'here-and-now' of first-person experience and to mentally integrate 'identities' across space and time and person is what anosognosic patients lack as regards their affected body. In the words of Merleau-Ponty about both anosognosia and phantom limb symptoms (1945/1962, p. 82):

> In the case under consideration, the ambiguity of knowledge amounts to this: our body comprise as it were two layers: that of the habit body and that of the body in this moment. In the first appear manipulatory objects that have disappeared from the other and the problem how I can have the sensation of still possessing a limb I no longer have amounts to finding out how the habitual body can act as quarantee for the body at

this moment. How can I perceive objects as manipulatable when I can no longer manipulate them? The manipulatable must have ceased to be what I am now manipulating, and become what one can manipulate; it must have ceased to be a thing manipulatable for me and become a thing manipulate in itself. Correspondingly, my body must be apprehended not only in an experience which is instantaneous, peculiar to itself and complete in itself, but also in some general aspect and in the light of an impersonal being.

Thus, anosognosic patients seem to have lost the ability to perceive their affected body parts in an 'impersonalised' way (in a whole-object relation in psychoanalytic terms). They can only perceive them in a personal, first-person (narcissistic) way. Indeed, psychoanalysis reminds us that when we relate to our 'objects' (other people and internalised others) in a split way, we also relate to ourselves in a similar way. Indeed, when the above understanding of 'impersonalised' perception is applied to the perception of one's own body, one notices an inevitable tension in the mind. The first-person, egocentric perspective (spatial and mental) remains fundamental for the perception of the body as mine, as under my volitional control, affectively personalised by interoception and as separate from other objects in the world (e.g. Damasio, 1994). In other terms, although the body can be perceived (impersonalised and objectified) as a kind of social, impersonal, unique object, it is also always the subject of all experiences. According to our dynamic understanding of this tension, typically in adults the more 'impersonalised' or more 'integrated' appreciation of the body needs to dominate to a degree the more egocentric (or, narcissistic) experience of the body when we need to be realistic about our body and its abilities. Of course, as we know from psychoanalysis, this dominance and inhibition is merely dynamic, i.e. it can be undone due to many reasons. We believe anosognosia represents a neurological example of this undoing of the integration of first-person, egocentric experience of the self and more 'whole-in-themselves', impersonalised views on the self.

We have recently shown that anosognosic patients are not impaired in third-person, visuospatial or verbal perspective taking itself (see also above), but they have a selective impairment in mentalising (reading the mental states of others) in allocentric mode (Besharati et al., 2016). Specifically, while patients were able to read other people's mental states when they had to take the perspective of other people in brief stories that also involved themselves (mentalisation from an egocentric stance; see Figure 12.2), they were unable to read other people's mental states when the stories read out to them did not involve them at all, i.e. they were stories referring to the relationship between two other people (mentalisation from an allocentric stance; Besharati et al., 2016). Indeed, in the field of autism, other researchers have noted that perspective taking may simply involve the transposition of the egocentric

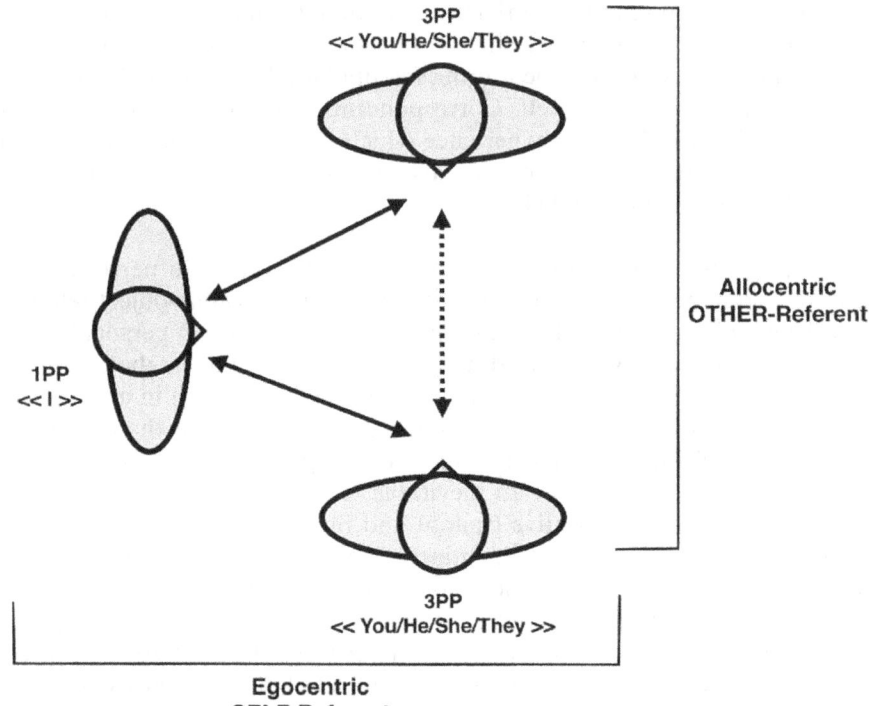

Figure 12.2 Synthesis of social and spatial cognition. The social world involves a first-person perspective (1PP) that can be transposed to another person with whom we are in the second-person relation, when we take a third-person perspective (3PP) to think about that person or ourself from their perspective (looking back at ourselves from the perspective of another person). However, in allocentric relations, there is no self-reference, in the sense that we have to imagine a relation between two other agents, irrespective of the self. Thus, egocentric (self-referent) mentalization involves perspective taking when the other (3PP) is *related* to the self, whereas allocentric (other-referent) mentalization is when the other (3PP) is completely *unrelated* to the self.

stance in a different location (a third-person perspective can remain egocentric and self-referent), whereas an allocentric stance acknowledges a relation between other minds that is completely independence of one's own egocentric perspective (Frith & de Vignemont, 2005; Vogeley & Fink, 2003). Interestingly, in our study, only their performance in the later, allocentric task and none of the other mentalisation and perspective-taking conditions correlated with severity of unawareness in our sample. Thus, there was a specific association between anosognosia and allocentric mentalisation; the worse patients were in allocentric mentalisation, the more severe was their anosognosia.

More generally, our prior and current empirical investigations focus on understanding further the psychological and neural nature of these impairments in allocentric and prospective beliefs about the self. For example, we are finding that in anosognosia allocentric errors (Besharati et al., 2016) and prospective errors (Kirsch et al., in preparation) relate not only to damage to limbic and premotor areas as aforementioned but also to disconnections of the ventral attention network (i.e. connections between temporo-parietal junction and ventral frontal cortex), through the superior longitudinal fasciculus (Pacella et al., 2019), which at least some authors have linked to post-perceptual processes involved in contextual updating and adjustments of top-down expectations (Geng & Vossel, 2013).

In summary, we have seen how the complex syndrome of anosognosia can be caused by patients' expectations about their first-person sense of (motor) agency and their first-person feelings of body ownership that cannot be updated because brain damage has affected how new information is processed in both sensorimotor and emotional domains. Importantly, patients cannot use third-person beliefs or feedback to update their beliefs either, as it appears that the higher order processes that typically allow the integration of subjective, first-person perspectives, and objective, third-person perspectives on the self are also affected by disconnection between the relevant brain areas. However, as we will argue below, one of the major contributions of psychoanalysis is to highlight that such high-order cognitive abilities are not mere cognitive acquisitions in development. Instead, they are also socio-affective processes that depend on the quality of care infants received in early childhood. We believe this intersubjective aspect of anosognosia has not been sufficiently covered in the original work by Kaplan-Solms and Solms (see also Ciaunica & Fotopoulou, 2017; Fotopoulou & Tsakiris, 2017). We outline these processes and their relevance to anosognosia below.

8 The second-person body: the emotional glue of the subjective and the objective body

The question of whether our mental life is initially and primarily shaped by embodied dimensions of the singular individual or by interpersonal relations has been debated in many fields such as psychology, philosophy and psychoanalysis. For example, these fields have extensively debated whether bodily or social drives are the primary motivator of the mind and whether bodily or social experience is the primary organiser of the self (see also Ciaunica & Fotopoulou, 2017; Fotopoulou & Tsakiris, 2017). In recent decades, proponents of the idea that an early distinction between self and other necessitates the development of 'mentalization' abilities have debated whether understanding other minds and one's own is achieved by 'simulation' and 'analogy' with one's first-person, embodied perspective (e.g. Gallese, 2005) or by cognitive inference from a third-person perspective (e.g. Morton & Frith, 1995). A similar debate exists regarding how we come to know our own mind. Indeed, mirroring the above sections on anosognosia, there are two major views in cognitive and affective neuroscience on how one comes to know one's (embodied) mind: one through integrating multimodal signals, including interoceptive signals into an egocentric reference frame and assigning the first-person perspective (Blanke, Slater & Serino, 2015; Damasio, 1994; Solms, 2013; Vogeley et al., 2001). Another through the cognitive ability to disengage from the embodied 1PP and adopt another person's, third-person perspective on your experience, the so-called theory of mind (ToM) or self-referent, or mentalising or metacognitive ability (Frith & Frith, 2007). We referred to the relevance of both aspects to anosognosia and thus self-awareness in the preceding sections.

Interestingly, more recently a number of intermediate positions have been put forward, notably interaction theory (Fuchs & De Jaegher, 2009; Gallagher, 2000; Gallagher & Frith, 2003) and second-person approaches (Ciaunica & Fotopoulou, 2017; Fotopoulou & Tsakiris, 2017; Reddy, 2008; Schilbach et al., 2013). These emphasise neither the first- nor the third-person view on understanding other minds and one's own, but instead put forward the idea that early, reciprocal interactions and emotional engagements with caregivers (the kind that Winnicot had in mind) are fundamental to our sense of self and the development of the distinction between self and other. We cannot do justice to all these positions and debates here, and their relevance to psychoanalysis, but we present the relevance of these notions to anosognosia and particularly the relevance of parental and psychotherapeutic responsiveness in the integration of the subjective and the objective body.

The aforementioned dissociation between the appreciation of the body from a first-person perspective versus a third-person perspective, as, e.g. observed in the difference between direct and mirror self-observation (see Figure 12.1), is reminiscent of how young infants do not realise that the image of the infant they see in the mirror actually 'corresponds' to themselves, or reversely that the felt body is also the body seen in the mirror, by both the self and others, *i.e. the internal and external 'appearance' of the body corresponds to one entity, the self.* It is typically around the age of two years that the infants can immediately recognise that mirror images of themselves refer back to their own body as experienced from a first-person perspective. Yet, as psychoanalysis first highlighted and several developmental studies now attest, this relatively late instant of physical mirroring is embedded in rich history of social, affective mirroring (e.g. Winnicot, 1972), in which good-enough parents are responding to an infant's bodily needs with bodily care, emotional sensitivity and cognitive (e.g. language) specification so as to facilitate the infant to progressively organise and regulate their minds. Indeed, a crucial feature of infants' early interactions with caregivers is the timing and appropriateness of caregiver actions relative to infant needs and actions. For example, infants and caregivers engage in sequences of mutually contingent patterns of looking, smiling and vocalising by one to three months or earlier (Kärtner et al., 2008; Kaye & Fogel, 1980). Recently, one of us (KF) has argued that such "sensitive" (Cassidy & Shaver, 2008), "contingent" (Gergely & Watson, 1999), "attuned" (Stern, 1985) or "mentalizing" (Fonagy, Gergely, Jurist & Target, 2002) social environments have an even more potent role than previous thought. Namely, they are necessary for the 'mentalization of homeostasis', which is the transition from the registration of interoceptive sensations in the infant's body to the formation of integrated, mental categories (predictive models) of embodied experiences of interoceptive needs and the corresponding actions towards or away from certain physical or social objects that would satisfy them. Typically, such mental categories are called emotions. We unpack below how anosognosia reveals that this developmental transition is also fundamental for the integration of the subjective (interoceptive, egocentric and narcissistic) experience of the body with third-person (exteroceptive and metacognitive) experiences of the same body.

Specifically, contrary to theories that argue that the sense of our bodily self primarily arises from the individual's interoceptive or emotional experience of their own body (Craig, 2009; Damasio, 1994; Critchley et al., 2004; Seth, Suzuki & Critchley, 2012; Solms, 2013) and also contrary to theories that view the development of mentalisation as a purely cognitive module (e.g. Brothers & Ring, 1992), it appears that in humans interpersonal interactions are necessary in determining the developmental emergence of mentalisation of self and others, including the mentalisation of affective states. The most fundamental reason for this socially mediated emergence in development seems to be the motor immaturity of human infants. Indeed, human infants are born without a fully matured motor system, and hence, they cannot fully regulate their own homeostasis unaided, beyond some minor forms of self-soothing (e.g. thumb sucking). A young infant cannot position and balance itself, feed itself, thermoregulate or protect itself from tissue damage (e.g. skin burns, bone fractures, etc.). Thus, in the case of such interoceptive modalities, *no movement on the part of the infant alone can change certain key neurophysiological states relating to homeostasis*. Put in simple terms, the infant can suck a dummy or his/her their fingers to regulate neurophysiological states. But in order to change states related to food intake, or temperature regulation, and build predictive models regarding the *mental causes* of such physiological changes (i.e. hunger and satiation, changes in temperature), *someone else* needs to be in proximity, interacting to offer the breast or the bottle. Thus, the unaided infant cannot use action to collect evidence about the causes of its interoceptive experiences, and thus, it cannot test its interoceptive predictions against the world. Instead, the infant's autonomic and motor reflexes in response to unpredicted physiological states (e.g. crying and kicking when hypothalamic function detects that glucose levels are not within the predicted viable range) can elicit the attention of the caregiver and ensure that the caregiver tries to change the physiological state of the infant (e.g. by feeding it or raping it in a blanket) until the homeostatic needs are met (i.e. glucose levels or body temperature is within the predicted range). Thus, updating interoceptive predictions in infants includes information regarding the reaction of caregivers to infants' initial autonomic and proprioceptive predictions. Therefore, it is the adult's actions and reactions, their frequency and multisensory characteristics that will generate changes in interoceptive states and hence ultimately contribute to the 'mentalization' of physiological states in the infant. It is exactly because a human infant depends on the caregiver to regulate her homeostasis that the interaction with caregivers is woven into the very emergence of the emotional self (and the emotional understanding of others). In the terminology of neuroscience, the origins of interoceptive active inference are always, by necessity, social, and thus, core subjective feelings such as hunger and satiation, pain and relief and cold or warmth have actually social origins.

Moreover, in good-enough caregiving environments, such caregiving behaviors are met, not only by facial expressions and other "mentally" attuned responses but – and crucially – with a variety of proximal, *embodied* responses, such as soothing touch, holding and many 'marking' behaviours, which can themselves produce further changes in the infant's physiology (e.g. heart-rate reductions). Thus, basic caregiving behaviours are the source of multisensory input (e.g. auditory, tactile, olfactory and visual bundles of experience) and amodal properties such as rhythm, frequency, synchrony and other such contingency variables (see also Stern's vitality affects, 1985).

Crucially, parental responsiveness and mirroring are never 'precise' or without uncertainty; they are 'good enough', playful (Winnicot, 1972) and 'marked' (Fonagy et al., 2002). Marking, gradual frustrations and incongruences, instances of asynchrony and distance, deliverable role-playing, pretense play and prohibitions by the parents during intersubjective interactions progressively allow infants not only to mentalise their own body with the help of their caregivers but also to strengthen the self-other distinction (i.e. to progressively start attributing the mentalised states either to the self or to the other, irrespective of appearances and their own bodily needs; see also above). Other bodies and their actions therefore stand right in the midst of all embodied mentalisation processes of the infant, helping it to detect imperfect contingencies between how it feels from the inside and what the world may offer and hence progressively learn both 'what' the body feels and 'whose' is that feeling body, their own or the 'good-enough' caregiver's. Thus, this caring but playful, imperfect and marked mirroring between infant and caregiver establishes a zone of *uncertainty* between the subjective and the objective of experience that makes learning and their integration possible. This concept of uncertainty is increasingly important in neuroscientific theories (e.g. Friston, 2010), including in anosognosia (Fotopoulou, 2015). Sadly, further coverage escapes the scope of the current chapter, but interested readers can refer to the neuroscientific concepts of 'precision' and the tolerance of uncertainty and the role of disambiguation in other writings of the topic (Fotopoulou, 2013, 2015). Here, we focus instead on the clinical role of this second person relating to anosognosia.

As we described above, anosognosic patients seem unable to form a realistic, metacognitive appreciation of their paralysis without feedback, but they are also unable to integrate third-person feedback, e.g. mirror or social feedback, with their first-person experience *of their body* and hence update their beliefs *about the body*. Could we use the above developmental considerations and reflect on how caregivers' mirroring facilitates the integration of the interoceptively felt and the exteroceptively observed self? Could we thus facilitate a proper self–other distinction in a safe, second-person context? Indeed, we would argue that 'good-enough' therapists can provide exactly this kind of context, as Kaplan-Solms and Solms (2000) have also demonstrated (see also Fotopoulou, 2010, for a case study). Within such safe, psychotherapeutic context, therapists can validate the emotions of the patients without caring too much about the precise 'cognitive contexts' that they appear (a form of adult pretense play, perhaps; see Case example 6) and they can also gently introduce integration opportunities between the patient's perspective and their own; see Case example 10). Sometimes though, particularly in diseases such as stroke, that early interventions can have much stronger effects than late interventions, the acute stroke ward may not be the right time and place for building psychotherapeutic rapport or may simply not be available by the system, as it is sadly the case in most acute rehabilitation stroke wards in the British National Health System. In this context, we have recently explored whether a psychotherapeutic attitude could be combined with some more basic, second-person, embodied interventions.

We selected social, affective touch. Recent neurophysiological, neuroimaging and behavioural studies suggest that certain tactile experiences, such as gentle caress-like strokes, are processed by at least two separate neurocognitive systems. First, as it has been known for decades, tactile stimuli are processed in terms of their exteroceptive, discriminatory processes in classical peripheral pathways and somatosensory cortical areas. Second, it was recently demonstrated that a specialised peripheral and central system codes for the *affective*, *interoceptive* properties of the same tactile stimulus (Case et al., 2016; Löken, Wessberg, Morrison, McGlone & Olausson, 2009; Morrison, Bjornsdotter & Olausson, 2011). Thus, while gentle, stroking-like touch originates from outside the body, it appears to simultaneously convey information about the state of the body itself (e.g. pleasure from the skin and reductions in physiological arousal) and the external world (e.g. sensation of skin stimulation of some density and softness characteristics, slow speed and little friction). Moreover, the system supporting affective touch has been found to respond optimally to touch of human temperature rather than colder robot-based touch (Ackerley et al., 2014). This and related findings (for reviews and the so-called social touch hypothesis, see Ciaunica & Fotopoulou, 2017; Gentsch, Panagiotopoulou & Fotopoulou, 2015; Morrison, Loken & Olausson, 2010) suggest that this system may be specialised for not only processing affective touch but also specifically social affective touch. Thus, we recently reasoned that this type of affective, social affective touch may be an optimal modality for facilitating the integration of the subjective and the third-person body. We hypothesised that given that a single tactile stimulus that elicits both interoceptive and exteroceptive signals occurring, by necessity, at the same time and place (thus they are characterised by the amodal properties of temporal and spatial congruency that bind modalities together and create predictions and generative models of their causes; Fotopoulou & Tsakiris, 2017), they are progressively mentalised as one experience. In other terms, the caregiver's touch contributes directly to the integration of the infant's interoceptive and exteroceptive bodily experiences, possibly helping the infant experience the skin as the boundary between her body and external world (see Anzieu, 1989, for related psychoanalytic ideas about the Skin Ego).

Could affective touch help re-personalise signals in the affected body parts of anosognosic individuals? As part of an ongoing experimental study, we have recently applied gentle, slow affective touch, following the properties of the aforementioned interoceptive system, as well as other types of emotionally 'neutral' touch, in a series of patients with anosognosia and deficits of body ownership at the acute stage of their recovery. In different instances, we also showed patients how to do the same with their intact arm (self-touch). We are still gathering data on the experiment, so our findings are preliminary at this stage, and in all cases, this was an experimental study rather than a clinical intervention, so care should be taken when interpreting our data. Nevertheless, we have made some promising observations in patients we first piloted this experiment. First of all, although right hemisphere patients have a degree of sensory deficit following their stroke, and indeed they perceived the intensity of strokes as less strong on their affected than their unaffected arms, most of the patients were able to perceive the pleasantness of slow, gentle touch equally in their affected and non-affected arms. Most interestingly, when we asked patients questions about the ownership of their affected arm, before and after affective and neutral touch, they showed acceptance of their paralysed arm to a greater degree after affective than other neutral touch. One patient who used to called her left arm, her 'alienated arm' in the first days following her stroke, told us that after the affective touch experiment, she would use her right, intact arm, to stroke her left arm and speaking to it, she said, 'come, correspond to me'. Another patient somewhat similarly told us a few days after the experiment:

> I woke up and I called this arm 'a beast'. It was not my arm, I did not want it, it was some foreign fellow. But then you touched it and I caress

it as you said and I decided to love it again. I said 'Come, I accept you. I welcome you back'... We have been through a lot together...

We believe these are preliminary indications of how caring, affective, embodied signals in an appropriate social or therapeutic context could allow patients to first relate to their own paralysed body in the second person (as embodied, subjective frustrations were once regulated and soothed by the body of 'good-enough' caregivers) and then from this self-caring stance they can progressively integrate their first-person expectations about their body with third-person perspectives on the body. Ultimately, the various stances are integrated and the body can again be perspective by the more balanced and realistic, impersonalised perspective of the reflecting, more narrative and less narcissistic self, as the patients in the two examples above so beautifully describe. Their arm may no longer be the functioning arm they wanted to be able to rely on, but it is still the same arm that they 'have been through a lot together' and hence indeed the arm that 'corresponds' to them, the arm that belongs to all the times and spaces of their lives.

9 Conclusion

In this chapter, we have revisited the classic neuropsychoanalytic insights of Kaplan-Solms and Solms about the role of the right hemisphere in the realistic appreciation of the self. We have used clinical examples and systematic, empirical investigations to show that patients are indeed unable to update their metacognitive beliefs about their body, because of a functional disconnection between brain areas that would typically allow new emotional and sensorimotor signals from the 'here-and-now' of the body to be integrated with more abstract, cognitive beliefs about the self across time, space and person. Moreover, simply attempting to 'train' patients' higher order abilities of thinking of the self across different temporal, spatial and social instances is ineffective, as the first-person (subjective) and the third-person (objective) self are indeed experienced as two separate beings. Instead, attempting to relate to patients in a second-person way allows a re-integration of split-off parts of the self into one's life narrative and ultimately in a more realistic, reflective and less narcissistic stance towards their body.

Acknowledgements

The authors would like to thank the patients and their families for their participation and the Neuropsychoanalysis Foundation for its continued support. This work was funded by a European Research Council (ERC) Starting Investigator Award for the project 'The Bodily Self' N_313755 to AF. The support of the DST-NRF Centre of Excellence in Human Development at the University of the Witwatersrand, Johannesburg, in the Republic of South Africa towards this research is hereby acknowledged to SB.

References

Ackerley, R., Backlund Wasling, H., Liljencrantz, J., Olausson, H., Johnson, R. D., & Wessberg, J. (2014). Human C-tactile afferents are tuned to the temperature of a skin-stroking caress. *Journal of Neuroscience, 34*, 2879–2883.

Anzieu, D. (1989). *The skin ego*. (Chris Turner, Trans.). New Haven, CT: Yale University Press.

Babinski, J. (1914). Contribution e l'etude des troubles mentaux dans hemiplegie organique cerebrale (anosognosia) [contribution to the study of mental disorders in hemiplegia (anosognosia)]. *Revue Neurologique, 27*, 845–848.

Barrett, L. F., & Simmons, W. K. (2015). Interoceptive predictions in the brain. *Nature Reviews. Neuroscience, 16*, 419–429.

Berti, A., Bottini, G., Gandola, M., Pia, L., Smania, N., Stracciari, A., & Paulesu, E. (2005). Shared cortical anatomy for motor awareness and motor control. *Science, 309*, 488–491.

Besharati, S., Crucianelli, L., & Fotopoulou, A. (2014). Restoring awareness: A review of rehabilitation in anosognosia for hemiplegia. *Revista Chilena de Neuropsicología, 9*, 31–37.

Besharati, S., Forkel, S. J., Kopelman, M., Solms, M., Jenkinson, P. M., & Fotopoulou, A. (2014). The affective modulation of motor awareness in anosognosia for hemiplegia: Behavioural and lesion evidence. *Cortex, 61*, 127–140.

Besharati, S., Forkel, S. J., Kopelman, M., Solms, M., Jenkinson, P. M., & Fotopoulou, A. (2016). Mentalizing the body: Spatial and social cognition in anosognosia for hemiplegia. *Brain, 139*, 971–985.

Blanke, O., & Metzinger, T. (2009). Full-body illusions and minimal phenomenal selfhood. *Trends in Cognitive Science, 13*, 7–13.

Blanke, O., Slater, M., & Serino, A. (2015). Behavioral, neural, and computational principles of bodily self-consciousness. *Neuron, 88*, 145–166.

Blass, R. B., & Carmeli, Z. V. I. (2007). The case against neuropsychoanalysis: On fallacies underlying psychoanalysis' latest scientific trend and its negative impact on psychoanalytic discourse. *The International Journal of Psychoanalysis, 88*, 19–40.

Blass, R. B., & Carmeli, Z. V. I. (2015). Further evidence for the case against neuropsychoanalysis: How Yovell, Solms, and Fotopoulou's response to our critique confirms the irrelevance and harmfulness to psychoanalysis of the contemporary neuroscientific trend. *The International Journal of Psychoanalysis, 96*, 1555–1573.

Brothers, L., & Ring, B. (1992). A neuroethological framework for the representation of minds. *Journal of Cognitive Neumsdence, 4*, 107–118.

Cappa, S., Sterzi, R., Vallar, G., & Bisiach, E. (1987). Remission of hemineglect and anosognosia during vestibular stimulation. *Neuropsychologia, 25*, 775–782.

Case, L. K., Čeko, M., Gracely, J. L., Richards, E. A., Olausson, H., & Bushnell, M. C. (2016). Touch perception altered by chronic pain and by opioid blockade. *Eneuro, 3*(1), 1–10.

Cassidy, J., & Shaver, P. R. (Eds.). (2008). *Handbook of attachment: Theory, research, and clinical applications* (2nd ed.). New York: Guilford Press.

Ciaunica, A., & Fotopoulou, A. (2017). The touched self: Psychological and philosophical perspectives on proximal intersubjectivity and the self. In C. Durt, T. Fuchs, & C. Tewes (Eds.), *Embodiment, enaction, and culture investigating the constitution of the shared world* (pp. 173–192). Cambridge, MA: MIT Press.

Clarac, M., Massion, J., & Smith, A. M. (2008). History of neuroscience: Joseph Babinski (1857–1932). *International Brain Research Organization*. Available at: http://ibro.info/wp-content/uploads/2012/12/Babinski-Joseph.pdf.

Cocchini, G., Beschin, N., Fotopoulou, A., & Della Sala, S. (2010). Explicit and implicit anosognosia or upper limb motor impairment. *Neuropsychologia, 48*, 1489–1494.

Craig, A. D. B. (2009). How do you feel--now? The anterior insula and human awareness. *Nature Reviews Neuroscience, 10*, 59–70.

Craig, A. D. B. (2010). The sentient self. *Brain Structure and Function, 214*, 563–577.

Critchley, H. D., Wiens, S., Rotshtein, P., Öhman, A., & Dolan, R. D. (2004). Neural systems supporting interoceptive awareness. *Nature Neuroscience, 7*, 189–195.

Critchley, M. (1955). Personification of paralysed limbs in hemiplegics. *British Medical Journal, 2*, 2284–2286.

Damasio, A. (1994). *Descartes' error: Emotion, reason, and the human brain*. New York: G.P. Putnam's Sons.

Davies, M., Davies, A. A., & Coltheart, M. (2005). Anosognosia and the two-factor theory of delusions. *Mind and Language, 20*, 209–236.

Feinberg, T. E. (1997). Anosognosia and confabulation. In T. E. Feinberg & M. J. Farah (Eds.), *Behavioral neurology and neuropsychology* (pp. 369–390). New York: McGraw Hill.

Flavell, J. H. (1979). Metacognition and cognitive monitoring: A new area of cognitive–developmental inquiry. *American Psychologist, 34*(10), 906.

Fleming, S. M., & Dolan, R. J. (2012). The neural basis of metacognitive ability. *Philosophical Transactions of the Royal Society B, 367*, 1338–1349.

Fonagy, P., Gergely, G., Jurist, E. L., & Target, M. (2002). *Affect regulation, mentalization, and the development of the self*. London: Karnac.

Fotopoulou, A. (2010). The affective neuropsychology of confabulation and delusion. *Cognitive Neuropsychiatry, 15*, 38–63.

Fotopoulou, A. (2012a). Illusions and delusions in anosognosia for hemiplegia: From motor predictions to prior beliefs. *Brain, 135*, 1344–1346.

Fotopoulou A. (2012b). The history and progress of Neuropsychoanalysis. In A. Fotopoulou, M. Conway, & D. Pfaff (Eds.), *From the couch to the lab: Trends in psychodynamic neuroscience* (pp. 12–23). Oxford: Oxford University Press.

Fotopoulou, A. (2012c). Towards psychodynamic neuroscience. In A. Fotopoulou, M. Conway, & D. Pfaff (Eds.), *From the couch to the Lab: Trends in psychodynamic neuroscience* (pp. 25–47). Oxford: Oxford University Press.

Fotopoulou, A. (2013). Beyond the reward principle: Consciousness as precision seeking. *Neuropsychoanalysis, 15*, 33–38.

Fotopoulou, A. (2014). Time to get rid of the 'Modular' in neuropsychology: A unified theory of anosognosia as aberrant predictive coding. *Journal of Neuropsychology, 8*, 1–19.

Fotopoulou, A. (2015). The virtual bodily self: Mentalisation of the body as revealed in anosognosia for hemiplegia. *Consciousness and Cognition, 33*, 500–510.

Fotopoulou, A. (2018). *Unawareness of paralysis following stroke: An existential-phenomenological inquiry into the paradox of anosognosia*. Doctorate Thesis. Middlesex University Research Depository.

Fotopoulou, A., Jenkinson, P. M., Tsakiris, M., Haggard, P., Rudd, A., & Kopelman, M. D. (2011). Mirror-view reverses somatoparaphrenia: Dissociation between first-and third-person perspectives on body ownership. *Neuropsychologia, 49*, 3946–3955.

Fotopoulou, A., Pernigo, S., Maeda, R., Rudd, A., & Kopelman, M. A. (2010). Implicit awareness in anosognosia for hemiplegia: Unconscious interference without conscious re-representation. *Brain, 133*, 3564–3577.

Fotopoulou, A., & Tsakiris, M. (2017). Mentalizing homeostasis: The social origins of interoceptive inference. *Neuropsychoanalysis, 19*, 3–28.

Fotopoulou, A., Tsakiris, M., Haggard, P., Vagopoulou, A., Rudd, A., & Kopelman, M. (2008). The role of motor intention in motor awareness: An experimental study on anosognosia for hemiplegia. *Brain, 131*, 3432–3442.

Friston, K. J. (2009). The free-energy principle: A rough guide to the brain? *Trends in Cognitive Sciences, 13*, 294–301.

Friston, K. J. (2010). The free-energy principle: A unified brain theory? *Nature Reviews Neuroscience, 11*, 127–138.

Friston, K. (2013). Life as we know it. *Journal of the Royal* Society *Interface, 10*(86), 20130475

Friston, K. J. (2018). Am i self-conscious? (or does self-organization entail self-consciousness?). *Frontiers in Psychology, 9*, 579.

Frith, C. (2000). Explaining the symptoms of schizophrenia: Abnormalities in the awareness of action. *Brain Research Reviews, 31*, 357–363.

Frith, C. D., Blakemore, S. J., & Wolpert, D. M. (2000). Abnormalities in the awareness and control of action. *Philosophical Transactions of the Royal Society of London, Series B. Biological Sciences, 355*, 1771–1788.

Frith, C. D., & Frith, U. (2007). Social cognition in humans. *Current Biology, 17*(16), R724–R732.

Frith, U., & de Vignemont, F. (2005). Egocentrism, allocentrism, and asperger syndrome. *Consciousness and Cognition, 14*, 719–738.

Fuchs, T., & De Jaegher, H. (2009). Enactive intersubjectivity: Participatory sense-making and mutual incorporation. *Phenomenology and the Cognitive Sciences, 8*, 465–486.

Gallagher, H. L., & Frith, C. D. (2003). Functional imaging of "theory of mind." *Trends in Cognitive Sciences, 7*, 77–83.

Gallagher, S. (2000). Philosophical conceptions of the self: Implications for cognitive science. *Trends in Cognitive Sciences, 4*, 14–21.

Gallese, V. (2005). "Being like me": Self-other identity, mirror neurons and empathy. In S. Hurley & N. Chater (Eds.), *Perspectives on imitation: From cognitive neuroscience to social science* (Vol. 1, pp. 101–118). Cambridge, MA: MIT Press.

Geng, J. J., & Vossel, S. (2013). Re-evaluating the role of TPJ in attentional control: Contextual updating?. *Neuroscience & Biobehavioral Reviews, 37*(10), 2608–2620.

Gentsch, A., Panagiotopoulou, E., & Fotopoulou, A. (2015). Active interpersonal touch gives rise to the social softness illusion. *Current Biology, 25*, 2392–2397.

Gergely, G., & Watson, J. S. (1999). Early socio-emotional development: Contingency perception and the social-biofeedback model. *Early social cognition: Understanding others in the first months of life, 60*, 101–136.

Gerstmann, J. (1942). Problem of imperception of disease and impaired body territories with organic lesions. *Archives of Neurology and Psychiatry, 48*, 890–913.

Jenkinson, P. M., & Fotopoulou, A. (2014). Understanding Babinski's anosognosia: 100 years later. *Cortex, 61*, 1–4.

Jenkinson, P. M., Haggard, P., Ferreira, N. C., & Fotopoulou, A. (2013). Body ownership and attention in the mirror: Insights from somatoparaphrenia and the rubber hand illusion. *Neuropsychologia, 51*, 1453–1462.

Kaplan-Solms, K. L., & Solms, M. (2000). *Clinical studies in neuropsychoanalysis.* London: Karnac Books.

Karnath, H.-O., Baier, B., & Nägele, T. (2005). Awareness of the functioning of one's own limbs mediated by the insular cortex? *The Journal of Neuroscience, 25*, 7134–7138.

Kärtner, J., Keller, H., Lamm, B., Abels, M., Yovsi, R. D., Chaudhary, N., & Su, Y. (2008). Similarities and differences in contingency experiences of 3-month-olds across sociocultural contexts. *Infant Behavior & Development, 31*(3), 488–500.

Kaye, K., & Fogel, A. (1980). The temporal structure of face-to-face communication between mothers and infants. *Developmental Psychology, 16*, 454.

Kinsbourne, M. (2000). How is consciousness expressed in the cerebral activation manifold?. *Brain and Mind, 1*, 265–274.

Kirsch, L. P., Besharati, S., Papadaki, C., Crucianelli, L., Bertagnoli, S., Ward, N., ... & Fotopoulou, A. (2020). Damage to the right insula disrupts the perception of affective touch. *Elife, 9*, e47895.

Langer, K. G., & Levine, D. N. (2014). Babinski, J. (1914). *Contribution to the study of the mental disorders in hemiplegia of organic cerebral origin* (Anosognosia). Translated by KG Langer & DN Levine: Translated from the original Contribution à l'Étude des Troubles Mentaux dans l'Hémiplégie Organique Cérébrale (Anosognosie). *Cortex: A Journal Devoted to the Study of the Nervous System and Behavior.*

Levine, D. N. (1990). Unawareness of visual and sensorimotor defects: A hypothesis. *Brain and Cognition, 13*, 233–281.

Levine, D. N., Calvanio, R., & Rinn, W. E. (1991). The pathogenesis of anosognosia for hemiplegia. *Neurology, 41*, 1770–1770.

Löken, L. S., Wessberg, J., Morrison, I., McGlone, F., & Olausson, H. (2009). Coding of pleasant touch by unmyelinated afferents in humans. *Nature Neuroscience, 12*, 547–548.

Malabou, C. (2015). Phantom limbs and plasticity: Merleau-Ponty and current neurobiology. *Chiasmi International, 17*, 41–52.

Marcel, A. J., Tegnér, R., & Nimmo-Smith, I. (2004). Anosognosia for plegia: Specificity, extension, partiality and disunity of bodily unawareness. *Cortex, 40*, 19–40.

Martinaud, O., Besharati, S., Jenkinson, P. M., & Fotopoulou, A. (2017). Ownership illusions in patients with body delusions: Different neural profiles of visual capture and disownership. *Cortex, 87*, 174–185.

Merleau-Ponty, M. (1945). *Phénoménologie de la perception.* Paris: Éditions Gallimard. English translation: C. Smith. *Phenomenology of Perception*, London: Routledge and Kegan Paul, 1962.

Merleau-Ponty, M. (1960). *Les relations avec autrui chez l'enfant.* Paris, France: Cours de Sorbonne, trans. by W. Cobb, "The child's relations with others", in M. Merleau – Ponty (1964), The Primacy of Perception And Other Essays on Phenomenological Psychology, the Philosophy of Art, History and Politics, J. M. Edie (Ed.), Evanston, IL: Northwestern University Press, pp. 96–155.

Morin, C., Pradat-Diehl, P., Robain, G., Bensalah, Y., & Perrigot, M. (2003). Stroke hemiplegia and specular image: lessons from self-portraits. *The International Journal of Aging and Human Development, 56*(1), 1–41.

Moro, V., Pernigo, S., Zapparoli, P., Cordioli, Z., & Aglioti, S. M. (2011). Phenomenology and neural correlates of implicit and emergent motor awareness in patients with anosognosia for hemiplegia. *Behavioural Brain Research, 225*, 259–269.

Moro, V., Scandola, M., Bulgarelli, C., Avesani, R., & Fotopoulou, A. (2015). Error-based training and emergent awareness in anosognosia for hemiplegia. *Neuropsychological Rehabilitation, 25*, 593–616.

Morrison, I., Bjornsdotter, M., & Olausson, H. (2011). Vicarious responses to social touch in posterior insular cortex are tuned to pleasant caressing speeds. *The Journal of Neuroscience, 31*, 9554–9562.

Morrison, I., Loken, L. S., & Olausson, H. (2010). The skin as a social organ. *Experimental Brain Research, 204*, 305–314.

Morton, J., & Frith, U. (1995). Causal modeling: Structural approaches to developmental psychopathology. In D. Cicchetti & D. Cohen (Eds.), *Developmental psychopathology* (pp. 357–390). New York: Wiley.

Nardone, I. B., Ward, R., Fotopoulou, A., & Turnbull, O. H. (2007). Attention and emotion in anosognosia: Evidence of implicit awareness and repression? *Neurocase, 13*, 438–445.

Pacella, V., Foulon, C., Jenkinson, P. M., Bertagnoli, S., Avensani, R., Fotopoulou, A., Moro, V., & Thiebaut De Schotten, M. Anosognosia for hemiplegia is a disconnection syndrome. *Elife, 8*, e46075.

Pezzulo, G., Rigoli, F., & Friston, K. (2015). Active inference, homeostatic regulation and adaptive behavioural control. *Progress in Neurobiology, 134*, 17–35.

Prigatano, G. P. (2010). *The study of anosognosia*. Oxford: Oxford University Press.

Prigatano, G. P. (2014). Anosognosia and patterns of impaired self-awareness observed in clinical practice. *Cortex, 61*, 81–92.

Prigatano, G. P., & Schacter, D. L. (1991). *Awareness of deficit after brain injury: Clinical and theoretical issues*. Oxford: Oxford University Press.

Prigatano, G. P., & Weinstein, E. A. (1996). Edwin A. Weinstein's contributions to neuropsychological rehabilitation. *Neuropsychological Rehabilitation, 6*(4), 305–326.

Ramachandran, V. S. (1995). Anosognosia in parietal lobe syndrome. *Consciousness and Cognition, 4*, 22–51.

Reddy, V. (2008). *How infants know minds*. Cambridge: Harvard University Press.

Romano, D., Gandola, M., Bottini, G., & Maravita, A. (2014). Arousal responses to noxious stimuli in somatoparaphrenia and anosognosia: clues to body awareness. *Brain, 137*, 1213–1223.

Ronchi, R., Rode, G., Cotton, F., Farnè, A., Rossetti, Y., & Jacquin-Courtois, S. (2013). Remission of anosognosia for right hemiplegia and neglect after caloric vestibular stimulation. *Restorative Neurology and Neuroscience, 31*, 19–24.

Schacter, D. L. (1990). Towards a cognitive neuropsychology of awareness: Implicit knowledge and anosognosia. *Journal of Clinical Experimental Neuropsychology, 12*, 155–178.

Schilbach, L., Timmermans, B., Reddy, V., Costall, A., Bente, G., Schlicht, T., & Vogeley, K. (2013). Toward a second-person neuroscience 1. *Behavioral and Brain Sciences, 36*, 393–414.

Seth, A. K. (2013). Interoceptive inference, emotion, and the embodied self. *Trends in Cognitive Science, 17*, 565–573.

Seth, A. K., Suzuki, K., & Critchley, H. D. (2012). An interoceptive predictive coding model of conscious presence. *Frontiers in Psychology, 2*, 1–16.

Solms, M. (2013). The conscious Id. *Neuropsychoanalysis, 15,* 5–85.

Stern, D. N. (1985). *The interpersonal world of the infant: A view from psychoanalysis and developmental psychology.* London: Karnac Books.

Thibierge, S., & Morin, C. (2013). Identification, recognition and misidentification syndromes: A psychoanalytical perspective. *Frontiers in Psychology, 4,* 835.

Turnbull, O. H., Fotopoulou, A., & Solms, M. (2014). Anosognosia as motivated unawareness: The "defence" hypothesis revisited. *Cortex; A Journal Devoted to the Study of the Nervous System and Behavior, 61,* 18–29.

Turnbull, O. H., & Solms, M. (2007). Awareness, desire, and false beliefs: Freud in the light of modern neuropsychology. *Cortex, 43,* 1083–1090.

Vocat, R., Staub, F., Stroppini, T., & Vuilleumier, P. (2010). Anosognosia for hemiplegia: A clinical-anatomical prospective study. *Brain, 133,* 3578–3597.

Vuilleumier, P. (2004). Anosognosia: The neurology of beliefs and uncertainties. *Cortex, 40,* 9–17.

Vogeley, K., Bussfeld, P., Newen, A., Herrmann, S., Happé, F., Falkai, P., & Zilles, K. (2001). Mind reading: Neural mechanisms of theory of mind and self-perspective. *NeuroImage, 14,* 170–181.

Vogeley, K., & Fink, G. R. (2003). Neural correlates of the first-person-perspective. *Trends in Cognitive Sciences, 7,* 38–42.

Vogeley, K., May, M., Ritzl, A, Falkai, P., Zilles, K., & Fink, G. R. (2004). Neural correlates of first-person perspective as one constituent of human self-consciousness. *Journal of Cognitive Neuroscience, 16,* 817–827.

Winnicot, D. W. (1972). Basis for self in body. *International Journal of Child Psychotherapy, 1,* 7–16.

Wolpert, D. M. (1997). Computational approaches to motor control. *Trends in Cognitive Sciences, 1,* 209–216.

Yeates, G., Henwood, K., Gracey, F., & Evans, J. (2006). Awareness of disability after acquired brain injury: Subjectivity within the psychosocial context. *Neuropsychoanalysis, 8*(2), 175–189.

Yovell, Y., Solms, M., & Fotopoulou, A. (2015). The case for neuropsychoanalysis: Why a dialogue with neuroscience is necessary but not sufficient for psychoanalysis. *The International Journal of Psychoanalysis, 96*(6), 1515–1553.

Chapter 13

Locked-in syndrome

The challenges of disentangling cognitive and dynamic factors

Amy Duncan

1 Introduction

Neuropsychology contains many relatively familiar categories of patient presentations: traumatic brain injury (TBI), stroke, dementia, etc. However, as a field it is always helpful to explore the boundaries of rare and under-investigated neurological conditions. One reason they are under-investigated is that they present a number of technical challenges to the common practice of the neuropsychologist. This chapter offers the description of one of these cases, by describing the investigation of a patient with locked-in syndrome (LIS). A key element of working with LIS patients is the adaptation and flexibility of the neuropsychologist in modifying the way in which they relate to, and assess, these patients.

There are several ways in which the complexity of working with these patients presents itself: the adaptation of assessment instruments, the exploration of mental status and the development of a therapeutic relationship. These adaptations allow us to explore the complexity of separating and integrating cognitive and emotional/dynamic elements in a patient presentation. This case also emphasizes the extent to which the clinician must tolerate ambiguity regarding elements that are imperfectly understood, and perhaps ultimately beyond full explanation. In addressing challenging cases like this, neuropsychoanalysis can expand its theoretical borders into places where other approaches are less willing to explore.

2 The pathology of LIS

Although vascular episodes, such as stroke or haemorrhage, are the most frequent cause of a patient becoming "locked in" (Dollfus, Milos, Chapuis, et al., 1990; Smith & Delargy, 2005), this syndrome can result from a number of other medical conditions, including brain trauma, demyelinating diseases (multiple sclerosis), infectious disease or progressive neurological diseases (amytrophic lateral sclerosis) (Birbaumer, Ghanayim, Hinterberger, et al., 1999; Smith & Delargy, 2005). The main features of LIS are a complete paralysis of the body, combined with anarthria – an inability to articulate speech – with preservation of only vertical eye movements, upper eyelid control and blinking (Bauer, Gerstenbrand & Rumpl, 1979; Smith & Delargy, 2005). There are patients where other movements are present. In such cases, the LIS is described as incomplete (Bauer et al., 1979; Smith & Delargy, 2005). LIS can be transient or chronic. The pathology usually involves a lesion of the brainstem, more specifically the ventral pons, but the lesion can also be in the central part of the pons or in the mesencephalic region, mainly at the level of the cerebral peduncles (Bauer et al., 1979; Dollfus et al., 1990; Kenny & Luke, 1989). It has been described that such lesions might interrupt the pyramidal and corticobulbar tracts, the descending motor pathways, the supranuclear fibres for horizontal gaze and the postnuclear oculomotor fibres (Bauer et al., 1979; Kenny & Luke, 1989).

Regardless the type of LIS, patients are often conscious and aware of their surroundings, probably due to the sparing of the upper pontine tegmentum above the level of the trigeminal nucleus (Kenny & Luke, 1989). They also generally have preserved hearing, but can present with other impairments such as diplopia or blurred vision, as well as vertigo, insomnia and emotional lability (Casanova, Lazzari, Lotta, et al., 2003; León-Carrión, van Eeckhout, Domínguez-Morales, et al., 2002). With regard to cognitive functioning, there is evidence reporting undisturbed cortical function on electro-encephalogram (EEG) and preserved the ability to communicate complex ideas in LIS patients (Bauer et al., 1979; Smith & Delargy, 2005). However, other studies have also noted that perception, attention, visual and verbal memory, executive function and intellectual ability in general can present some level of impairment in this population (Garrard, Bradshaw, Jäger, et al., 2002).

3 The case of Mr P

Mr P was a single, 30-year-old male. He acquired LIS due to a TBI, caused by a road traffic accident. Mr P was cycling alone early one morning, when a car driving inside the cycle lane hit him from behind. He was taken to a trauma hospital unconscious. He regained consciousness ten days after the accident once sedation was stopped. Mr P sustained multiple traumas including a partial dislocation of his left acromioclavicular joint, bilateral haemothoraces with multiple rib fractures, a fracture of his right fibula and multiple skull fractures. As a consequence of the TBI, Mr P presented with diffuse axonal injury, a parietal subarachnoid haemorrhage, a post traumatic cerebral aneurysm (which was treated with coiling) and an intraventricular haemorrhage with brainstem contusion. Data from a magnetic resonance imaging (MRI) scan taken two years after the accident suggested the involvement of the pons as well as signs of head trauma, with encephalomalacia in the right temporal and frontal lobes.

Immediately after the accident, Mr P was completely locked in, not being able to move any part of his body. He was also anarthric and suffered from dysphagia – a difficulty swallowing – and nystagmus – uncontrolled movement of the eyes. Eye response of looking up for "yes" and down for "no" started after four months. After approximately seven months, after intensive rehabilitation, Mr P was finally able to press his right thumb down and squeeze his right fist. The capacity to raise his right thumb up appeared nine months post-accident. Following this there was a slow motoric recovery of his right fingers, hand and foot. Almost three years after his accident, following intensive rehabilitation, Mr P became able to lift his lower right leg, roll his right leg in and out, move his left arm and leg slightly and turn his head from side to side while lying or sitting. Speech and the capacity to generate voice sounds did not improve with time. Thus, Mr P could be described as having incomplete LIS (Bauer et al., 1979). It is important to note that all these movements were carried out after external command only, as Mr P *never* moved spontaneously.

In relation to Mr P's cognition, due to the LIS it was not possible to comprehensively assess whether there were any deficits associated with the injury. It has been described in the literature that some patients with LIS do experience neuropsychological impairment (Garrard et al., 2002). In consequence, considering the extent of Mr P's injuries, there was a strong possibility that his cognitive functioning was not completely intact. Nevertheless, due to the lack of improvement of speech but an increased ability to use his residual motoric capacities to communicate, Mr P's carers believed that he could benefit from talking with someone regarding his subjective experience, an intervention that could also shed some light regarding the state of his cognitive functioning. In consequence, 18 months post-accident I was included as part of his rehabilitation team as a neuropsychologist.

I began to see Mr P regularly, once per week, for approximately 50 minutes, at his home, as he was largely bedridden. In contrast to his reaction to other therapies, where he was often reluctant and disengaged due to pain and frustration, Mr P appeared to develop a positive therapeutic relationship with me. This was affirmed by his mother, and also by the fact that he never missed a session. Nevertheless, it is also important to underscore that he never expressed the need to see a psychologist to discuss his difficult life situation. While he seemed to enjoy the company, he never presented any complaints regarding his situation and rarely presented topics he wanted to talk about. He seldom spoke about his mood, even when the topic was raised by me, and did not consider himself to be depressed – although he had been medically treated with antidepressants since approximately one year post-accident.

4 A brief history

Mr P had a mother, stepfather and a sister. His mother and biological father were divorced when Mr P was about three years old, and his father moved overseas shortly thereafter. His father was not very present in his life, although Mr P would travel to see him every two or three years. Mr P's mother remarried when Mr P was about five years old, and she said that Mr P had had a good relationship with his stepfather. Mr P grew up with his mother, stepfather and sister, and left home to attend university and complete a four-year degree with two majors. He was described by his mother as a very positive, confident person, never depressed. He was an excellent sportsman at school and university and represented his province and country on a number of occasions. After university he worked in the sports industry and was an internationally successful sportsman, often described by his mother as stubborn, extremely driven and focussed, demanding an extremely high standard from himself. His mother described him as always having had a greater focus on the outdoors than on his internal world and feelings. She said, for example, that although she felt he had unresolved feelings about his biological father, he didn't like the idea of talking to a psychologist about them.

At the time of his accident, he had moved overseas and was still a sportsman representing his country at various events. He was living with his long-term girlfriend in a country different from that of both his family and his biological father. After the accident, Mr P's family found that caring for him in the country in which the accident had occurred was difficult, so they made the decision to move back to the country in which he grew up. His long-term girlfriend moved with them, but became overwhelmed by the situation and made the decision to move back overseas with her parents.

5 Technical challenges to communicating

Given the severe motoric impairment of LIS patients, their communication with the outside world is often drastically compromised. However, alternative communicative methods have been developed to facilitate communication, allowing them to select predefined replies, make decisions, communicate their thoughts and even use the Internet. Examples of such technological methods include measuring pupil responses (Stoll, Chatelle, Carter, et al., 2013), changes in the pH of saliva in response to certain stimuli (Wilhelm, Jordan & Birbaumer, 2006), using alphabet boards to spell out words where the patient responds to rows and columns with a slight movement (Smith & Delargy, 2005; Söderholm, Meinander & Alaranta, 2001) and a variety of patient–computer interfaces (Söderholm et al., 2001).

Before I met Mr P, attempts had been made by his speech therapists to implement a patient–computer interface, where he would be able to select, among other things, pre-programmed replies quickly and more efficiently than spelling them out. However, the software was first based on eye gaze which was virtually impossible and very frustrating, given his nystagmus. They then adapted the program so that Mr P might be able to select options with a button, but this required quite a bit of thumb pressure and much concentration, and approximately two years after his accident, he decided not to pursue this any further. When I began seeing Mr P, we experimented with an alphabet board of letters in rows and columns to make selecting a specific letter faster. Rather than waiting until the end of the alphabet to select "Y", for example, one could select it by saying columns 1, 2, 3, 4, "5", rows 1, 2, 3, "4". However, Mr P's nystagmus and his extreme headaches made this difficult, and he preferred not to use it. Thus, communication with Mr P was almost solely via the use of his right thumb. I would ask yes/no questions to which he would raise his thumb if he meant "yes" and not move it if he meant "no". However, this method was not straightforward, since a lack of movement could also mean "I don't know", "I don't want to answer", "I haven't had enough time to think about it", etc. In order to address this difficulty, his "no" responses were constantly checked to confirm their meaning. When discussing more complex topics, I would also ask open-ended questions after which I would ask, "Are you ready?", and he would raise his thumb indicating "yes". I would then go through the alphabet, and Mr P would raise his thumb when I got to the letter he wanted. I would then repeat the letters he had already given me and say, "next letter", and then go through the alphabet again until he spelt out the word he was looking for. This was obviously time consuming, but for the most part it worked well. Most often, though, Mr P would give one-word answers, and importantly he *never* spontaneously volunteered any information or asked any question.

Later in our sessions I began to rely on non-verbal communication as a source of information. Even though his facial expressions were limited, he could cry, smile and laugh (by inhaling). He would also acquire a "serious" look that would flash across his face for certain topics and a "naughty" look in and around his eyes if he was teasing me. In the beginning, I did not notice these as easily, but later I began to use them in my interpretation of our conversations. Although, at times, our methods of communication were unusual and unique, what was revealed during our sessions was even more fascinating and raised some interesting and important questions regarding the inner life of a patient such as Mr P.

6 Neuropsychological presentation

In our very first session, Mr P was assessed by a clinical neuropsychologist consultant (Prof Mark Solms). Mr P was orientated to place, but not to time.

On questioning, he thought it was 2011 (in reality it was 2014), and he was unsure of the month or the day of the week. His vision was found to be intact, although further examination indicated that he felt unsteady or unbalanced much of the time due to his nystagmus. On questioning, Mr P replied that he sleeps well, but does not dream at all. When enquired, Mr P denied any type of memory difficulties. When given a list of yes/no answer-based questions regarding his daily activities (e.g. "did you have a bath today?", "did the physio come today?"), he answered all ten questions correctly. However, he was not able to remember how long ago the accident was. Incidental memory was assessed by asking Mr P if he remembered Prof Solms's name. Initially he did not. He was given my name along with two others and selected my name correctly. Prof Solms told Mr P his name again and asked Mr P if he thought he would remember, to which he indicated that he would. Prof Solms also told Mr P the correct date. Prof Solms then asked Mr P what his name was via multiple choice and Mr P answered correctly. Given multiple-choice answers for the day, month and year, he selected the correct day (Wednesday), but the incorrect month and year (April 2011). Prof Solms asked Mr P, "Do you remember me telling you it's not 2011?". Mr P said yes and selected the correct year (2014) from five multiple-choice answers. At this point his mother asked him if he was teasing by saying the incorrect date and Mr P said yes. This brief examination offered some initial insights into Mr P's neuropsychological functioning, but raised some questions regarding his orientation and memory.

After the initial assessment, further examinations were performed in order to explore Mr P's executive abilities. Two adapted tasks were used for this purpose. Firstly, a go-no go task was used to assess inhibition and set shifting. Mr P was instructed to push his thumb down for red and lift it up/ release the pressure for green. In general, he was able to perform this task well, but his "twitchy" thumb interfered. In order to determine if the movement of this thumb was related to the motoric impairment or to impulsivity, further training in the task was provided. After obtaining a more reliable performance, the rule was changed to press for green and release for red. Mr P performed this task correctly immediately, suggesting a preserved ability to inhibit previous learning and flexibly change behaviour according to contextual demands. A modified "similarities" task was also used to assess Mr P's executive abilities, in particular, abstract thinking. Here, his performance was also spotless, thus not showing signs of concrete thinking. He gave the following answers: circle and square= SHAPE; apple and banana= FRUIT; jacket and pants= CLOTHES; painting and song= ART; rough and smooth= TEXTURE; love and hate= FEELINGS; capitalism and socialism= MONEY. In conclusion, and based on the limited neuropsychological exploration allowed by his motoric impairments, Mr P did not appear to present with a marked dysexecutive syndrome.

7 Disentangling the cognitive and dynamic

7.1 Amnesia and disorientation

A perplexing aspect of Mr P's presentation was his unusual and inconsistent memory. In our sessions, we began speaking about topics such as his accident, his girlfriend who had left him and moved back with her parents, the losses he'd experienced, his experience of life now and his thoughts regarding his various therapies. He would be able to (correctly) tell me the names of his carers, therapists and details from his and their recent lives, but he would never remember us talking about either his accident or the fact that his girlfriend had left him. If I went through the details with him again, it would be as if he was hearing them for the first time since his accident. Late into our relationship, he even claimed that he did not know he had been in an accident and had no idea why he was unable to communicate or move.

However, on testing, his memory appeared to be intact. On one occasion, I assessed his memory with the four hidden objects test (Strub & Black, 2000). Instead of using four objects, I showed him three as I felt spelling out four might be a bit taxing for him. I asked him to name them. He spelt PEN, KEYS and PHONE (correct). I then hid these items and asked him to recall them. He was able to do so. I then hid each in a different hiding place (the pen under the chair, the phone near the door and the keys near the fan). He remembered two of the items (PHONE and KEYS), but only one hiding place, which he got correct. I went over it again and he got all three items and all three hiding places correct. Thus, with a bit of practice, he did not demonstrate any problems with immediate recall.

We then went on to speak about other things, and at the end of the session I asked about the items again. He correctly recalled the number of items and recalled that the phone was near the door. He also correctly recalled the keys, but said that the fan had been one of the items (it was one of the hiding places). He was adamant that the fan was an item, but when asked if there was a third item, he replied yes and spelt KEYS and said that the keys were near the FAN. When asked again whether the fan was an item or a hiding place, he replied that it was a hiding place. He therefore correctly recalled two of the three items in their correct hiding places after a delay of approximately 25–30 minutes.

At the beginning of our next session, I asked Mr P if he remembered that I had shown him some items the week before. He said that he did remember. When I asked how many there had been, he replied that there were three (correct). He recalled KEYS (correct), WALLET (incorrect) and PEN (correct). I mentioned that wallet was incorrect, but he couldn't recall the third item. However, even though one item was incorrectly recalled, his performance indicated a largely intact ability to store and recall new information – even over the period of one week.

Some months later, I again used the hidden object test, but this time with four items. Mr P was able to name them: PEN, NOTE (money), CRÈME (hand cream, spelt incorrectly) and GLASSES. This time he was able to correctly remember all four items and their hiding places. At the end of the session, I asked him what the items were that I had asked him to remember. He recalled that there had been four items and correctly named the items and their hiding places (after a delay of approximately 25 minutes). I asked him if he remembered something from the last session that we had spoken about and he replied SEX (correct). I asked if there had been anything else we spoke about that he remembered and he answered YEAR (also correct). The following conversation ensued:

ME: What year is it now?
MR P: 2014 (correct)
ME: Do you really believe it's 2014?
MR P: No
ME: You just remember me telling you?
MR P: Yes
ME: What year does it feel like for you?
MR P: 2011
ME: It really feels like 2011 for you?
MR P: Yes

In another session, sometime later, I verbally gave Mr P three words (apple, pen, table) to remember at the beginning of the session. Forty minutes later, I asked him what those words were. He answered DOG, TABLE, PEN (two out of three correct), but he was unsure about "dog". On receiving a number of multiple-choice answers, he correctly recognised "apple".

The interactions above offer some insight into his apparent disorientation. They demonstrate that rather than being disorientated Mr P "feels" as though it is 2011, the year before his accident, but is aware of what year everyone around him believes it to be. Even when our sessions continued into the next year, this disconnect between "his" and "our" time continued, and he remained orientated to both. A possible explanation for this disconnect could be due to a large period of post-traumatic amnesia, which would be consistent with Mr P's neuropathology. However, additional ideas are explored later in this chapter that perhaps better explain this perplexing symptom. What the interactions and his cognitive performance on testing don't explain, however, is his lack of memory for the emotionally charged events of his accident and the loss of his girlfriend, since his ability to learn information since the accident appears to be intact. A likely explanation for this inconsistent presentation would rather be that his amnesia is motivated by psychodynamic factors and that he would rather forget than remember these painful experiences. He once even alluded to this in a conversation.

We had been speaking about how his girlfriend was his only reason for living and that he didn't have a future without her, and I shared with him that I wished there was a way I could help him to hold on to the information I had shared with him (about her needing to leave), so that he could process it. The below conversation followed:

ME: So, you're just waiting and hoping, not knowing [where she is]?
MR P: Yes
ME: How does that feel for you?
MR P: SHIT
ME: Does it feel shit when you wonder where she is and you don't know?
MR P: Yes
ME: Do you feel like "Okay, she's [me, the Neuropsychologist] told me, I want to try to hold on to that?"
MR P: No
ME: Or do you feel like, "This is awful news. I just want to forget about it."
MR P: Yes

In this example, Mr P appeared to prefer to wait, not knowing, than to embrace the information and assimilate it into his conscious experience. This idea of waiting was a recurrent one that was often accompanied by a lack of motivation to seek out or volunteer information, communication and so on.

7.2 Adynamia

Adynamia or apathy is defined as a lack of initiative to start an activity or to keep going to finish an activity. It refers to a loss of motivation and drive, an indifference or lack of concern about oneself and a loss of interest in and a lack of enjoyment of activities that previously caused joy. It can also involve an absence of subjective distress, flat affect and a general lack of responsiveness to positive or negative events (Brown & Pluck, 2000). Apathy can be a consequence of damage to the brain, particularly the frontal cortex and subcortical structures, as well as striato-thalamo-cortical circuits (Brown & Pluck, 2000) and the anterior cingulate region and ventral striatum (Le Heron, Apps & Husain, 2018). This symptom has been found to correlate with executive dysfunction (McPherson, Fairbanks, Tiken, et al., 2002) as well as TBI (Andersson & Bergedalen, 2002; Rao & Lyketsos, 2000).

Due to certain features of Mr P's clinical presentation, a question that emerged early in the treatment was whether or not he presented with adynamia/apathy and whether or not this was as a consequence of his TBI. In addition to information from his mother regarding his lack of physical movement without instruction, in our interactions he would answer any question I asked without reservation, but I was struck by how he would not spontaneously offer any additional information. He would never ask a question or raise a topic and would answer only what was asked of him – no more, sometimes less – and would mostly use one-word answers, which he justified as a strategy to make the process of spelling a sentence easier. I would begin each session by asking him if there was something he would like to talk about that day, and each session he would answer "no". If I followed that by asking if I must pick something to talk about, he would always answer "yes".

Once, I asked him to tell me about his best triathlon race using as much detail as possible. His reply was "[VENUE]. SWIM WAS OKAY. FINISHED THE BIKE FIRST. RUN WAS OKAY. WON". When I questioned him about the lack of detail and emotion, he replied that, in his opinion, there was nothing missing and nothing more to the story. As mentioned, he did indicate that it was easier to answer with short responses, but I did not always feel that was the whole answer and felt, at times, that he either could not answer me or was influenced by this idea of adynamia that affected his generativity of both thoughts and actions.

More evidence pertaining to a lack of motivation can be found even in relation to his attitude towards recovery, where although he is concerned, his response lacks a sense of drive:

ME: Are you worried that this [his amount of recovery thus far] is it?
MR P: Yes
ME: How would you feel if this is it?
MR P: NOT GOOD
ME: What else?
MR P: WAIT
ME: If this is it, you'll wait for it to get better?
MR P: Yes

Sometimes this apparent adynamia even affected his well-being. Mr P commonly experienced debilitating migraines. Although the cause was largely unknown, a likely trigger appeared to be lying on his stomach, with his head to one side, for too long without being turned. I had spoken with him about this, and Mr P had answered, on questioning, that one of his night nurses was not turning him and that this was the cause of his headaches. Even though this problem had apparently been discussed before between him, his mother and the night nurse, Mr P did not take the initiative to inform his mother of his "proof" so that she could discuss it with the nursing staff:

ME: He [the nurse] is adamant that he turns you?
MR P: Yes
ME: Is that a lie?
MR P: Yes
ME: If your mom put a camera in here, she would catch him out?
MR P: Yes

ME: Do you think he likes giving you headaches?

MR P: No

ME: Do you think he doesn't turn you on purpose?

MR P: Yes

ME: Why?

MR P: SLEEP

ME: He doesn't turn you because he's asleep?

MR P: Yes

ME: Has he told you?

MR P: No

ME: Are you guessing?

MR P: No

ME: Do you know he's asleep?

MR P: Yes

ME: How?

MR P: SNORES

ME: So, you can hear him snoring?

MR P: Yes

ME: Have you told your mom?

MR P: No

ME: Why not?

MR P: DUNNO

ME: But you have told her that you don't like him (Yes), that he doesn't turn you (Yes) and that he gives you a headache (Yes). Can I tell your mom?

MR P: Yes

ME: But why can't you?

MR P: DOESN'T ASK

ME: But when I was chatting to your mom now, it sounds like you will bring up a conversation with her?

MR P: No

ME: You only talk about what she asks?

MR P: Yes

ME: But if you've got her attention and she's looking at your hand, why not bring it up?

MR P: DON'T KNOW

I was also struck by Mr P's neutral emotional state, never showing passion, anger, intense sadness or elation. He would mostly use words such as "OKAY", "HAPPY" or "SAD", and when questioned about this, he replied that he had never been a particularly emotive person. But even in response to his feelings regarding his current situation, he would offer the same limited range of emotion. For example, in response to questions about how he felt about being in pain, his situation and his difficulties in communicating, he would reply with words such as "SUCKS", "FRUSTRATING", "NOT GOOD" and "IRRITATING".

In order to explore the hypothesis of apathy, Mr P's generativity was assessed using a modified version of the Controlled Oral Word Association Test (COWAT; Benton, Hamsher & Sivan, 1994). In this task, Mr P was asked to spell out three words that begin with the letter F as quickly as he could. He spelt FISH, then after about 20–30 seconds FROM, then after one to two minutes FROM again. It is interesting to note here that during the task Mr P was considerably slower than when spelling answers for other types of questions. A few months later, the same modified task was used again, this time asking him to generate as many words beginning with the letter F, A and S with three minutes per letter to allow for spelling time. Mr P lit up and appeared completely engaged in the task. In three minutes, he was able to spell out FISH, FRIDGE, FROG, FAN, FRY and FOG. In the next three minutes, he spelt ABACUS and ALBATROSS, and then became stuck. In the last three minutes, he spelt SUGAR, SWEET, SOMEONE and SAW. Later on, his semantic fluency was also assessed, and Mr P was asked to generate as many names of animals as possible in three minutes. He spelt out the following animals: ANT, LION, BEAR, BIRD, FISH, CHICKEN and FROG. This was unexpected as he appeared to generate a high number of words in a relatively short period of time, and although this was inconsistent with his first performance, his output argued against the hypothesis of apathy. Although one may argue that this is a more forced (i.e. not spontaneous) form of generativity, and that it may not be representative of his true ability, letter fluency provides a closer representation of spontaneous generativity than semantic fluency, and his performance provides evidence that he is able to generate ideas. As a matter of interest, he commented, on questioning, that he had enjoyed this test.

Another example not in keeping with an adynamic state came from a session. Although I would often ask open-ended questions and ask him if there was anything he wanted to talk about or ask me, this was the very first (and last) time he ever asked me a question:

ME: Can you tell me a sentence?
MR P: HOW ARE YOU?
ME: Can you tell me another sentence?
MR P: WHAT CAR DO YOU DRIVE?
ME: I drive a … It's very underpowered going up a hill.
MR P: [laughed]
ME: Can you tell me about a feeling you're having?
MR P: I MISS MY MOM
ME: Can you tell me another feeling?
MR P: WHY DID THIS HAPPEN TO ME?

His presentation in the excerpt of the session above, as well as his performance on the second trial of COWAT, is in vast contradiction to Mr P's usual appearance, but more importantly does not support the hypothesis of apathy being the underlying mechanism of his behaviour. It seems unlikely, therefore, that his adynamic presentation could be the result of a neurological consequence of his TBI as if this were the case his presentation would remain consistent. Could there, perhaps, be something else going on?

While apathy is strongly correlated with depression, although not formally assessed, Mr P denied any feelings of depression and had been on antidepressants, as a precautionary measure, since approximately one year post-accident. Could his apathy then be motivated by psychodynamic reasons, for example the expression of a defence mechanism in order to cope with an emotionally unbearable situation? Dudzinski (2001), in her paper regarding Jean Dominque Bauby, the famous locked-in patient who told his story through the book *The Diving Bell and The Butterfly*, speaks of "kinaesthetic flows" and the "capacity to act" and how that is linked to "feel[ing] that action in one's body" (p. 35). One wonders what almost complete paralysis must do to a person's ability to be the agent of their own action, to their capacity to act when they can no longer feel the action expressed in their body. This same question has been, for example, formulated by case studies of tetraplegic patients, where the capacity of the organisms to voluntarily act upon the environment is altered (see, e.g., Salas, 2010).

7.3 Wishful thinking or delusion?

The above symptoms, although inconsistent at times, were initially considered to be plausible, given his TBI and the dramatic changes and losses he had experienced. However, something entirely unexpected happened next.

I saw Mr P for approximately 18 months, and about 9 months into our treatment he surprised me by sharing ideas about a "dream" – he had reported before that his dreaming had stopped. On questioning, it was uncovered that he believed that his present experience was a dream. It is not unheard of for a locked-in patient to feel *as though* they are trapped in a dream or nightmare (see Chisholm & Gillett, 2005). However, Mr P believed it was currently 2011, and he was asleep in bed, next to his girlfriend, and had dreamed everything that had happened to him since he began laying down new memories following his accident. He was upset that his biological father hadn't warned him that such a dream could take place. On exploring ideas about his dream, he provided further evidence. He remembered his last day before falling asleep and recalled what he had done before going to bed. He had been walking and talking and was perfectly healthy. It was 2011. Thus, how could it suddenly be 2014 and could he not walk or talk? On the morning of that day, he had also had a training session with a female friend of his who was single. Yet all of a sudden, she was married with a baby. He said that people had recently told him he had completed a major sporting event (which he did in 2012), but that he had never done so (since he believed it was 2011). When I tried to explain the concept of post-traumatic amnesia, he was unable to accept it as a possible explanation for these inconsistencies and could only believe that these things were not real, that I was not real.

These thought processes may have been a representation of derealisation, which can occur following trauma and represent a coping mechanism to deal with the affective intensity of a traumatic event (Mayo Clinic, 2017; Simeon, 2004). In derealisation, the external world is altered and seems unreal, and it can be accompanied by emotional dampening, another symptom displayed by Mr P.

Later in our sessions, he told me that this dream he was having was a premonition and it then took on purpose. One such purpose was to teach him that "riding [his] bike in the fog was a bad idea" and to warn him of what could happen should he ride his bike on that particular day. He asked me the date on which the accident occurred and explained that he wanted to know so that he could avoid riding that day and prevent having the accident in the future, after he had woken up. Another purpose of the dream was the confirmation that he would marry his girlfriend, although he did not (or could not) explain this idea further.

Mr P's belief that his locked-in reality was a dream appeared to be an irrational way of thinking. However, our communication difficulties and his inability or unwillingness to explain ideas in depth made me question whether these beliefs were irrational, or just wishful thinking.

There were, however, other thoughts that also appeared irrational in nature, particularly in relation to a paranoid idea of persecution by a male character. The first was the belief that his night male nurse was causing Mr P's headaches by not turning him. While Mr P did not appear to believe that the nurse was doing this on purpose, to try to hurt him, he nevertheless held this belief adamantly. Importantly, he did not have any belief of this sort in relation to his female carers. The second was a belief in relation to his stepfather that he *was* trying to hurt Mr P on purpose:

ME: Who do you have negative feelings about?
MR P: DAD
ME: Your stepfather?
MR P: Yes
ME: What sort of feelings do you feel?
MR P: FRUSTRATED
ME: Why?
MR P: ONLY LIKES THINGS THAT HURT ME
ME: What do you mean? What kind of things?
MR P: EVERYTHING
ME: Can you give me a specific example?
MR P: PHYSIOTHERAPY

Mr P explained that his stepfather watches him while he has physiotherapy, which is often a painful and emotionally negative experience for Mr P, and that his stepfather would only give him attention when he was having physiotherapy. He also gave another example where he described that his stepfather will come into his room and put him on his side which is a very uncomfortable position, and sometimes even painful. He will do this in the morning while not speaking to Mr P, and then leave the room, leaving Mr P in pain, in that position until his carer comes in to check on him.

Mr P's mother insisted that these two situations were not true. She investigated the night nurse and would check on Mr P at varying times of the night – he would always be asleep and his position would have been turned at the appropriate time interval. Additionally, the night nurse would also be awake. With regard to his stepfather, she said he doesn't even know how to turn Mr P (as there are special techniques they use), and he had always had a wonderful relationship with Mr P until the accident. Since then, she had noticed a change in Mr P, for he was no longer interested in sharing any experiences with him. She commented that this had been getting progressively worse and was emotionally painful for them.

This collateral information is compelling and strengthens the idea that Mr P may be demonstrating delusional thinking; however, there remains a chance that these incidents were, in fact, taking place. What is undeniably delusional, however, is the following.

Mr P held two beliefs about his biological father. One was that he was the root cause of Mr P's headaches, due to genetics, and that Mr P had somehow inherited them, even though he acknowledged that to his knowledge his father had not had headaches and that the headaches began after his accident. The other was that his biological father had not warned him that this dream would happen, and that on some level he was to blame for this.

Furthermore, these irrational thoughts appeared to develop over time. At first, Mr P said that his night nurse simply "did not believe in turning him". Later this changed into an idea of negligence on the part of the nurse, suggesting possible paranoid ideas. Changes in his relationship with his stepfather also appeared to worsen as time progressed. At first Mr P's mother had just noticed a change. Two years following his accident, Mr P wouldn't allow his stepfather to watch television with him or keep him company, and would not interact with him by choice.

The other area in which there appeared to be a development is slightly more complex. When I first met Mr P, his mother had mentioned that he had asked her whether this (his present life) was a dream. Six months into our sessions, it came up again in relation to feelings about his biological father. I asked him whether he felt his life "was like a dream" and "as if it wasn't real" to which he replied yes. Later he told me "THIS IS ONE BAD DREAM". Later still, he considered the dream to be a premonition. The reason that this last example is more complex is due to our way of communicating. Firstly, I often asked yes/no answers, so his affirmative answer to my asking him if it "feels like a dream" may not be completely representative of what he was thinking. Further, while his mother noted that he had asked her if this was a dream, when I began our sessions, we concentrated on history and topics that developed through our conversation. Thus, this topic wasn't addressed until later in our sessions together. I, therefore, cannot be certain of whether he first wished this was a dream or whether he believed it was a dream from the beginning. My qualitative feeling is, however, that the belief that this IS a dream (as opposed to wishing it were a dream or wondering if it's a dream) only developed later, and certainly the idea that it is a premonition was an idea that was only brought up months into treatment.

Mr P's dream delusion prompted the reconsidering of his other symptoms and irrational ideas in a new light. His apathy and disorientation could be alternatively explained in terms of his dream reality. His amnesia was found to be only for emotionally negatively charged events he would far rather not remember, but could also be interpreted in terms of his dream as one wouldn't need to remember something sad or scary if it is not real. Further, there appeared to be a sense of development to Mr P's ideas. Together, these supported the likelihood that Mr P presented some form of psychotic thinking pattern, which may represent a psychotic reactive episode to his drastic circumstances.

8 Neurological or psychodynamic? A case formulation

This case emphasizes the extent to which the clinician must tolerate ambiguity regarding elements of the patient presentation that are imperfectly understood, and perhaps ultimately beyond full explanation. In addressing challenging cases like this, neuropsychoanalysis can expand its theoretical borders into places where other approaches are less willing to explore.

It was initially suspected that Mr P's disorientation, memory loss and apathy/adynamia could all be the result of his extensive brain damage due to the traumatic nature of his head injury, and a neuropsychological hypothesis for his presentation was tested. However, as time went on, inconsistencies in these symptoms began to be revealed, and it became apparent that a simple dichotomy between cognition and psychodynamic factors seemed difficult to sustain. It gradually became clear that other accounts, different from the cognitive ones, were playing a substantial role in the patient presentation and were necessary to generate a comprehensive case formulation: loss of agency due to changes in the interaction between body/mind and environment, mourning for a wide range of losses and psychodynamic elements related to caring figures.

It has been reported that while quality of life in locked-in patients has been found to be similar to that of healthy controls, those who use a yes/no means of communication report a significantly lower quality of life than their counterparts (Rousseau, Baumstark, Alessandrini, et al., 2015). Furthermore, those who employ problem-orientated coping strategies such as seeking for information demonstrate a more successful psychological adjustment to the disease (Lulé, Zickler, Häcker, et al., 2009). While I tried as much as possible to ask open-ended questions and to use spelling in our conversations, Mr P told me that his interactions with everyone else was limited to a yes/no response. It is possible that his lack of agency and ability to affect any action on the world, coupled with his further stunted or limited means of communicating with the world, resulted in the development of a psychosis and an elaborate inner process perhaps originally based on wishful thinking.

The fact that Mr P's symptoms were better explained from a psychodynamic perspective, than a neurological/cognitive one, is of significant importance. For example, in this case, one may ask "why be the agent in your life if it's not real?" and, more importantly, "why take part in rehabilitation if you're just waiting to wake up?" These are issues that can significantly impact on treatment and rehabilitation, and if Mr P was treated only from a neurological (and not a psychological) perspective, we may never have understood potential mechanisms underlying his behaviour.

The inner psychodynamic world of neurological patients is often not considered by mental health and rehabilitation professionals, but the revelations learned about Mr P provide us with evidence as to the importance of such work, for such knowledge may be applicable to others too, and it is only by delving into the inner mind of patients that we can gain an understanding of the person and how their beliefs, resistances and mechanisms of coping impact on their functioning and rehabilitation. One may even argue that the need for psychological support for neurological patients may be even greater than those without neurological deficit, and this extends to all neurological patients, not only to those with LIS.

9 Countertransference

In my final remarks regarding Mr P, I would also like to raise the relevance of countertransference in this case. This rehabilitation team appeared to get unusually involved with this patient, each having an extraordinarily personal connection with him. While this is not necessarily a negative thing, one needs to be aware of one's personal goals and wishes interfering with what is best for the patient. Not being able to perform the tasks that were so enthusiastically wanted of him, for example being able to mobilise particular parts of his body or being able to use the communication device, was a completely negative experience for Mr P. Even in his pseudo-adynamic, going-with-the-flow, neutral-emotion way of being, he chose to fire one of his speech therapists that pushed him beyond things he could achieve by giving her the middle finger (which is significant as voluntary movement in Mr P was almost unheard of, and movement of his middle finger was very difficult for him).

They, and his mother for a long time, would also appear to assume that Mr P could do more than he actually could, or that he would be able to do more in the future. Rather than being a beacon of hope in his life, their need for him to improve as a way of them being able to cope with their own emotional reactions may have negatively impacted on him and may too not have been in the best interest of the patient.

There are obvious benefits to psychological work with neurological patients, but there are also times where not all aspects of psychanalytical work with such patients are explicitly beneficial or clear. For example, Mr P was of the belief that reality was a horrible dream, that he was still fast asleep next to his beloved girlfriend and that if only he would wake up everything would be back to normal. Is it ethical to tell such a patient that his reality is not real and that in fact his dream is a nightmare from which he will never wake up? Is it ethical to tell a tetraplegic patient they will never walk again? In other words, is our job to confront patients with reality? Some psychoanalysts would argue it is: being able to confront reality allows us to process it and come to terms with it, making acceptance possible. He may be able to process the losses of his girlfriend, his mobility, his speech and his life, and would, in time, perhaps come to find new interests that challenge his mind rather than his body. But does being in touch with his reality really offer him a better way of living? Being such a competitive sportsman, so physically focussed and to a large extent lacking in introspective thought, the idea of being trapped inside an immobile vessel with only one's mind to keep one company may be terrifying. Is it not kinder and more psychologically supportive to allow this defence?

While my therapeutic stance was to never entertain the idea that his delusion was reality, my own personal view is mixed, and I feel it is dependent on time. If Mr P was guaranteed a long life with little prospect of further recovery, I feel it would be a waste to spend his whole life waiting to wake up and feeling persecuted by certain characters in his story, and that this may place a larger burden on those who care for and love him. Even though he is such an outdoorsy person with a far greater focus on things outside of him than inside, he may find new interests which he could pursue that could bring him a sense of fulfilment and accomplishment. However, if Mr P's life expectancy was only a few more years, why not let him create a reality that allows him to cope with such an unimaginable situation. Before passing judgement, try lying down on a bed and not moving for ten minutes. Do you have an itch? Has a fly just landed on your nose? Are you perhaps thirsty? Attempting such an experiment can give us an idea of what it might feel like, but in the back of your mind you know you can still escape, scratch, shoe away the fly, call out or get up for that glass of water (and you are probably counting down the seconds until you do these things). But he can't. And he is unlikely to ever be able to. In such a case, I feel that to be complicit in his delusion may be offering the most humane form of therapy and support. But I also believe that this is completely case dependent and is a hugely contentious issue.

10 Conclusion

As can be seen in the previous sections, patients of this sort (LIS + TBI) present enormous challenges in developing a case formulation. Firstly, if we want to understand subjective experience, communication is at the heart of what clinicians do, and there are numerous challenges faced by clinicians in achieving such understanding with these types of patients. The second issue is assessment. Neuropsychology has well-established tools, but these must inevitably be adapted when working with LIS patients, undercutting psychometric validity. This is perhaps one of the reasons why the number of studies reporting the neuropsychological status of these patients is discrete (for a review, see Wilson, Hinchcliffe, Okines, et al., 2011). Neuropsychoanalysis, on the other hand, has always been aware of the complexity of neurological patients and the need to connect neuropsychological data and psychodynamic observations. This case study attempts to be an example of such an approach, combining a flexible hypothesis-driven neuropsychological exploration and the consideration of dynamic factors that may play a role in the patient presentation. It is my belief that neuropsychoanalytic minded clinicians/neuropsychologists are in a unique position to provide neurological patients with the care they need, for they have been trained to work in the realm of both mind and brain, and have a great responsibility to fill the gap so obviously seen in medical settings. I would like to thank Mr P for our time together and for the opportunity to share our interactions in this chapter.

References

Andersson, S., & Bergedalen, A.-M. (2002). Cognitive correlates of apathy in traumatic brain injury. *Neuropsychiatry, Neuropsychology, and Behavioral Neurology, 15*(3): 184–191.

Bauer, G., Gerstenbrand, F., & Rumpl, E. (1979). Varieties of the locked-in syndrome. *Journal of Neurology, 221*(2): 77–91.

Benton, A. L., Hamsher, K. D., & Sivan, A. B. (1994). *Multilingual Aphasia Examination.* Lutz, FL: Psychological Assessment Resources, Inc.

Birbaumer, N., Ghanayim, N., Hinterberger, T., Iversen, I., Kotchoubey, B., Kübler, A., Perelmouter, J., Taub, E., & Flor, H. (1999). A spelling device for the paralysed. *Nature, 398*(6725): 297–298.

Brown, R. G., & Pluck, G. (2000). Negative symptoms: the 'pathology' of motivation and goal-directed behaviour. *Trends in Neurosciences, 23*(9): 412–417.

Casanova, E., Lazzari, R. E., Lotta, S., & Mazzucchi, A. (2003). Locked-in syndrome: improvement in the prognosis after an early intensive multidisciplinary rehabilitation. *Archives of Physical Medicine and Rehabilitation, 84*(6): 862–867.

Chisholm, N., & Gillett, G. (2005). The patient's journey: Living with locked-in syndrome. *British Medical Journal, 331*(7508): 94–97.

Dollfus, P., Milos, P. L., Chapuis, A., Real, P., Orenstein, M., & Soutter, J. W. (1990). The locked-in syndrome: A review and presentation of two chronic cases. *Paraplegia, 28*(1): 5–16.

Dudzinski, D. (2001). The diving bell meets the butterfly: Identity lost and remembered. *Theoretical Medicine and Bioethics*, *22*(1): 33–46.

Garrard, P., Bradshaw, D., Jäger, H. R., Thompson, A. J., Losseff, N., & Playford, D. T. (2002). Cognitive dysfunction after isolated brain stem insult. An underdiagnosed cause of long term morbidity. *Journal of Neurology, Neurosurgery, and Psychiatry*, *73*(2): 191–194.

Kenny, D. J., & Luke, D. A. (1989). 'Locked-in' syndrome. Occurrence after coronary artery bypass graft surgery. *Anaesthesia*, *44*: 483–484.

Le Heron, C., Apps, M. A. J., & Husain, M. (2018). The anatomy of apathy: A neurocognitive framework for amotivated behaviour. *Neuropsychologica*, *118*(B): 54–67.

León-Carrión, J., van Eeckhout, P., Domínguez-Morales, M. del, R., & Pérez-Santamaria, F. J. (2002). Survey: The locked-in syndrome: a syndrome looking for therapy. *Brain Injury*, *16*(7): 571–582.

Lulé, D., Zickler, C., Häcker, S., Bruno, M. A., Demertzi, A., Pellas, F., Laureys, S., & Kübler, A. (2009). Life can be worth living in locked-in syndrome. *Progress in Brain Research*, *177*: 339–351.

Mayo Clinic (16 May 2017). *Depersonalization-derealization disorder.* Retrieved from https://www.mayoclinic.org/diseases-conditions/depersonalization-derealization-disorder/symptoms-causes/syc-20352911 10 July 2019.

McPherson, S., Fairbanks, L., Tiken, S., Cummings, J. L., & Back-Madruga, C. (2002). Apathy and executive function in Alzheimer's disease. *Journal of the International Neuropsychological Society*, *8*: 373–381.

Rao, V., & Lyketsos, C. (2000). Neuropsychiatric sequelae of traumatic brain injury. *Psychosomoatics*, *41*(2): 95–103.

Rousseau, M.-C., Baumstark, K., Alessandrini, M., Blandin, V., de Villemeur, T. B., & Auquier, P. (2015). Quality of life in patients with locked-in syndrome: evolution over a 6-year period. *Orphanet Journal of Rare Diseases*, *10*: 88.

Salas, C. (2010). Naturaleza Muerta. Transformaciones psíquicas en un caso de Tetraplejia. *Revista Chilena de Neuropsicología*, *5*(2): 160–169.

Simeon, D. (2004). Depersonalisation disorder: A contemporary overview. *CNS Drugs*, *18*(6): 343–354.

Smith, E., & Delargy, M. (2005). Locked-in syndrome. *British Medical Journal*, *330*(7488): 406–409.

Söderholm, S., Meinander, M., & Alaranta, H. (2001). Augmentative and alternative communication methods in locked-in syndrome. *Journal of Rehabilitation Medicine*, *33*(5): 235–239.

Stoll, J., Chatelle, C., Carter, O., Koch, C., Laureys, S., & Einhäuser, W. (2013). Pupil responses allow communication in locked-in syndrome patients. *Current Biology*, *23*(15): 647–648.

Strub, R. L., & Black, F. W. (2000). *The mental status examination in neurology* (4th edition). Philadelphia: F. A. Davis Company.

Wilhelm, B., Jordan, M., & Birbaumer, N. (2006). Communication in locked-in syndrome: Effects of imagery on salivary pH. *Neurology*, *67*(3), 534–535.

Wilson, B. A., Hinchcliffe, A., Okines, T., Florschutz, G., & Fish, J. (2011). A case study of locked-in-syndrome: Psychological and personal perspectives. *Brain Injury*, *25*(5), 526–538.

Closing

Chapter 14

Final thoughts

The contribution of neuropsychoanalysis to neuropsychological rehabilitation

Christian Salas and Oliver Turnbull

The relationship between psychoanalysis and neuropsychological rehabilitation has never been simple. Some from the field have even raised concerns as to whether psychoanalysis has *any* role and is even 'compatible', with the rehabilitation of people with acquired brain injury (Wilson, 2014). However, such views are rare. A more common, evidence-based, perspective is that psychoanalytic ideas have been present in the development of rehabilitation since its inception, particularly in relation to the understanding and treatment of the psychological consequences of brain damage. We might choose many examples of this. Kurt Goldstein, arguably the father of neuropsychological rehabilitation, used psychodynamic concepts such as anxiety and defence mechanisms to explain survivors' reactions to their deficits (Goldstein, 1965). Importantly, he also suggested a more *general* account of the therapeutic relationship, as a tool to enhance the patient's adherence to treatment (Goldstein, 1954). A more recent strand, inspired by Goldstein's ideas, might be George Prigatano's introduction (in the 1990s) of psychoanalytic concepts into the formulation of holistic rehabilitation. He was especially focused on the relevance of psychohistory and attachment in shaping the idiosyncratic experience of loss found in brain injury survivors (Prigatano, 1986, 1999).

Clinical neuropsychologists have also developed these ideas further in the psychoanalytic domain. Examples include using Kohutian concepts to explain changes in the cohesion and continuity of the self (Klonoff & Lage, 1991; Klonoff, Lage & Chiapello, 1993). We see Jungian ideas used to address the existential challenges of adjusting to life after brain damage (Prigatano, 2012). And we see relational concepts used to shed light on the *interpersonal* changes generated by the injury (Freed, 2002; Lewis, 1999; Pepping, 1993; Salas, 2008, 2012; Yeates, 2013). The original *Clinical Case Studies* book was a pioneer in contributing to this endeavour, proposing various ways in which brain damage generated changes in the regulation of drives and in the structure of personality (Kaplan-Solms & Solms, 2000). What then is the 'common thread' amongst these psychodynamically minded clinical neuropsychologists? It has always been a profound interest in the 'depth psychological' consequences of brain injury and how it changes the 'inner world'. This was not a common theme in the early moments of neuropsychological rehabilitation, and it seems fair to suggest that a psychodynamic approach has played a key role in expanding the scope of the field beyond the cognitive realm (Turnbull & Solms, 2004).

The neuropsychological rehabilitation of individuals with brain damage has been described as a complex task, requiring a broad 'theoretical spectrum'. To achieve this, one needs to knit together models and methodologies from neuropsychology, and also from cognitive and behavioural psychology (Wilson, 1997). The chapters contained in this book offer abundant evidence that classic and modern psychoanalysis is becoming a key actor in this dialogue. This is particularly relevant if we consider the recent shift in neuropsychological rehabilitation, placing emotion and identity at the centre of case formulations and rehabilitation efforts (Wilson & Gracey, 2010; Ylvisaker & Feeney, 2000). It is widely accepted today in neuropsychological rehabilitation that interventions that target only *cognitive* performance and functionality are not enough. Instead, the field also needs to focus on two further elements: firstly, how impairments and functional problems are *signified* and interpreted by survivors, and secondly, how survivors manage and elaborate the feelings generated by the injury and its consequences. In other words, this recent shift in rehabilitation requires clinicians to develop models that explain the complex relationship between emotion, grief and identity. For decades, this has been, in fact, one of the main areas of contribution that psychoanalysis has had to the field of neuropsychological rehabilitation. The diversity of the chapters in this book is a testament to the breadth of that influence.

To say that motor and cognitive deficits are individually signified would be a commonplace today in neuropsychological rehabilitation. However, this was not the case in the 1980s, when rehabilitation efforts were predominantly focussed on cognitive retraining and work re-entry. One might mark a historical turning point here two decades ago, when Prigatano (1999) proposed his 13 principles: the first of them suggesting that any rehabilitation effort should begin by entering the *phenomenological* field of the patient. If we read this principle literally, it means that we should attempt to understand how survivors experience the world, and themselves, after the injury. However, viewed through a psychoanalytic lens, an interpretation of that principle might be more complex. After all, brain injury survivors are profoundly influenced by their personal, and especially their *attachment* history. We are increasingly aware of how attachment history shapes their experience of the world, and themselves, and how it leads them to signify their injury. Let us take a few concrete examples. The same memory impairment can be signified in completely different ways: by an individual who has developed a lifelong capacity to tolerate imperfection, compared to someone that has developed psychological mechanisms to avoid feelings of vulnerability. Similarly, individuals may be happy to request and receive help from staff and family to manage their memory impairment. But only if they have previously developed a sense of trust in others, especially in moments of distress (Yeates & Salas, 2019). These ideas are still a matter of debate (Salas, 2014), but they have slowly been incorporated into neuropsychological rehabilitation thinking. However, they often arrive from *other* theoretical frameworks that have adopted psychodynamic ideas, for example the attachment system in compassion-focused therapy (Ashworth, Gracey & Gilbert, 2011).

Another perspective on Prigatano's principle is that, from a psychodynamic perspective, survivors can signify their injury and its consequences without being aware of the meanings attributed to them, or indeed how those meanings are connected to their previous life experience. Of course, this is a psychoanalytic axiom: that human behaviour is motivated (through emotions) by the relational history of an individual. Today, neuroscience frames this idea by proposing that the brain is a 'predictive machine' that uses the past to prepare for the future (Bar, 2011). It seems clear that the influence of unconscious mental life remains a conceptual and cultural challenge for neuropsychological rehabilitation. In part this is due to a strong behavioural and neo-behavioural tradition that remains in the cognitive zeitgeist of the field. With a few exceptions (Gracey, Longworth & Psaila, 2016; Ylvisaker & Feeney, 2000), emotion still lacks a proper theoretical framework – one that conceives emotion and cognition as dynamically interacting forces. Notably, this has been the object of study of psychoanalysis for over a century, but has not impacted on many aspects of neuropsychological rehabilitation.

We can now focus on the contribution that psychoanalysis has made to the *management* of emotion after by the injury. A common problem observed by clinicians working with survivors is that the neural and neurocognitive 'machinery' that allows humans to deal with loss, and develop a mourning process, is often compromised after brain damage (Coetzer, 2003). In other words, the same attentional, memory, language and executive impairments that hinder individuals' capacity to be functional in life can *also* impede survivors' ability to think about what they feel and how feelings are related to their injury and losses. In modern psychoanalysis, this regulatory ability is called mentalizing and refers to the use of mental representations to regulate feelings (Bateman & Fonagy, 2012). Authors in the field of neuropsychological rehabilitation have described how mentalizing can be altered after brain injury, compromising the capacity to use thoughts to self-regulate, as well as regulating emotional interactions with others (Salas, 2012; Yeates, 2013). Interestingly, it appears that specific profiles of cognitive impairment can change mentalizing ability in different ways (Kaplan-Solms & Solms, 2000; Yeates, 2013). This model has important clinical consequences, for it allows clinicians to generate dense case formulations, where standard neuropsychological information can be linked with changes in emotional experience and emotion regulation, at both intrapersonal and interpersonal levels (Salas et al., 2014; Salas & Yuen 2016). Such understanding can offer conceptual and diagnostic tools to develop psychological interventions. It can especially help to scaffold the mentalizing abilities that are necessary for the mourning process.

A related technical implication of this view is the consideration of how the therapeutic process (and its components; see Orlinsky, 2009) can be differentially affected by specific cognitive and affective impairments. In general, the literature on technical adaptations of psychological interventions has been rather superficial. They have often focused on changes to the *format* in which psychotherapy is delivered: the length of sessions, the use of memory compensatory strategies, etc. (for a review, see Gallagher, McLeod & McMillan, 2019). In contrast, using a mentalizing approach makes it possible to consider how different aspects of the therapeutic process (therapeutic contract, therapeutic operations, therapeutic bond, in-session impacts) can be challenged by *specific* profiles of cognitive impairment. Viewed in this light, one can see how the necessary adaptations of the therapeutic process can be developed (for an example of modifications to the therapeutic process to accommodate psychological interventions with patients with concrete behaviour, see Salas, Vaughan, Shanker & Turnbull, 2013).

A common limitation of brain injury services today across the world is the lack of support *beyond* the first year of rehabilitation, despite the well-known fact that psychological needs last a lifetime. In this context, longer term provision of emotional and relationship support for survivors (and their significant others) is needed to offset negative psychosocial outcomes. However, such support is rarely available. As discussed above, a neuropsychoanalytic approach appears *particularly* suited to contribute to interventions for brain injury survivors and their relatives (Coetzer et al., 2018). This is true, theoretically and technically, during assessment, case formulation and the development of interventions. It is specifically relevant for the *archetypical* challenges faced by this population, such as identity re-construction, emotional adjustment and the negotiation/preservation of relationships.

The chapters in this book are a breadth of examples of these possibilities. They also portray the wide and diverse range of psychoanalytic perspectives that can be applied to the rehabilitation of brain-injured patients. We have a range of hopes and aspirations for these chapters: that they will allow clinicians to become familiar with modern psychoanalytic thinking and technique, that they will stimulate the clinical and scientific exploration of the possibilities of psychoanalytic ideas and perhaps that they may inspire others to go *beyond* our present boundaries in supporting survivors of brain injury. We would like a pool of knowledge that is deeper, that is more familiar and that encourages others to take the discipline to new places. We await these future developments with interest.

February, 2020
Papudo, Chile/Bangor, Wales

References

Ashworth, F., Gracey, F., & Gilbert, P. (2011). Compassion focused therapy after traumatic brain injury: Theoretical foundations and a case illustration. *Brain Impairment*, *12*(2), 128–139.

Bar, M. (ed.). (2011). *Predictions in the brain: Using our past to generate a future*. Oxford: Oxford University Press.

Bateman, A. W., & Fonagy, P. E. (2012). *Handbook of mentalizing in mental health practice*. Arlington: American Psychiatric Publishing, Inc.

Coetzer, B. (2003). Grief following traumatic brain injury. *Grief Matters: The Australian Journal of Grief and Bereavement*, *6*(2), 31.

Coetzer, R., Evans-Roberts, C., Turnbull, O. H., & Vaughan, F. (2018). Neuropsychoanalytically-informed psychotherapy approaches to rehabilitation: The North Wales Brain Injury Service – Bangor University experience 1998–2018. *Neuropsychoanalysis*. *20*(1), 3–13.

Freed, P. (2002). Meeting of the minds: Ego reintegration after traumatic brain injury. *Bulletin of the Menninger Clinic*, *66*(1), 61–78.

Gallagher, M., McLeod, H. J., & McMillan, T. M. (2019). A systematic review of recommended modifications of CBT for people with cognitive impairments following brain injury. *Neuropsychological Rehabilitation*, *29*(1), 1–21.

Goldstein, K. (1954). The concept of transference in treatment of organic and functional nervous disease. *Psychotherapy and Psychosomatics*, *2*(3–4), 334–353.

Goldstein, K. (1995[1965]). *The organism a holistic approach to biology derived from pathological data in man*. Notes. New York: Zone.

Gracey, F., Longworth, C., & Psaila, K. (2016). A provisional transdiagnostic cognitive behavioural model of post brain injury emotional adjustment. *Neuro-Disability and Psychotherapy*, *3*(2), 154–185.

Kaplan-Solms, K., & Solms, M. (2000). *Clinical studies in neuro-psychoanalysis: Introduction to a depth neuropsychology*. New York: Routledge.

Klonoff, P. S., & Lage, G. A. (1991). Narcissistic injury in patients with traumatic brain injury. *The Journal of Head Trauma Rehabilitation*, *6*(4), 11–21.

Klonoff, P. S., Lage, G. A., & Chiapello, D. A. (1993). Varieties of the catastrophic reaction to brain injury: A self psychology perspective. *Bulletin of the Menninger Clinic*, *57*(2), 227.

Lewis, L. (1999). Transference and countertransference in psychotherapy with adults having traumatic brain injury. In K. Langer, L. Laatsch and L. Lewis (eds.) *Psychotherapeutic interventions for adults with brain injury or stroke: A clinician's treatment resource*, pp. 113–130. Madison, CT: Psychosocial Practice.

Orlinsky, D. E. (2009). The "Generic Model of Psychotherapy" after 25 years: Evolution of a research-based metatheory. *Journal of Psychotherapy Integration*, *19*(4), 319.

Pepping, M. (1993). Transference and countertransference issues in brain injury rehabilitation: implications for staff training. In C. J. Durging, N. D. Schmidt & L. J. Fryer (eds.) *Staff development and clinical intervention in brain injury rehabilitation*, pp. 87–103. Maryland: Aspen Publication.

Prigatano, G. P. (1986). *Neuropsychological rehabilitation after brain injury*. Baltimore, MD: Johns Hopkins University Press.

Prigatano, G. P. (1999). *Principles of neuropsychological rehabilitation*. New York: Oxford University Press.

Prigatano, G. P. (2012). Jungian contributions to successful neuropsychological rehabilitation. *Neuropsychoanalysis*, *14*(2), 175–185.

Salas, C. E. (2008). Elementos relacionales en la rehabilitación de sobrevivientes de lesión cerebral adquirida. Alianza de trabajo, transferencia y contratransferencia, usos de terapeuta (Relational elements in the rehabilitation of survivors of acquired brain injury. Working alliance, transference, countertransference, psychotherapist' uses. *Revista Psiquiatría Universitaria*, *4*(2), 214–220.

Salas, C. E. (2012). Surviving catastrophic reaction after brain injury: The use of self-regulation and self-other regulation. *Neuropsychoanalysis*, *14*(1), 77–92.

Salas, C. E. (2014). Identity issues in neuropsychoanalysis. *Neuropsychoanalysis*, *16*(2), 153–158.

Salas, C. E., Radovic, D., Yuen, K. S., Yeates, G. N., Castro, O., & Turnbull, O. H. (2014). "Opening an emotional dimension in me": Changes in emotional reactivity and emotion regulation in a case of executive impairment after left fronto-parietal damage. *Bulletin of the Menninger Clinic*, *78*(4), 301–334.

Salas, C., Vaughan, F., Shanker, S., & Turnbull, O. (2013). Stuck in a moment: Concreteness and psychotherapy after acquired brain injury. *Neuro-disability and Psychotherapy*, *1*(1), 1–38.

Salas, C. E., & Yuen, K. S. (2016). Revisiting the left convexity hypothesis: Changes in the mental apparatus after left dorso-medial prefrontal damage. *Neuropsychoanalysis*, *18*(2), 85–100.

Turnbull, O. H., & Solms, M. (2004). Depth psychological consequences of brain damage. In J. Panksepp (ed.) *Textbook of biological psychiatry*, pp. 571–595. New Jersey: Wiley-Liss.

Wilson, B. A. (1997). Cognitive rehabilitation: How it is and how it might be. *Journal of the International Neuropsychological Society*, *3*(5), 487–496.

Wilson, B. (2014). Are psychoanalysis and neuropsychology compatible? In S. Cooper & K. Ratele (eds.). *Psychology serving humanity. Proceedings of the 30th international congress of psychology*, pp. 84–90. New York: Psychology Press.

Wilson, B., & Gracey, F. (2010). Towards a comprehensive model of neuropsychological rehabilitation. In B. Wilson, F. Gracey, J. Evans & A. Bateman (eds.) *Neuropsychological rehabilitation. Theory, models, therapy and outcome*, pp. 1–21. New York: Cambridge University Press.

Yeates, G. (2013). Towards the neuropsychological foundations of couples therapy following acquired brain injury (ABI): A review of empirical evidence and relevant concepts. *Neuro-disability and Psychotherapy*, *1*(1), 108–150.

Yeates, G., & Salas, C. E. (2019). Attachment-based psychotherapies for people with brain injury. In G. Yeates & F. Ashworth (eds.) *Psychological therapies in acquired brain injury*, pp. 109–131. London: Routledge.

Ylvisaker, M., & Feeney, T. (2000). Reconstruction of identity after brain injury. *Brain Impairment*, *1*(1), 12–28.

Index

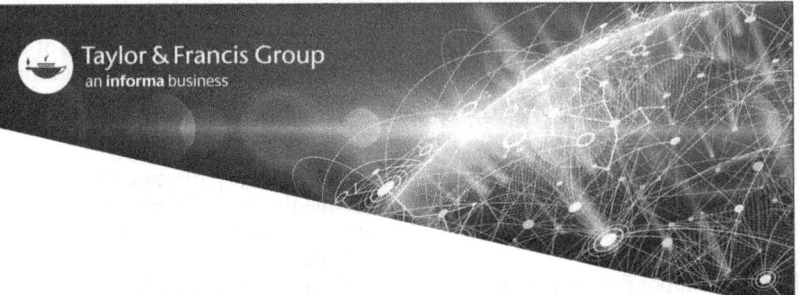
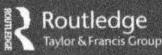
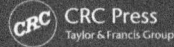